SITUATIONAL ANALYSIS IN PRACTICE

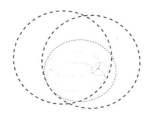

For Anselm . . .

SITUATIONAL ANALYSIS

in Practice

Mapping Research with Grounded Theory

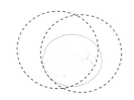

Adele E. Clarke
Carrie Friese
Rachel Washburn
editors

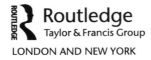

Routledge
Taylor & Francis Group

LONDON AND NEW YORK

First published 2015 by Left Coast Press, Inc.

Published 2016 by Routledge
2 Park Square, Milton Park, Abingdon, Oxon OX14 4RN
711 Third Avenue, New York, NY 10017, USA

Routledge is an imprint of the Taylor & Francis Group, an informa business

Library of Congress Cataloging-in-Publication Data

Situational analysis in practice : mapping research with grounded theory / Adele E. Clarke, Carrie Friese
and Rachel Washburn, editors.
    pages cm
Includes bibliographical references and index.
 ISBN 978-1-62958-106-4 (hardback : alk. paper) —ISBN 978-1-62958-107-1 (pbk. : alk. paper)
 —ISBN 978-1-62958-108-8 (institutional ebook) —ISBN 978-1-62958-109-5 (consumer ebook)
 1. Grounded theory. 2. Social sciences--Methodology. I. Clarke, Adele. II. Friese, Carrie. III. Washburn,
Rachel, 1975-
 H61.24.S58 2015
 001.4'2—dc23
                    2014047860

 ISBN 978-1-62958-106-4 hardback
 ISBN 978-1-62958-107-1 paperback

CONTENTS

FOREWORD

S ITUATIONAL ANALYSIS HAS come of methodological age. This book marks, demonstrates, and celebrates the commanding presence situational analysis now enjoys in qualitative research. Situational analysis has taken its rightful place as a recognized innovative method of this century. Adele Clarke made her cutting-edge statement of the method in the first edition of *Situational Analysis* only ten short years ago. Since then, the method has gained substantial attention within and across diverse disciplines and professions. The past few years have shown a remarkable increase in the number of studies that situational analysis has generated. *Situational Analysis in Practice* testifies to its varied topics, range of analyses, theoretical reach, and growing number of proponents.

What makes situational analysis innovative and distinctive? The method not only addresses the messiness of the empirical world, but moreover acknowledges the messiness of conducting research. This simple but profound axiom guides the entire process: The situation of inquiry itself becomes the fundamental unit of analysis. The assumptions we hold, the actions we take, the data we generate, and the analyses we construct all reside within the situation of inquiry. No longer can researchers hide behind data and present their findings as objective facts separate from the conditions of their production. Every study develops within a situation and likely is transformed by multiple situations throughout inquiry.

Yet situational analysis does more than acknowledge the complex nature of the empirical world and the limitations of the methods on which social scientists have traditionally relied. Situational analysis provides a way out. A major strength of this approach is that it offers a considered and rigorous way out of research conundrums. The method fosters interpretive theoretical understandings of situations while simultaneously subjecting them to rigorous scrutiny—throughout the research process. Situational analysis offers methods that make the hidden and chaotic visible and comprehensible. The method's explicit emphasis on language and discourse prompts researchers to examine nuances of meanings and of silences—ours as well as those of our research participants. Situational analysis fosters learning about implicit meanings, tacit actions, and assumptions embedded in discourses. In short, the research situation merges with the process and product.

Situational analysis was built on theoretical and methodological alliances and oppositions. The method endorses methodological strategies of earlier versions of grounded theory but opposes the quest for disembodied and unanchored generalizations. Like constructivist grounded theory with which this method is aligned, situational analysis builds on Anselm Strauss's legacy of pragmatist philosophy and grounded theory methods and takes his legacy into the 21st century. Situational analysis, however, gives Strauss's legacy new form that transcends 20th-century perspectives and practices. Similarly, situational analysis draws on diverse sources—feminist theory, postmodernist critiques, epistemological debates, and science and technology studies, to name a few—but synthesizes, integrates, and transforms them to produce an original statement and a unique method.

The chapters in this book explain the essentials constituting the method and exhibit products of it. In one short volume, readers new to situational analysis will be able to understand its theoretical and methodological underpinnings, see how select researchers have put the method to practice, and, moreover, be able to apply the lessons gained to their studies. *Situational Analysis in Practice* takes the method from its experts and gives it to all qualitative researchers.

Kathy Charmaz, author of *Constructing Grounded Theory*

ACKNOWLEDGMENTS

OOKS ARE COMPLEX ENDEAVORS, and we owe debts of gratitude to many people. We thank them here especially for their generosity of spirit, a precious attribute. Special thanks go to Norm Denzin, who suggested that Adele Clarke organize a session on situational analysis for the 2013 meetings of the International Congress of Qualitative Inquiry in Urbana/Champaign, Illinois. That session became the core of this book. All the presenters offered early versions of their reflections on using situational analysis, now revised and published here with their original research articles. As editors, we are delighted to include them and express our gratitude to them for being ideal contributors—prompt, thoughtful, courteous, really smart, and fun! Norm has created a particularly vibrant qualitative community at the International Congresses of Qualitative Inquiry. Discussions there with many people over the past decade have deeply enriched our understandings and strengthened our perspectives.

Supportive colleagues and faculty make major differences in our lives. For decades of remarkable collegiality, we thank the qualitative teaching faculty at UCSF from nursing and sociology: Kit Chesla, Carol Dawson-Rose, Janice Humphreys, Holly Kennedy, Susan Kools, Ginnie Olesen, Howard Pinderhughes, Roberta Rehm, Janet Shim, Lenny Schatzman, and Carolyn Wiener. Everyone has gone far out of their way to encourage the development of situational analysis. UCSF anthropologists have also been a haven of support and intellectual stimulation, and we thank Vincanne Adams, Deborah Gordon, Sharon Kaufman, Barbara Koenig, and Ian Whitmarsh. Staff and students at UCSF have also been terrific. Brandee Woleslagle, Cynthia Mercado-Scott, and Regina Gudelunas have kept Adele Clarke and the whole Department of Social and Behavioral Sciences purring along despite cutbacks. Doctoral student Megan Dowdell provided excellent bibliographic and indexing support. And sociology and nursing doctoral students in the qualitative courses since 1990 have all contributed to the forging and polishing of situational analysis in countless ways. They were willing guinea pigs for this extension of grounded theory and taught us how to use it, teach it, and make it better and better.

Special thanks also go to thoughtful colleagues from around the globe who have discussed, commented on, and supported situational analysis workshops over the years: Stine Willum Adrian, Gabriela Alonso-Yanez, Warwick Anderson, Paul Atkinson, Isabelle Baszanger, Geof Bowker, Stacy Carter, Lisa Cartwright, Monica Casper, Daniel Cefaï, Kathy Charmaz, Amanda Coffey, Lars Dahlgren, Suzanne de Castell, Annie Dugdale, Maria Emmelin, Ulrike Felt, Mary Margaret Fonow, Ulrike Froschauer, Daiwe Fu, Andrea Hagn, Bente Halkier, Peter Hall, Donna Haraway, MarySue Heilemann, Lene Koch, Charlotte Kr--kke, Patti Lather, Joanna Latimer, Merete Lie, Reiner Keller, Katie King, Marjorie MacDonald, Ray Maietta, David Maines, Reuben Message, Guenter Mey, Jan Morse, Katja Mruck, Michelle Murphy, Carrie Sanders, Susan Leigh Star, Jörg Strübing, Mette Nordahl Svendsen, Angela Wroblewski, and Chia-ling Wu. Monica, Kathy, Reiner, and Jörg truly went the distance in providing superb comments.

Presses vary widely, and it is our great good fortune to be publishing this volume with Left Coast Press, Inc. and to be working with Mitch Allen and Stephanie Adams. Mitch was an early supporter of grounded theory and situational analysis, and working with him feels like coming home. Notably, Left Coast also published *Developing Grounded Theory: The Second Generation* on the full range of grounded theory approaches.

Carrie Friese thanks Stephanie Miller for steadfast support and expresses profound appreciation to Hazel (now eight months old) for being awe inspiring and life changing. Rachel Washburn thanks Peter Davidson for his patience, love, and unwavering support. For caring and sustaining friendship, Adele Clarke thanks Monica Casper, Pam Mendelsohn, Jenny Ross, and Dan Doyle. Since 1971, Allan Regenstreif has always "been there" and assumed she could accomplish whatever she wanted—even doing this book in three months. So this one, too, is for Allan, without whom. . . .

PART I

INTRODUCING SITUATIONAL ANALYSIS

CHAPTER 1

INTRODUCING SITUATIONAL ANALYSIS

Welcome to this volume on the qualitative research method called situational analysis (hereafter, SA). It includes an ambitious introductory essay that situates SA in the historic renaissance of qualitative inquiry since the 1960s, several previously published papers focused on the method itself, and five exemplars—excellent examples—of SA research. Also included are reflections by those researchers on the process of using this method in the empirical projects on which these papers are based. SA is an extension of grounded theory (hereafter, GT), transnationally the most popular form of qualitative analysis in the social sciences and humanities today (e.g., Clarke & Charmaz 2014). SA has also been widely taken up and now merits its own edited volume.

GT was developed by Barney Glaser and Anselm Strauss in 1967 and has been elaborated over the years by a number of scholars, especially Kathy Charmaz (1995, 2000, 2006, 2014 [2006]; Morse et al. 2009). GT's roots are in sociology (e.g., Strauss & Corbin 1997), and it quickly spread to nursing (e.g., Schreiber & Stem 2001). Soon, GT was also taken up in organization and management studies (e.g., Locke 2001); education (e.g., Cresswell 2007); library and information science (e.g., Star & Bowker 2007), counseling psychology (e.g., Fassinger 2005); computer and information science (e.g., Bryant 2002; Urquhart 2007); social work (e.g., Oliver 2012); public health (e.g., Dahlgren, Emmelin, & Winkvist 2007); science, technology, and medicine studies (e.g., Clarke & Star 2008); and queer studies (e.g., Plummer 2005). Over the past almost five decades, GT has grown to merit its own hefty *Handbook of Grounded Theory* (Bryant & Charmaz 2007) and major new

Situational Analysis in Practice, edited by Adele E. Clarke, Carrie Friese, and Rachel Washburn
11–75 © 2015 Taylor & Francis. All rights reserved.

texts (e.g., Birks & Mills 2011; Charmaz 2014 [2006]; Corbin & Strauss 2014; Dey 1999).

After using and teaching GT for over twenty years, Adele Clarke, who studied with Anselm Strauss, developed SA by extending GT modes of analysis to include an array of poststructural and other contemporary concerns (Clarke 2003, 2005, 2007). For Clarke, GT itself is a "theory/methods package" that incorporates symbolic interactionism and pragmatist philosophy (Clarke 2005:2–5; Clarke & Star 2008; Star 1989). Both GT and SA are there-fore rooted in social constructionism and seek to explore the multiplicity of perspectives and the processual and contingent nature of social life through a relational ecological framework. Over the years, Clarke had generated a critique of GT and she developed SA to explicitly address what she saw as shortcomings of the method. This includes its positivist tendencies, a lack of reflexivity, oversimplification instead of addressing differences, and a lack of analysis of power (see Clarke 2005:11–16).

SA specifically addresses these shortcomings by acknowledging the embodiment and situatedness of the researcher, grounding qualitative analysis in the broader situation of inquiry, attending carefully to differences, complexities, and range of variation in the data, including discourse data and analyses, and taking nonhuman elements (material things such as animals and technologies) into analytic account. In SA, *the situation of inquiry itself broadly conceived becomes the key unit of analysis.* This differs radically from traditional GT, which centers on the main social processes—human action—in the area of inquiry (Clarke 2005:19–31). In SA, the situation of inquiry is *empirically* constructed through making three kinds of maps (situational, social worlds/arenas, and positional) and through doing analytic work with the maps. Such work includes writing analytic memos of various kinds about each map, examining relations among the elements, and often updating the maps to reflect one's evolving analysis of the situation.

The roots of SA in GT include especially the ecological orientation of symbolic interactionism, Strauss's social worlds/arenas theory (1978, 1982a, 1982b, 1984, 1993), and pragmatism (e.g., Denzin 1996; Koopman 2009; Rorty 1979, 1982). Its new roots include Foucault's (e.g., 1972, 1973, 1978) emphasis on discourse, Foucault's (1975, 1991) concepts of the "conditions of possibility" and "dispositive," Deleuze and Guattari's (1987) work on assemblages and rhizomes, and science and technology studies. Clarke was also inspired by C. Wright Mills's (1940) concern with situatedness, Denzin's (2009 [1989/1970]) pioneering efforts at situating qualitative research, and Haraway's

(1991) concept of "situated knowledges." SA integrates poststructural assumptions and strategies of inquiry with those of symbolic interactionist social theory and offers strong emphases on analyzing discourses (narrative, visual, and historical), elucidating differences, including nonhuman elements in analysis and analyzing relations of power. Reflecting its theoretical orientation, Clarke's (2005) book was titled *Situational Analysis: Grounded Theory after the Postmodern Turn*.[1]

Today, both social theory and research methods are increasingly transdisciplinary and travel widely (Barry & Born 2013). As a methodological advance in GT, SA, too, has been widely recognized in qualitative methods (e.g., Clarke 2006, 2007, 2009, 2011, 2012; Clarke & Friese 2007; Clarke & Keller 2014; Morse et al. 2009), including a German translation of the book and several articles (Clarke 2011, 2012; Clarke & Keller 2011, 2014). A second edition is in progress (Clarke, Friese, & Washburn Forthcoming 2016).[2] It is most gratifying that SA is already being taken up in research outside the United States and across varied disciplines and professional venues. Demonstrating its transdisciplinarity, SA research has to date appeared in journals of counseling and psychotherapy, education, family studies, health policy, library and information science, public health, nursing, science and technology studies, social work, sociology, and others and is taught in urban planning and architecture. SA has also been traveling transnationally. In addition to the United States, we know that it has been taught in Sweden, Norway, Denmark, Germany, Austria, France, Canada, New Zealand, Australia, Taiwan, and Japan.

Situational Analysis Strategies

The main strategies of SA are the three maps that researchers do across the full trajectory of the research project from the earliest design stages to preparation of publications. The first maps, *situational maps*, lay out *all* the major human, nonhuman, discursive, historical, symbolic, cultural, political, and other elements in the research situation of concern. Ideally, this map is initially made during the early design phase, laying out everything about which at least some data should be gathered and gaining a tentative sense of possibly important relations among them. This is helpful in guiding data collection and can also help researchers develop stronger proposals for funding their research. Downstream in the research, situational maps are used to provoke analysis of relations among the different elements, called relational mapping. Working *against* the usual simplifications in particularly postmodern and potentially feminist and critical ways, these maps capture and provoke discussion of the many and heterogeneous elements, their relations to one another, and the messy complexities of the situation (Clarke 2005:83–108). Relationalities and complexities have come to the forefront of concerns across the social sciences and humanities in this century (e.g., Lather 2007; Law 1999, 2004, 2007; Law & Mol 2002; Taylor 2005), and SA explicitly addresses such issues (e.g., Clarke & Keller 2014).

Second, the *social worlds/arenas maps* lay out all of the *collective* actors and the arena(s) of commitment within which they are engaged in ongoing discourses and negotiations. Such maps offer *interpretations* of the broader situation, taking up its social organizational, institutional, and discursive dimensions (Strauss 1978).[3] They invoke distinctively poststructural assumptions: We cannot assume directionalities of influence; boundaries are open and porous; negotiations are fluid; discourses are multiple and potentially contradictory. *Negotiations* of many kinds from coercion to bargaining are the "basic social processes" that construct and constantly destabilize social worlds' relations and arenas maps (Clarke in prep.; Strauss 1979). Symbolic interactionism tells us that things could always be otherwise—not only individually but also collectively, organizationally, institutionally, and discursively. These maps portray such poststructural possibilities. The flipside of social worlds/arenas maps are discourse/arenas maps. That is, social worlds are themselves "universes of discourse," routinely producing discourses about themselves, about other social worlds, and about issues of concern in the arena (Strauss 1978). Such discourses can be positionally mapped and analyzed in various ways (see Clarke 2005:109–124).

Third, *positional maps* lay out the major positions taken, and *not* taken, in the data vis-à-vis particular axes of variation and difference, focus, and controversy found in the situation of concern. The discursive data can include interviews, observations, media discourse materials, websites, and so on. Perhaps most significantly, positional maps are *not* articulated with persons or groups but rather seek to represent the full range of *discursive* positions on key issues in the broad situation of concern. They allow multiple positions and even contradictions to be articulated. Discourses are thus disarticulated from their sites of production, decentering them and making analytic complexities more visible. Complexities are themselves heterogeneous, and we need the improved means of representing them that SA offers (see Clarke 2005:125–136).

In doing SA, researchers also code data and write memos as in GT (e.g., Charmaz 2014 [2014:109–191]), including memoing about each map. Researchers make situational and social worlds/arenas maps early in the project and then make them again after major waves of data collection and analysis. Positional maps are usually done quite late in the project once most or all of the data have been collected. While situational maps are rarely included in write-ups, both social worlds/arenas and positional maps commonly are, and most of the exemplars offered in this volume include such maps.

Distinctive Strengths and Contributions of Situational Analysis

Compared to GT, what is new about SA includes:

+ doing the three kinds of analytic maps and working with them;
+ enhanced reflexivity of the researcher;
+ attention to elucidating differences and varied perspectives in the data;
+ moving beyond the knowing subject of interviews to include analyses of discourses;
+ "helping silences speak" by analyzing absent positions in positional maps of discourses;
+ elucidating important nonhuman elements in the situation of inquiry (technologies, buildings, animals, etc.) and their relations in the situation;[4] and
+ pursuing analyses of power, especially through analyzing implicated actors (discussed below).

(All of these issues are discussed in detail in Clarke's article "From Grounded Theory to Situational Analysis: What's New? Why? How?" included in Part II of this volume.)

A particular strength of SA is that it can be done with interview, ethnographic, historical, narrative, visual, and/or other discursive materials. Public and institutional discourses are growing in importance due to wide and fast electronic access. SA's capacities for analyzing such discourses are excellent, making the method especially useful for multi-site research where several different kinds of data are gathered. For example, one might gather data through interviews with software designers, websites describing their programs, and ethnographic observational materials from conferences. With

SA, the researcher has the alternatives of analyzing all the data together or separately and comparing the outcomes (see also Keller 2011, 2012b, 2013).

Mapping *all* the actors and discourses in the situation *regardless of their power* also ruptures taken-for-granted hierarchies and promotes *epistemic diversity*—an enhanced understanding of the varied perspectives present in the situation that are often rooted in different assumptions about epistemology—*how* we can know and understand (e.g., Pascale 2011). Historically, there have been highly stratified hierarchies in terms of the valuation of different kinds and bases of knowledge. A key feature of poststructuralist and interpretive approaches, as well as postcolonial and indigenous approaches to knowledge, often involves ignoring such tired and exclusive hierarchies and instead seeking to represent the full array of interpretations and understanding present in the situation. This produces epistemic diversity in the analysis.

Implicated actors are actors silenced or only discursively present in situations. In discourse data, they are usually constructed by others for others' purposes. There are at least two kinds. The first, while physically present, are silenced, ignored, or made invisible by those having greater power in the situation. Second are those *not* physically present but *solely* discursively constructed by others, usually disadvantageously. *Neither* kind of implicated actor is actively involved in self-representation. This concept provides a means of analyzing the situatedness of less powerful actors and some of the consequences of others' actions for them.[5]

Using Situational Analysis

Here we briefly introduce the uses of SA in qualitative research in general qualitative inquiry, in participatory action research, in policy research, and in feminist and other critical qualitative research. (For fuller discussions, please see the SA texts by Clarke [2005] or Clarke, Friese, & Washburn [Forthcoming, 2016].)

SA in General Qualitative Inquiry

SA is a method of analysis that can be used in the full array of qualitative research endeavors. It is commonly used in interview-based studies, but also in ethnography, narrative and visual discourse analysis, and historical studies. It is especially useful in multi-site or multi-modal research that can draw together different kinds of data about a particular phenomenon or sets of data about different sites, or both. To date, SA has been used in qualitative research across the wide variety of disciplines and specialties noted above (see also the Appendixes of this volume and the SA website www.situational analysis.com for listings of works using SA).

Outstanding examples of SA in qualitative research in addition to those in this volume include one on psychotherapy. Strong and colleagues (2012) studied how counselors responded to the DSM-IV-TR, a highly contested psychiatrically oriented administrative set of classifications of mental problems required to receive insurance coverage for therapy services. The authors offer situational, relational, and two different positional maps of their data that were innovatively generated through an online survey of counselors, invited contributions to a website blog, and in-depth interviews. They chose the SA method because of its strengths in elucidating differences and helping researchers specify the array of positions taken in a discourse, their focus of interest. Indeed, they found a wide array of positions about the DSM-IV-TR and many and divergent strategies used by counselors to deal with the "administrative fact" of being forced to use it in order to be paid for their work. Particular tensions were found among counselors who practice psychotherapy from non-psychiatric frames such as family systems or feminist approaches.

Another general SA research paper by Martinez (2013) challenges ethnocentric myths about acculturation and dietary change among Latino immigrants. The myth has been that when "at home" in Latin America, people ate more healthily because foods were more local, less processed, and usually prepared in the home. In sharp contrast, in her innovative SA interview and participant observation study that included home visits to cook with families, Martinez found that the modernization of food production and consumption—even huge tortilla factories and McDonalds—had long been part of the Latin nutritional landscape (e.g., Pilcher 2012). What worsened immigrants' diets once in the United States was food insecurity due to a combination of their undocumented status, arduous work with irregular hours, inadequate kitchen facilities, poor health care, and overall impoverishment.

SA in Participatory Action Research and Policy Research

SA has been innovatively used by Genat (2009 and this volume) to develop an interactionist approach to participatory action research (PAR) that is also relevant to policy research. Genat draws deeply on symbolic interactionism and feminist standpoint epistemologies and situated knowledges, and he aligns his approach with postcolonial theory (e.g., Gandhi 1998) and decolonizing methodologies (e.g., Denzin, Lincoln, & Tuhiwai Smith 2008; Mertens, Cram, & Chilia 2014; Tuhiwai Smith 2012 [1999]). Genat's approach to PAR is based on social worlds/arenas mapping and seeks to enable researchers and their local research partners to foreground *shared local understandings* in order to both critique more dominant discourses originating elsewhere and to generate locally based statements of need on which policy positions to improve the local situation can be founded. (Genat's article is introduced in more detail in the Introduction to Part II.)

Similarly, some years ago, Samik-Ibrahim (2000) argued that GT methodology was a really strong research strategy for use in developing countries because of its bottom-up, inclusive approach to data gathering and analysis. And several studies in Botswana have used it, including in needs assessment (e.g., Seboni 1997; Seloilwe 1998; Shaibu 2002). Because of its parallels to GT and its inclusion of things and discourses, SA is also well suited to policy development and needs assessment projects where formulation of local goals and concerns is central. Situational maps that lay out what is actually in the situation can be especially useful, and can help analysts discern what is *not* in the situation that might address local needs.

Situational Analysis in Policy Research

In policy research, social worlds/arenas mapping strategies are particularly important as they can help in carefully delineating *all* the "stakeholders" or interested parties (both individual and organizational or institutional) whom policies might affect. This is a very important aspect of the policy development process. Among the most common errors in policy development is failure to consider the breadth of the consequences of changing a policy or instituting a new policy captured in the sad term "unintended consequences." For example, Newbury (2011) views SA as appropriate for social work policy development as that discipline focuses on developing human services policies for what she calls "centerless systems," the wide-open ecologies of community settings in which social work must operate and where policies should be effective.

Policy research might also draw on situational maps to assess the full range of elements that a particular policy should be capable of addressing. In a project that contributes to policy analysis, organization studies, medical sociology, and science and technology studies, Chen (2011) analyzed the development of harm reduction policies in Taiwan to prevent HIV/AIDS by reducing needle sharing among injection heroin users. He used SA to analyze how harm reduction policy was recently imported into Taiwan in this multi-sited project. Historically, "activism in the streets" was the originating impetus for promoting free access to clean needles—in New York City and Sydney in the late 20th century. In contrast, Chen shows how the bureaucratic and/or legislative office is today becoming a new site for assembling various harm reduction policy options developed and packaged elsewhere and now traveling transnationally. Local officials can select and adapt from the available options to address distinctive national and local conditions, needs, and goals by drawing on precedents, introducing local expertise, and transplanting skills and know-how (see also Reid 2005).

Further, in terms of policy research, positional maps offer fresh perspectives on the contested issues in the situation in which policies might engage (whether intentionally or not). For example, Carder (2008) analyzed the different positions taken about the challenging problem of managing medication distribution in assisted living settings. While some people assert that such settings should promote the independence, choice, and privacy of residents, these goals also create predicaments in terms of medications. Based on data from a five-year ethnographic study in six different settings in Maryland, Carder interestingly analyzed how two concerns, safety and autonomy, dominate the discourse, displacing other important issues (such as reasonableness and offering individual choice rather than rigid institutional policies for all residents) by demanding more attention than deserved in such settings.

SA in Feminist and Other Critical Qualitative Research

Feminist qualitative research has been another common site for the use of SA, and Clarke's "Feminisms, Grounded Theory, and Situational Analysis" in this volume discusses the use of SA in an array of such endeavors. The excellent "how-to-do-SA" article by Fosket (this volume) is also on a feminist topic—the innovative use of chemotherapy as a *preventive* strategy for women at high risk of breast cancer.[6] Elsewhere, Fosket (2004) analyzed the construction of a website-based breast cancer risk assessment tool to screen women for eligibility for chemoprevention.

In another feminist qualitative project, Khaw (2012) used both GT and SA to theorize the process of leaving an abusive partner. She first did a classic situational map and later, with more data, generated project-focused maps including only those elements relevant to perceptions of changing family boundaries in the process of leaving—which assuredly was a process and not an event (e.g., Lempert 1996). From this, Khaw developed a family-level theory of boundary ambiguity that could allow leaving. She noted: "The practical and theoretical utility of situational analysis to supplement traditional grounded theory methods is immense, which makes the method highly adaptable to fit the needs of various qualitative research endeavors" (Khaw 2012:138).

Another use of SA that demonstrates its facility for the analysis of power relations is in *critical* qualitative research projects. Several authors have found SA particularly useful in social justice and critical qualitative research projects (e.g., Pérez & Cannella this volume, and 2013).[7] "We are critical in the sense that what we research matters. We believe that research is a socially theoretical act and that it must be headlined by a socially just and equitable practice. We believe that research must be contextual and is tentative in its surroundings" (Steinberg 2012:ix). Such projects typically question the assumptions not only of positivism but also of neoliberalism (e.g., Lave, Morowski, & Randalls 2012), attempting to grasp the complexities of new forms of political economic entanglements including disaster capitalism (e.g., Adams 2012; Canella & Lincoln 2009; Klein 2007).

Critical qualitative projects are often hybrid and may also analyze through feminist (e.g., Naples 2003; Sprague 2005), anti-racist and intersectional (e.g., Schulz & Mullings 2006), postcolonial (e.g., Gandhi 1998), indigenous (e.g., Denzin, Lincoln, & Tuhiwai Smith 2008; Genat this volume; Mertens, Cram, & Chilia 2014; Tuhiwai Smith 2012 [1999]), LGBT/queer (Phellas 2012; Plummer 2005), or other liberatory lenses. SA was incubated in critical, feminist, and science and technology studies worlds where Clarke works as a scholar and was designed to lend itself to such projects.

Specifically, SA lends itself to critical, feminist, anti-racist, and related projects in several important and very intentional ways. These include first, its distinctive emphasis on elucidating complexities and diversities of the elements and positions in the situation under examination. One of the most common patterns in both qualitative and quantitative research is focusing on commonalities and erasing or not attending to most everything else—including people and positions working against "the way things are." Minority people, minority disciplinary positions, minority voices, and other things at the margins simply do not appear. In short, most research is done (however inadvertently) from "the top down" because of unexamined assumptions about hierarchies of importance. In very sharp contrast, SA advocates articulating *all* elements, *all* positions, *all* voices. It offers tools to help the researcher work not only "from the bottom up" but also "from the outside in" to capture and represent what and who is at the margins of the situation, especially helpful in questioning extant power hierarchies. It not only does not focus on the dominant, but attempts to upset and displace tacit hierarchies.

Second, by attending to nonhuman actors and elements in the situation of inquiry, SA blurs the human/nonhuman distinction so fundamental to Enlightenment thought and so deeply limiting in multiple ways. At basic levels, whether or not people have things such as food, housing, toilets, running water *matters*. Whether things like bombs and guns and tanks are in their daily lives *matters*. Whether people have things like cell phones, computers, and Internet connections *matters*. One of the ways social stratification is instantiated and reproduced across generations is through access to things, and access is typically highly gendered, racialized, classed, and so on (e.g., Schwalbe 2008). Yet things have by and large been "missing in action" from qualitative research. In sharp contrast, SA demands that researchers include all the important things in the situation they are studying on their situational maps and analyze their interrelations with other elements. It is not only people who matter in analyzing situations and what Foucault (1975) called "conditions of possibility."

Third, by acknowledging researchers' own embodiment and situatedness in the research project per se, the researcher's own positionality in terms of background and potential privilege (or disadvantage) is clarified and can more easily be taken into account. That is, analyzing the possible consequences of the researcher's position and perspectives is a fundamental aspect of reflexivity that SA emphasizes (see Clarke 2005:12–21). Moreover, attempting to dissolve the hierarchical relation of researcher and researched by situating oneself as the learner in critical inquiry can shift the tenor of the research itself in valuable ways. As science and technology studies (STS) scholars, we do not assume that those we study will have less power or authority than we do, though that is the tacit assumption of much if not most writing on qualitative inquiry. We encourage "studying up" as well as "across" or "straight ahead."[8] We are all experts on our own lives. This is especially important to grasp in critical projects.

Last, mapping *all* the actors and discourses in the situation regardless of their power (e.g., instead of only "the master discourse") also ruptures taken-for-granted hierarchies and promotes epistemic diversity. By *not* analytically recapitulating the power relations of domination, analyses that represent the full array of actors and discourses turn up the volume on the less powerful, the quiet, the silent, and the silenced.[9] Moreover, some voices/discourses/things are empowered through representational processes that recognize and acknowledge their presence and contributions. The powerful may matter a lot, but other things and people also really matter to some and good research should reveal *all* the key issues.

In sum, pushing ourselves and others to be open to new ways of seeing and knowing; listening carefully to the full array of voices and positions in the situation; legitimating and promoting epistemic diversity (knowledge production by differently situated producers); and working against epistemic violence that erases or silences minor voices and perspectives are each and all important. These *intentional* research processes of SA can facilitate feminist, critical, anti-racist, indigenous, and other efforts toward social justice.

We include several critical articles with post-research reflections on using SA by the authors in Part III Exemplars of Situational Analysis Research: one from education (Pérez & Cannella 2011), another from public health nursing (Gagnon, Jacob, & Holmes 2010), one from sociology and organizations (French & Miller 2012), and one from science and technology studies (Washburn 2013).[10]

Situating Situational Analysis
as an Interpretive Qualitative Method[11]

For those who have moved out from under a narrow scientificity, other practices are being rehearsed toward changing the social imaginary about research. Moving beyond the normalized apparatuses of our own training, a social science more answerable to the complications of our knowing is beginning to take place. (Lather 2007:19)

Readers, students, and workshop attendees have repeatedly asked us: "How does SA fit into the contemporary research methods scene?" This section offers an answer, briefly situating SA historically as well as methodologically, especially in the United States but also in Europe and in other English-speaking sites where similar trends have prevailed.[12] After the early background, we describe the rise of the culture of research post-WWII and the dramatic expansion of both higher education and funded research in the

United States. We discuss the emergence of GT in 1967, nearly fifty years ago, as the first manifesto of modern qualitative inquiry. We delineate the impacts of the civil rights, anti-war, and feminist movements and the rise of cultural studies on the academy and in qualitative inquiry. We then trace the renaissance of qualitative inquiry and all the "turns" (narrative, postmodern, poststructural, practice, etc.) undertaken and their often contested consequences over the next half century. These led to both the growth of transdisciplinary qualitative methods and to the wide array of approaches practiced today. We follow developments in GT since it was created, including the emergence of SA from GT, feminist, critical, and science and technology studies approaches. We conclude by delineating the range of issues confronting SA and other interpretive qualitative methods today.

Realizing that many readers will be new to qualitative inquiry while others are already old hands, knowledgeable about the history and current debates, we provide citations to the various literatures mentioned for further pursuit if desired. Not only do we each enter a discourse at different times, but also through different portals (disciplines, specialties, etc.) and with different backgrounds, all of which inflect our perspectives and all of which are in some senses "local."[13] Understanding the broader situation of qualitative research can strengthen our own practices within it. We conclude with explicit discussion of our own perspectives on various issues.

Early 20th Century

Ethnography, the name under which most early qualitative inquiry was pursued, has a deep history, extending back many centuries.[14] Early contributions were often Western travelers' accounts of non-Western locales and their peoples (e.g., Pratt 1992), described by Said (1978) as stories of "the Other," which often exoticized or "orientalized" them. Since the late 19th century, in both anthropology and sociology, (more or less) naive realist ethnographies professionalized such accounts. Denzin and Lincoln (1994:7) called this "the traditional period" of qualitative inquiry (1900–1950).[15] Scholarship here centered on a variety of "others," including "primitive" groups studied primarily by anthropologists (e.g., Malinowski's *Argonauts of the Western Pacific*), and Native Americans (e.g., Kroeber's *The Arapaho*). Sociologists focused largely on the city and "civic others" (Vidich & Lyman 1994:31), including minority communities (e.g., DuBois's *The Philadelphia Negro*; Frazier's *The Negro Family in the United States*), immigrants (e.g., Thomas & Znaniecki's

The Polish Peasant in Europe and America), deviants (e.g., Thrasher's *The Gang*), the poor (e.g., Sutherland & Locke's *Twenty Thousand Homeless Men*), and various subcultures (e.g., Cressey's *The Taxi-Dance Hall*). Much of this sociological work emerged from the University of Chicago and became known as the Chicago School (e.g., Bowden & Low 2013; Bulmer 1984; Fine 1995).[16] Vidich and Lyman (2000) generated the useful category "ethnography of assimilation" in which the Other continues to be othered, under lively critique today (e.g., Martinez 2013).

Early Chicago School ethnographic sociology was notable for recognizing and representing diversity, marginality, and racism, especially but not only in the United States. It coalesced under the name "symbolic interactionism" coined by Blumer (1969:1) in 1937. Interactionist work has sustained those early emphases (e.g., Reynolds & Herman-Kinney 2003),[17] and some strands are considered prescient about elements of postmodernism (e.g., Ferguson et al. 1990), including Stonequist's *The Marginal Man* (1961 [1937]), and Hughes's early work (1971).[18]

While the Great Depression and WWII slowed these developments, qualitative approaches continued to expand in subject matter including, for example, Sutherland's *White Collar Crime* and Vidich and Bensmans's *Small Town in Mass Society: Class, Power and Religion in a Rural Community*. At the same time, quantitative social science research was on the rise, especially at Harvard, Columbia, and (surprisingly) the University of Chicago (Abbott 1999; Bulmer 1997; Fine 1995).

Post-WWII, a new scientific era began to flourish, and research became "the name of the game" in academia and beyond—requisite not only across the natural and social sciences but also in the professions, humanities, and industry. Initially in the West but expanding transnationally, schools of education, nursing, medicine, social work, business, management, organizations, and emerging specialties/disciplines in universities such as communications, ethnic studies, cultural studies, and women's and gender studies each and all viewed research capacities as requisite for faculty and graduate students as well as for disciplinary and specialty advancement. For emergent areas of study, the need to set their own research agendas and to establish and legitimate their scholarship via research were pressing issues indeed.

During the Cold War, quantitative approaches held sway. Manicas (2007:7) subtitled his article on this history "The Rise and Fall of Scientism." With the rise of survey research and demography, and in the health sciences, the rise of epidemiology, scientism reigned in American social sciences. Quantitative functionalist sociology, dominated by survey research, had taken deep hold by the late 1930s and dramatically expanded post-WWII (Ross 1990). Market research also grew out of this foment, as we became consumption societies (e.g., Appadurai & Kopytoff 1986). But several enduring if marginal strands of anti-scientism in American social science kept interpretive alternatives alive: symbolic interactionism (e.g., Blumer's *Symbolic Interactionism* [1969]), C. Wright Mills's work (esp. *The Sociological Imagination* [1959]) (Manicas 2007:9), and newly emergent ethnomethodology (e.g., Garfinkle 1967).

The Modernist Phase

Then, from a medical sociology setting at UC San Francisco, a new manifesto for qualitative research appeared in 1967: Barney Glaser and Anselm Strauss's *Discovery of Grounded Theory: Strategies for Qualitative Research*.[19] Charmaz (2014 [2006]:7; see also 2008) asserts that it is difficult to overestimate the power of this intervention as a defense of and rallying cry for qualitative research: "Their book made a cutting-edge statement because it punctured notions of methodological consensus *and* offered systematic strategies for qualitative research practice." The book was a crucial turning point in what became the "qualitative revolution" still unfolding today (Denzin & Lincoln [2011 [1994, 2000, 2005]:ix). Over the next half century, GT became the most popular form of qualitative analysis on the planet, with literally thousands of dissertations, articles, and books using GT and on GT as method.[20] (We discuss the divergences of GT below and in Part II.)

Of course, GT was never the only qualitative approach in use. Ethnography and field research had continued, but their status had waned in the United States from the 1930s into the 1960s. Over the two decades following publication of *Discovery* in 1967, an array of older qualitative methods were reanimated and innovative new approaches generated. Denzin and Lincoln (2011 [1994, 2000, 2005]:8) aptly called the years from about 1950 to 1970 "the modernist phase." It included ethnography, field research, interview, and other studies (e.g., Atkinson et al. 2001; Spradley 1979; Van Maanen 1995). Grounded theorists also pursued ethnographic work (e.g., Charmaz & Mitchell 2001).[21] In anthropology, major debates were underway about what constituted "good" ethnographic work (e.g., Clifford & Marcus 1986; Rosaldo 1989). Numerous qualitative text books were published, including Schatzman and Strauss's (1973) *Field Research: Strategies for a Natural Sociology* (see also

Bogdan & Taylor 1975). One classic sociological monograph of the era was *Boys in White: Student Culture in Medical School* (Becker et al. 1961).

Fundamental to the qualitative renaissance, at about the same time, explicit social constructionism, triggered by publication of Berger and Luckman's (1966) classic *The Social Construction of Reality*, was widely taken up. Constructionism (or constructivism) assumes that people (*including* researchers) construct or interpret through their own situated perspectives the realities in which they participate. Further, constructionism assumes that there is no one "true" reality "out there" to be understood; partial accounts of the array of extant perspectives understood "through the eyes of the beholder" are the goal. These assumptions became the epistemological and ontological grounding of much if not of most qualitative inquiry by the end of the century (e.g., Pascale 2011). Largely constructionist-based methods alternatives were initially offered to address the challenges posed by various critiques of positivism and theoretical functionalism of the 1960s and 1970s.

Constructivism can be viewed as an early formulation of the interpretive paradigm recently framed by Knoblauch, Flick, and Maeder (2005:5, emphasis added) as:[22]

> based on theories like symbolic interactionism, phenomenology, hermeneutics, ethnomethodology etc.—positions that stress the importance of investigating action and the social world *from the point of view of the actors themselves*. In a Kuhnian sense, this interpretive paradigm was supposed to substitute for the "normative paradigm," represented by structural functionalism or Rational Choice theories. Qualitative research, as it exists nowadays, is supported by and dependent upon a line of thought that is orientated towards meaning, context, interpretation, understanding and reflexivity.

In the United States, manifestos for constructivism and the interpretive turn were published by Herbert Blumer in a series of papers published in the 1950s that developed the symbolic interactionist theoretical and interpretive methodological implications of the thought of pragmatist philosopher George Herbert Mead. Blumer's (1969) classic *Symbolic Interactionism: Perspective and Method* is a collection of these papers that triggered literally years of debate between, on the one hand, functionalist theorists and survey methodologists, and on the other hand (or side), interactionists and other interpretive sociologists—especially ethnomethodologists (a then emerging tradition) such as Garfinkel. Significant here, Blumer essentially argued that theory and method are inextricably entwined and nonfungible. Today, this would be described as co-constitutive and Star's (1989) concept of "theory/methods packages" circulates widely (e.g., Clarke & Star 2008; Jensen 2014), including in SA (see also Clarke 2005:2–5).

The uptake of constructionism was transdisciplinary and transnational. Holstein and Gubrium's (2007) *Handbook of Constructionist Research* provides a valuable overview of how constructionism was taken up and put to work across disciplines and substantive areas. Lynch (1998), an ethnomethodologist, offers a contructivist genealogy of social constructivism focused on qualitative methods and social studies of science (see also Lincoln & Guba 2013; Velody & Williams 1998).

Important to the later transnational renaissance of interpretive qualitative research, at about this time, papers by Blumer, Garfinkel, Cicourel, and others were translated and published in German as a two-volume reader titled *Everyday Knowledge, Interaction and Social Reality* (Arbeitsgruppe Bielefelder Soziologen 1973). This and other translations of the time constituted the first big push for the revival of qualitative research in Germany.[23] In one such paper, Wilson (1970:701) wrote, "in the interpretive view of social interaction, in contrast with the normative paradigm, . . . the meanings of situations and actions are interpretations formulated on particular occasions and . . . subject to reformulation."[24] Moreover, "much more careful attention needs to be given to the way in which a particular interaction is embedded in larger social contexts" (Wilson 1970:706), at the heart of SA. Some years later, interpretive German sociologist Soeffner (2004 [1983]), a close colleague of Strauss, differentiated between Cartesian [positivist] and hermeneutic [interpretive] perspectives, asserting that this was the fundamental distinction *within research*, rather than the distinction between quantitative versus qualitative approaches.[25] This assertion was, as we shall see, quite prescient.

Rejection of normative functionalist approaches was becoming widespread. In 1971, Goffman wholly dismissed the scientistic claims of positivist (especially quantitative) sociology, asserting: "A sort of sympathetic magic seems to be involved, the assumption being that if you go through the motions attributable to science then science will result. But it hasn't" (quoted in Vidich & Lyman 1994:40). Anthropologist Geertz argued in 1973 for "thick description" for example, and applauded that "the old functionalist, positivist, behavioral totalizing approaches to the human disciplines were giving way to a more pluralist, interpretive, open-ended perspective," while boundaries between social sciences and humanities were blurring as well (Denzin & Lincoln 2011 [1994:9, 2000, 2005]). In sum, this initially modernist qualitative revival gained momentum until there was a full-fledged "renaissance of qualitative research" (Gobo 2005), which involved an interesting series of intellectual turns.

The Interpretive Turn

The next twenty or so years, c1970–1990, were called the era of blurred genres by Denzin and Lincoln (2011 [1994:9, 2000, 2005]). We see it as an era of considerable change characterized by the coalescence of constructionism and the "interpretive turn" and a tsunami of critiques of traditional approaches to research and responses to them. First, let us clarify that the interpretive turn has historical roots in Kant, Nietzche, Marx, Freud, Dilthey, Weberian *verstehen*, and, we would add, in American pragmatist philosophy, especially the work of Mead (1964 [1927], 1962 [1934]) on perspective. The Thomas's (Thomas 1978 [1923]; Thomas & Thomas 1970 [1928]) proto-constructionist "theorem" that if things are believed (read interpreted) to be real, they are real in their consequences also contributed. Lye asserts that the interpretive turn has become a cultural force with several central ideas:[26]

+ meaning has been relocated from "reality out there" to "reality as experienced by the perceiver";
+ an observer is inevitably a participant in what is being observed;
+ interpretations must be situated;
+ cultures are networks of distinctive symbols and signifying practices;
+ interpretation per se is conditioned by cultural perspective and mediated by symbols and practices.

Thus, the interpretive turn is an inclusive term.

During the renaissance of qualitative inquiry more generally, an updated vocabulary of inquiry came into use.[27] Generally speaking, "positivist" here is understood as attempting to understand empirical relations in objective reality. "Constructivism" assumes that the real is subjectively and locally interpreted—that there is no single "reality" people share, rather we interpret (individually and collectively) what is "out there." "Postpositivism" draws gently on constructionism and assumes that reality can only be represented imperfectly. "Critical" projects (discussed next) critique social, economic, and political representational and other practices in hopes of social change.

"Interpretive" approaches assume both the subjective interpretation of others' understandings (constructionism) and may also feature aspects of critical and poststructuralist/postmodern approaches (discussed below). It is today the broader term and travels more widely.

Feminist and Other Critical Turns

Participants in the interpretive turn in qualitative inquiry also began taking the critiques of the politics of the 1960s and 1970s seriously. Civil rights, anti-war, feminist, and other social movements generated critiques of *both* qualitative and quantitative research on multiple grounds including, especially in the United States, having sexist, racist, classist, elitist, homophobic, and colonialist tendencies, among others. Some critiques overlapped with others and merged into an array of new interpretive approaches that attempted to address those problematics. Here we briefly address critical and feminist approaches and discuss postcolonial/indigenous research innovations below.

In the United Kingdom, the Centre for Contemporary Cultural Studies (CCCS) at the University of Birmingham, founded in the early 1960s, became a driving transnational and transdisciplinary force for the interpretive study of subcultures, marginalities, popular culture, and media. Its researchers included Stuart Hall, Maureen McNeil, Hazel Carby, Celia Lury, and Sarah Franklin. They are known for combining critical, feminist, poststructural, and critical race theorizing, founding cultural studies as a field (e.g., Grossberg, Nelson, & Treichler 1992), and for renovating qualitative sociology, especially ethnography (e.g., Lury & Wakeford 2012) and subculture studies (e.g., Gelder & Thornton 2005). The influence of the CCCS, especially the critical and often innovatively Gramscian work of Stuart Hall on identity and community, still echoes loudly despite its tragic closure under British neoliberalism.

The roots of critical research are commonly traced to the Frankfurt School, including Adorno, Horkheimer, Marcuse, and Habermas both pre- and post-WWII, and they emphasized qualitative research. Neo-Marxist and other critical approaches expanded dramatically after the 1960s, due in part to anti-war, feminist, and civil rights activism, all of which served to highlight the profound inequalities in the United States persisting despite the post-war boom. Critical social scientists have sought to document patterns of injustice, subjugation, the reproduction of inequalities, and the changing nature of capitalism and its consequences, an ongoing research and praxis agenda (e.g., Kincheloe & McLaren 1994; Cannella et al. 2015).

During the 1960s, for example, Herbert Marcuse (then at UC Santa Cruz), became "the philosophical voice of the New Left," concerned with political emancipation (Kincheloe & McClaren 1994:139). Jürgen Habermas's work integrated critical theory and pragmatism in Deweyan efforts to link communicative rationality and the public sphere, especially *On the Logics of the Social Sciences* (1967).[28] Another key contributor to critical endeavors at about this time was Pierre Bourdieu, especially his *Outline of a Theory of Practice* (1977 [1972]), and field theory (1975). Bourdieu founded a major research institute in Paris that has elaborated his approaches transnationally (discussed below).

Other critical approaches, broadly defined, have also gained ground since the 1970s. Vis-à-vis qualitative methods, Kincheloe and McClaren (1994:140) assert that despite deep differences *within* critical communities of practice, there is general accord that "mainstream research practices are generally, although most often unwittingly, implicated in the reproduction of systems of class, race and gender oppression." We heartily agree and further assert that shared critique was incredibly productive in generating a wide array of critically informed new approaches to research by feminist, anti-racist, LGTB, disability studies, and other scholars now extending across almost half a century.[29]

Feminist research became a major growth area in the 1970s, especially but not only because of the growth of women's studies and later gender studies. The adage that "the personal is political," or that lived experience matters, was a key early generator of research issues as well as consciousness-raising. In its early years, *Signs: A Journal of Women in Culture and Society*, founded in 1975, published many "feminist state of the discipline" articles clarifying transdisciplinary research concerns. Both major debates and research texts and readers soon emerged (e.g., Fonow & Cook 1983; Harding 1987). The nonfungibility of theory and method was clearly manifest in feminist work (Hekman 2007). Stanley's (1990) edited volume on feminist research even had a section on "Demolishing the 'Quantitative' v. 'Qualitative' Divide." This point was later echoed by Haraway (1999), who asserted that counting for feminist purposes (such as documenting infant mortality where such deaths were not being recorded for political reasons) mattered. Both qualitative and quantitative approaches to research could be appropriate (e.g., Sprague 2005).

While there were—and are—many contributors, two are of particular note vis-à-vis feminist qualitative inquiry. First, sociologist Dorothy Smith (1987) wrote a searing critique of the discipline, *The Everyday World as Prob-*

lematic, calling for a new feminist sociology using "experience as data" (e.g., Campbell 1998), and critiquing "ruling knowledges." Smith and collaborators then framed a method called institutional ethnography, especially useful for organizational and policy-oriented research (e.g., Campbell & Gregor 2002; Smith 2005).[30]

Another sociologist, Patricia Hill Collins (1990), published perhaps the major anti-racist feminist statement as *Black Feminist Thought: Knowledge, Consciousness, and the Politics of Empowerment* that still echoes across the social sciences and humanities. Her theoretically astute work was soon combined with that of law professor Kimberly Crenshaw (1989, 1991; Crenshaw et al. 1996) on the concept of intersectionality, asserting that race, class, gender, and other major identities (such as sexuality, disability, etc.) are simultaneous and embodied. They are nonfungible and co-constitutive, generative of distinctive lived experiences that should be understood as such through research. Part of broader black feminist thought and critical race theory, research that can grasp intersectionality became—and continues to be—a major feminist goal (e.g., Boylorn & Orbe 2013; Gunaratnam 2003; Schulz & Mullings 2006).[31]

In anthropology, *Women Writing Culture*, edited by Behar and Gordon (1995), was the feminist response to the almost complete absence of women's voices in *Writing Culture* (Clifford & Marcus 1986).[32] Visweswaran's (1994) brilliant *Fictions of Feminist Ethnography* brought postcolonial, cultural, and discourse concerns together with feminist research issues and continues to deserve attention. And *Feminist Dilemmas in Fieldwork* (Wolf 1996) attended to distinctive ethnographic challenges. In education, Lather's (1991) *Getting Smart: Feminist Research and Pedagogy With/In the Postmodern* and other work (e.g., Lather 1993, 1995) broke new ground, establishing a key center of gravity for feminist poststructural education research that has now seeded the country (e.g., Jackson & Mazzei 2012; St. Pierre & Pillow 2000). Gradually, the array of readers and handbooks on feminist research has grown increasingly transdisciplinary in seeking to "liberate method," also reflecting the strong transdisciplinarity of women's and gender studies (e.g., Devault 1999; Hesse-Biber 2013a).[33]

Poststructuralisms and Their Reception

Poststructuralisms continued to inform interpretive projects across the disciplines in the West and beyond as the work of Foucault, Derrida, Deleuze, and other theorists began traveling widely and rupturing taken-for-granted assumptions. A series of often overlapping turns were choreographing emergent scholarship including linguistic (e.g., Rorty 1967), deconstructive (e.g., Derrida 1978), critical (e.g., Marcus & Fisher 1986), feminist (e.g., Lather 1991), participatory action (Greenwood & Levin 1998), cultural (e.g., Clifford & Marcus 1986), narrative (e.g., Holstein & Gubrium 2012; Riessman 1993), practice (e.g., Schatzki, Knorr Cetina, & von Savigny 2001), and postmodern (e.g., Denzin 1991) (see also Lather 2007:1–3, 2013).

At this time, the term "human sciences" also began to be used to indicate the turn away from scientistic and behavioral approaches toward more contextualized (we would say situated) approaches to the centrality of meaning and meaning making.[34] "[I]t suggests a critical and historical approach which transcends [social science disciplines] and links their interests with those of philosophy, literary criticism, aesthetics, law and politics" (Editorial for the first issue of *History of the Human Sciences* 1988:1). At issue here is that "a 'social' science emphasizing 'prediction' and 'control' can too easily use the veil of 'objectivity' to hide a dehumanizing impulse" (Yanow & Schwartz-Shea 2013 [2006:388]). Both terms, social sciences and human sciences, are now in use and remain differently inflected.[35]

Additional critical challenges of this era were posed by the related crises of representation and reflexivity. Here anthropologists took the lead in articulating issues including researcher reflexivity and how gender, class, race, and other attributes are manifest within research processes, both in relations between researchers and those being studied as well as in research products. Rosaldo's (1989) remarkable *Culture and Truth: The Remaking of Cultural Analysis* altered the project of qualitative inquiry profoundly, calling for a new ethnographic candor (see also Clifford & Marcus 1986). In education and elsewhere, Lather's (1993) "Fertile Obsession: Validity after Poststructuralism" challenged the nonreflexive core of positivism and became iconic (see also 1991). In sociology, Clough's (1992) *The End(s) of Ethnography: From Realism to Social Criticism* captured what was at stake for qualitative researchers. In nursing, Morse (1989) placed "sticky issues" on the table and recruited outstanding qualitative nurse researchers to create "a contemporary dialogue" that opened many doors for the future. And Fine's (1994) still remarkable paper, "Working the Hyphens: Reinventing Self and Other in Qualitative Research," laid out both the need for and means of addressing the crisis of representation and the relentless presence of the researcher at *all* stages of the research process (see also Pascale 2008). Reiterating pragmatist George

Herbert Mead, Yanow and Schwartz-Shea (2013 [2006:38]5) reflexively note that "data are generated, not 'given.'" The title of a recent book on uses of big data captures this perfectly: *"Raw Data" Is an Oxymoron* (Gitelman 2013).[36]

The first edition of Denzin and Lincoln's huge and hugely successful *Handbook of Qualitative Research* in 1994 signaled "loud and clear" that the renaissance in qualitative research had arrived. Because it brought together a very wide array of older and newer approaches to qualitative inquiry, the *Handbook* drew many interpretive and revisioned qualitative approaches under a broad qualitative umbrella, placing once "distant cousins" in direct conversation. To us, this *Handbook* was the second manifesto of the qualitative revolution—urging engagement across different approaches and many disciplines to both broaden interpretive approaches to qualitative inquiry and to strengthen the position of qualitative research globally. We would argue that it forever changed the face of qualitative inquiry and the teaching of qualitative methods in the United States and beyond. It was no longer possible to wholly ignore the postmodern/poststructural/interpretive turn, though some continue to try, sustaining the "contested" character of the field.

The emergent sensibility of this era had at its core the poststructuralist "doubt that any discourse has privileged place, any method or theory a universal and general claim to authoritative knowledge" (Richardson quoted in Denzin & Lincoln 2011 [1994:2, 2000, 2005]). Today, interpretive scholars make that doubt generative by rethinking the work that doubt can do in the research process per se, in keeping with Locke, Golden-Biddle, and Feldman's (2008) proposal. Here doubt is used to question innocence and can thereby be ethically productive. The moral and ethical issues involved in understanding and acknowledging that representing *is* intervening (e.g., Hacking 1983) are complex and continue to demand attentive engagement. In fact, these issues are at the very heart of contemporary interpretive efforts, especially work that engages indigenous concerns (e.g., Bainbridge, Whiteside, & McCalman 2013; Battiste 2007; Christians 2011).

Before proceeding with further developments, we want to discuss the reception of the postmodern/poststructural/interpretive turn. Interpretations of this turn range(d) widely from grave skepticism about the very possibility of further research to viewing its possibilities for thinking usefully outside of modern paradigms as strong encouragement to reexamine methods and their assumptions. According to Spencer (2001), in Anglophone anthropology this turn was made manifest in *Writing Culture* (Clifford & Marcus 1986), which brought the threads of many critiques together, and was "an accident waiting to happen." That is, the confrontation was already overdetermined by critiques dating back to the 1970s, especially those posed by feminism and Said's *Orientalism* (1978), both of which addressed problematic anthropological representational practices of exoticization.

We would argue in parallel that Denzin and Lincoln's (1994) *Handbook of Qualitative Research* was the "revolution waiting to happen: in qualitative sociology, communications, cultural studies, education, and so on. As Spencer (2001:444) noted, "The models of phlegmatic orthodoxy which had dominated . . . had somehow ceased to carry conviction," and "much of the volume's early impact was heavily polarized, along more or less generational lines." Some interactionists have taken this turn, Clarke included, initially via science and technology studies (about which more below), while others have remained wedded to more traditional ethnographic approaches, creating serious schisms across qualitative worlds.[37] For example, Atkinson and Delamont (2006) described the debate about poststructuralism as located "in the roiling smoke" of the battlefield, while Hammersley (2008:11) claimed that "the future of qualitative research is endangered." Denzin (2009a) replied with a play about the contestation titled "Apocalypse Now," and accused them, per Foucault, of attempting to "discipline qualitative research" (Denzin, Lincoln, & Giardina 2006). In some places, such debates continue to haunt qualitative inquiry, but not everywhere nor consistently.[38]

Interpretation, poststructuralism, and postmodernism, however contested, became keywords. Scholars from the United States were rather late to incorporate European social science and theory (Manicas 2007:17), and the work of Foucault was especially rupturing. But by 2011, sufficient momentum had accrued to have a remarkable conference titled "Foucault across the Disciplines" at UC Santa Cruz (Koopman 2011b) and to a special issue of *Foucault Studies* on Foucault and Pragmatism (e.g., Koopman 2011a).[39] Baiocchi, Graizbord, and Rodríguez-Muñiz (2013) have even explored Foucault-influenced actor–network theory and the "ethnographic imagination." The Atlantic Ocean is finally intellectually becoming what the British have long called it—"the pond"—and much wading back and forth is occurring.

At the turn of this century, Charmaz (1995, 2000) argued specifically for a constructivist interpretive GT. Yet even constructionism, which had interactionist roots that date to the 1920s and had fostered many qualitative approaches, was still in and of itself quite provocative to some traditional researchers (e.g., Glaser 2002) and entered U.S. public discourse via the bitter "culture wars" of the 1980s and 1990s (e.g., Hilgartner 1997) that still echo loudly today. Clarke comments about the tenor of this period:

> In 1997, as I was beginning to formulate situational analysis, I was invited to speak on qualitative research at a major university with strong qualitative doctoral training. The title of my talk contained the word "postmodern" and students later told me they were not allowed to use that word in the department. Moreover, at my talk, only faculty were allowed to ask questions and my talk was cut short by the chair, I suspect because I was presenting an affirmative and rather matter-of-fact perspective on postmodern issues. I was neither extreme nor easily demonizable, but clearly attempting to understand the social changes postmodernism engaged and insights offered. Similarly, other colleagues later recommended that I not subtitle the first edition of the SA text *Grounded Theory after the Postmodern Turn*.

Clarke was far from alone in appreciating the Denzin and Lincoln (1994) *Handbook*. For example, Gubrium and Holstein (1997; see also 2002) made an early effort at mediating the debates by seeking renewed attention to "methods talk." They viewed postmodernism as one of four "new languages of qualitative method" deserving attention.[40] Gubrium and Holstein (1997:80) further asserted that sociologists were "lagging considerably behind their anthropologist kin," and cited works in science and technology studies (e.g., Latour & Woolgar 1979) as "empirical projects that retain sociological orientations and objectives within more-or-less postmodernist frameworks."[41] We heartily agree!

Postmodernism was also generating its own research audiences. Alvesson (2002), a business school professor, published *Postmodernism and Social Research* in the United Kingdom as a guide for master's and doctoral students across the social sciences. Some in critical research traditions have also welcomed poststructuralist interventions: "In our view, postmodern criticism does not so much weaken the Marxian tradition as help to expand the Marxian critique of capitalist social relations by addressing the ambiguity currently surrounding the reconstituted nature of classes and class consciousness and by interrogating 'the cultural logic of late capitalism'" (Kincheloe & McClaren 1994:142).

Meanwhile, the renaissance in qualitative research has continued to manifest elsewhere in the academy including "recent scholarly 'movements' seeking diversity in methodology, such as 'Perestroika' in U.S. political science and 'Post-autistic Economics' in European economics" (Yanow & Schwartz-Shea 2013 [2006:388]). After receiving a petition with over a thousand members' signatures, the American Political Science Association established a new Organized Section on Qualitative and Multi-Method Research in 2003 (Collier & Elman 2008).[42] The "Post-autistic Economics" reform movement has at its heart an understanding of social relations and humans as interpretive and agentic persons (which autistics often lack), rather than as aggregates or things as has been the core assumption of positivist "normal science" in economics. It is directed explicitly against neoclassical economics, which, they argue, has attempted to suppress all other forms of economic inquiry and theorizing.

There has also been a qualitative revolution in psychology where calls for greater methodological pluralism have been made since the 1990s. Here, Wertz (2011) found that the areas in which qualitative methods have become most strongly established included applied, feminist, and multicultural psychologies. Toward the end of this era, in a book titled *Interpretive Interactionism* intended to draw symbolic interactionism around the postmodern turn and respond to anthropologist Geertz's (1973) call for thick description, Denzin appropriately called for "thick interpretation."

From Grounded Theory to Grounded Theories

At about this juncture, Strauss and Corbin (1990; see also 1994) published the first edition of *The Basics of Qualitative Research: Grounded Theory Procedures and Techniques*, essentially a "how to" textbook largely in the constructionist interactionist tradition that became extremely popular. Later editions (1998; Corbin & Strauss 2008, 2014) were completed after Strauss's death in 1996. *The Basics* added to GT research strategies, including axial coding, but also provoked very serious rebuttals by Glaser (1992, 2002, 2006; Glaser with Holton 2004) who then began his sustained campaign for the purity of the original—now called classic or Glasserian—GT (e.g., Martin & Gylnnild 2011).

Glaser and Strauss had ceased publishing together on methods after the *Discovery* book in 1967, and each had later published articles and his own important book on methods: Glaser's (1978) *Theoretical Sensitivity* and Strauss's (1987) *Qualitative Analysis for Social Scientists*.[43] We and many others (e.g., Atkinson, Coffey, & Delamont 2003:150; Bryant 2002; Charmaz 2000, 2014 [2006]; Strübing 2007) have argued that Glaser has remained faithful to the positivist functionalist sociology of Merton and Lazarsfeld at Columbia with whom he originally trained.[44] The positivist character of Glaserian GT is vividly realist and naively empiricist. In sometimes sharp contrast, and reflecting his philosophical pragmatism, Strauss became increasingly constructivist in his thinking (Strauss 1987, 1991, 1993) and remained an interpretive symbolic interactionist all his life (Charmaz 2008; Clarke 2007, 2008a, 2008b; Schütze 2008; Strübing 2007).[45]

By the new millennium, then, several different emphases in GT were in active circulation: Glaser's (1978, 1992, 2006) as positivist and objectivist; Strauss's (1987) as constructivist, interactionist, and interpretivist; Strauss and Corbin's (1998 [1990]) as procedural and post-positivist/constructivist, and Charmaz's (1995, 2000) as fully interpretive constructivist. And more GT developments were in the offing—including SA.

The 21st Century

In a major millennial review in Europe, two main themes in current qualitative inquiry were discerned: diversity as the growth of different approaches and unity ,"since despite all the differences, the various ways of doing research are characterised by the interpretive paradigm, a way of 'doing' social sciences that builds on meaning, understanding and context" (Knoblauch, Flick, & Maeder 2005:Abstract). The use of the term "interpretive paradigm" is significant in terms of the globalizing acceptance of poststructuralisms. Knoblauch and colleagues (2005:Abstract) further asserted that "scientific enterprises such as qualitative research are imprinted by cultures—and not only by 'epistemic cultures,' but . . . also by their surrounding institutions, traditions and political as well as economic contexts" (regional and national cultures).

The concept of "epistemic cultures" (Knorr Cetina 1999) asserts that through their actual practices of working, different scientific disciplines, specialties, and approaches generate distinctive cultures based on their epistemic assumptions, theories, and the practices used in doing such research.[46] This concept is part of the "turn to practice" moving across the social sciences and humanities (e.g., Schatzki, Knorr Cetina, & von Savigny 2001). While developed around natural sciences, Knoblauch and colleagues (2005) used this concept regarding contemporary qualitative research, and we find it quite useful as epistemic cultures are kinds of "social worlds" (e.g., Cefaï Forthcoming; Clarke 1991, 2005; Strauss 1978). This new century is deeply characterized by a proliferation of qualitative research worlds, sometimes feuding and others happily co-habiting under shared umbrellas, as we shall see next.

In the twenty plus years since publication of the first edition of the *Handbook of Qualitative Research* (Denzin & Lincoln 1994), new ways of configuring *both* qualitative and quantitative research have crystallized in terms of positivisms, constructionisms, interpretation, and so on, across disciplines and transnationally. With Outhwaite and Turner (2007:2), we would assert that there is today "a new geography of knowledge." Despite heterogeneous refutations of positivism starting with Lenin in 1907 and later followed by Parsons, Adorno, and Gouldner, among others, it is amazingly easy to "track positivism's uncanny persistence in the human sciences up to the present moment" (Steinmetz 2005:2).[47] Wyly (2009:310), a geographer, finds major changes since the mid/late 20th century, "when positivist epistemology, quantitative methodology, and conservative political ideology seemed always to go hand in hand." Of course, as he notes, this neat alignment was always contingent and contextual. But still, many of us use(d) it as shorthand in methods discussions, positioning positivist quantitative approaches to research under a broad umbrella in direct contrast to constructivist qualitative approaches, asserting the above assumptions and highlighting the very different liberatory feminist, queer, social justice, postcolonial, indigenous, and related commitments more common among contemporary qualitative researchers.

But today, not only is the "qual versus quant" shorthand no longer apt (if it ever really was), it is also dangerously obfuscating. For quite diverse reasons, the political alignments of a research project must now be interrogated rather than assumed. One reason, Wyly (2009:310) argues, is that "Right-wing political operatives have coopted many of the epistemologies and methods traditionally associated with the postpositivist academic left." Progressive researchers are also *themselves* pursuing *both* quantitative and mixed methods research for various reasons, certainly including hoping to make a difference in terms of public policy around many issues including race, gender, class, and so forth. For example, progressive epidemiologists have led the way in quantitative health inequalities research (e.g., Krieger 2005). Critical geographers have recently adopted a "strategic positivism" to revitalize their policy relevance toward building emancipatory geographies (Wyly 2009; see also Schwanen & Kwan 2009).

Feminist sociologists are pursuing quantitative research, including biosocial studies, asserting that feminists must participate in such projects to have gender issues adequately addressed (e.g., Springer, Stellman, & Jordan-

Young 2012; see also Sprague 2005). In education, de Freitas and Sinclair (2014) have published *Mathematics and the Body: Material Entanglements in the Classroom*. And there has been a longstanding fundamental importance of quantitative research to reveal inequalities of all kinds—and to assess the effectiveness of specific interventions to reduce processes furthering inequalities such as racism (e.g., Haraway 1999; Williams & Mohammed 2013). Further, the very groundings of quantitative research have been interrogated and expanded. Walter (a Tasmanian sociologist) and Anderson (2013) (a Canadian professor of Native studies and editor of the journal *Aboriginal Policy Studies*) published *Indigenous Statistics* to engage native quantitative research on population concerns on their own terms. They take very seriously not only the questions "What and who counts?" and "To whom?" but also "What counts as counting?" and "How does counting happen?"[48]

Further, *within* qualitative methods worlds across disciplines and transnationally if unevenly, there are also reconfigurings. Specifically, the crystallization of *positivist* qualitative methods and *interpretive* qualitative methods under quite distinctive umbrellas has deepened significantly. Several triggering factors are in evidence. One is the remarkable success of qualitative research transnationally (if also unevenly) in establishing itself as legitimate, becoming increasingly professionalized and institutionalized in the research curricula of the social sciences, humanities, professional education, and beyond—even in computer and information science, the military, science education, and applied linguistics.[49] A wide array of new national and international organizations, annual conferences, journals, and the like has been established in many parts of the world.[50] Knoblauch (2014) thoughtfully draws our attention to the "costs" of such institutional success—on the one hand, a proliferation of new approaches to qualitative research (though not always valuable contributions), and on the other, the growing tendency toward standardization or formalization of qualitative approaches. He asserts that the broader "interpretivist project" (Keller 2012a) is *intrinsically* placed at risk by attempts at standardization because remaining analytically open is so deeply important and standards tend to promote premature closure, especially in the hands of anxious beginners.[51] We heartily agree. The costs of success can be very high!

A second and related factor dividing the qualitative world into distinctive positivist and interpretivist camps has been an array of neoliberal attempts to scientize qualitative approaches. Often called "evidence-based" research

(EBR) movements, these are versions of the standardizations and formalizations that Knoblauch (2014) finds worrisome. Lather (2013:635) wonderfully called such initiatives efforts to "discipline and punish," reminding us that research methods are always already historically situated. In the United States, such neoliberal attempts to scientize have occurred especially in education (e.g., Lather 2010, 2013; *Qualitative Inquiry* 10 Nos. 1 and 2, 2004) and the health professions (e.g., Daly 2005; Knaapen 2013; Mykhalovskiy & Weir 2004; Timmermans & Berg 2003; Timmermans & Mauck 2005). Many other disciplines and specialties have been similarly if less intensely affected, including sociology (Lamont & White 2005; Ragin, Nahgel, & White 2004).[52] In both the United Kingdom (Henwood & Lang 2005) and Germany (Flick 2005:15), national research organizations have been created that similarly urge "integrative curricular formations" of "proven" research methods for doctoral training and beyond. (While such decisions largely remain local and disciplinary in U.S. higher education, research and other funding patterns exert both methodological and theoretical constraints.)

Such EBR efforts often seek to marginalize innovative interpretive approaches, and lively responses and debates have ensued across many disciplines, including sociology and political science (e.g., Becker 2010; Yanow & Schwartz-Shea 2013 [2006]), among others. Sadly, neoliberal guidelines often control access to funding and generate and support new and older positivist qualitative efforts. Proven methods generally manifest realist ontological orientations and objectivist epistemologies, and mixed methods with common problems may also be advocated. For example, "[T]he ontological and epistemological groundings of interpretive methods are so different from and contradictory to those of methodologically positivist methods that the two approaches are incompatible, resulting, all too often, in the kind of subjugation apparent in the NSF report and elsewhere" (Yanow & Schwartz-Shea 2013 [2006:384]).[53]

At the same time (but largely regardless of funding), other qualitative communities of practice or epistemic cultures have coalesced into an array of distinctive and *non*overlapping configurations. For example, there is today a strong transnational critical Bourdieusian ethnographic tradition with major centers of gravity in France, the United States, the United Kingdom, and Germany, and in many publications in the journal *Ethnography*, among others. This work often empirically examines various forms and structures of inequality interpreted via Bourdieu's theoretical frames. Some Bourdieusians claim the high ground for their approaches over all others (e.g.,

Bourdieu with Wacquant 2002; Burawoy 1998, 2000; Wacquant 2002; for responses to their parochialism, see Adler & Adler 2005; Anderson 2002; Dunier 2002; Newman 2002). Other Bourdieusians, however, engage more widely and with issues such as the adequacy of qualitative interviews in the contemporary moment (e.g., Lamont & Swidler 2014; Savage & Burrows 2007). Interpretive scholars not within the Bourdieusian fold also draw on his concepts such as cultural capital (e.g., Shim 2010).

Some qualitative communities of practice have eschewed the postmodern/interpretive turn and engagement with poststructural, constructionist, feminist, or postcolonial social theories. They rely largely on neopositivist or post-positivist traditional ethnographic approaches with different historical roots in terms of qualitative research dwelling within and across disciplines. In the social sciences, for example, there is an annual Qualitative Analysis Conference in Canada, books (e.g., Puddephatt, Shaffir, & Kleinecht 2009), and journals that more or less maintain traditional approaches.[54] Glaserian classic GT fits comfortably under this loosely neopositivist qualitative umbrella (e.g., Martin & Gylnnild 2011).

In sharp contrast, the interpretive qualitative methods umbrella has been zestfully held up against positivist and neopositivist deluges, especially but not only by the Denzin and Lincoln *Handbooks of Qualitative Research* (2011 [1994, 2000, 2005]) and the International Institute of Qualitative Inquiry. Since 2005, the institute has hosted annual congresses every May in Urbana, Illinois, of about 1,600 people from about eighty countries with preconferences in different languages (Portugese, Turkish, Spanish, etc.).[55] These conferences are effective organizing devices for the transnational qualitative social movement now globalizing the legitimacy of qualitative research across the disciplines. There are related readers on *Qualitative Inquiry and Social Justice* (Denzin & Giardina 2009), a *Handbook of Critical and Indigenous Methodologies* (Denzin, Lincoln, & Tuhiwai Smith 2008), and new interpretivist journals including *Qualitative Inquiry*, the *International Review of Qualitative Research*, and *Cultural Studies/Critical Methodologies* as well as older journals that welcome interpretive work.

A remarkably wide range of interpretive approaches dwell under this broad interpretive umbrella, from autoethnography and phenomenology with their emphasis on lived experience to conversational analysis and ethnomethodology,[56] and arrays of feminist, critical and cultural studies approaches, Foucaultian, and other modes of discourse analysis (widely taken up in Europe).[57] Interpretive symbolic interactionism, constructionist GT (Charmaz 2000,

2014 [2006]) and, as we shall see in this volume, SA (Clarke 2005; Clarke, Friese, & Washburn 2016) all dwell very comfortably here.

The 21st century has also brought renewed energy to critical, feminist, anti-racist, and most recently to LGBT research, today increasingly hybrid traditions (Kincheloe, McLaren, & Steinberg 2011). Recent critical readers (e.g., Denzin & Giardina 2009; Steinberg & Cannella 2012) include attention to all of the above. An edited volume on *Researching Non-heterosexual Sexualities* (Phellas 2012) is distinctively transdisciplinary as well as addressing both qualitative and quantitative concerns. Contemporary texts combining critical and feminist work also attend to both qualitative and quantitative approaches (e.g., Hesse-Biber 2013a [2006a], 2013b [2006b]; Sprague 2005) and explicitly activist research (e.g., Naples 2003). And feminist research has been ambitiously assessed and reviewed (e.g., Fonow & Cook 2005; Hekman 2007; Kitzinger 2004; Olesen 1994, 2000, 2005, 2011).

Flyvberg's (2001) call for "a social science that matters" captures some of the motivations for such changes, seeking more democratic and inclusive approaches and less polemical and confrontational and more dialogical forms of engagement. Emerging in the 21st century from the "science wars" and "qualitative wars" of the late 20th, scholars called for social research that focused less on universals and prediction and more on context, practice, and putting experience to work. This is a juncture where critical practice traditions (e.g., Bourdieu and others) began blurring in research pursuits with pragmatist philosophical attention to practice (e.g., Dewey) and poststructural framings (e.g., the Dreyfuses and Foucault). Flyvberg captured this productive synthesis.

Perhaps the greatest push in such democratizing directions has been the rapid growth of both participatory action research and indigenous research, both of which involve various strategies for fuller participation by those whose lives are being studied. Again, these are also often hybrid approaches. Action research, participatory action research, and cooperative inquiry (multiple terms are used) have roots in critical traditions, Bateson's holism, Friere's liberationist educational strategies, and Habermasian communicative strategies (e.g., Reason 1994). Such approaches have also been fueled by the turn toward reflexivity in qualitative research that questions relations between researchers and those being researched, especially vis-à-vis power (e.g., Reason & Bradbury-Huang 2008 [2001]). They have been most extensively used in education (e.g., Noffke & Somekh 2009) and health (e.g., Genat 2009; Minkler 2012; Minkler & Wallerstein 2008).

Relations of power between researchers and those being studied have historically been particularly fraught in colonial and postcolonial sites with indigenous populations. Over the past two decades, an array of new "decolonizing" practices and strategies for participation and innovative approaches in such sites have appeared (e.g., Denzin & Giardina 2007; Denzin, Lincoln, & Tuhiwai Smith 2008; Tuhiwai Smith 2012 [1999]). This is due in no small part to the fact that indigenous people are now scholars themselves seeking to undertake research differently, including understanding and legitimating radically different local epistemologies and ontologies toward enhanced epistemic diversity in research worlds and elsewhere (e.g., Bainbridge, Whiteside, & McCalman 2013; Battiste 2007; Mertens, Cram, & Chilisa 2014).

Epistemic diversity relies on the explicit recognition in all research processes and products that there are many ways of knowing or "local epistemologies,"[58] such as different paradigms within the same discipline, across the sciences, and within and across cultures and subcultures. Decolonizing and indigenous approaches are particularly attentive to this issue. The implications are broader in that non-indigenous people also may share quite different epistemologies from the dominant cultures in which they dwell. Recognizing epistemological diversity is part of the broader move toward social justice (see also Battiste 2007; Dillard 2008; Meyer 2008; Verran 2001; Watson-Verran & Turnbull 1995).

The Emergence of Situational Analysis

During the first decade of this century, GT was greatly elaborated transnationally. Charmaz (2014 [2006]) produced her fully interpretivist constructionist text *Constructing Grounded Theory*, already in its second edition. The ambitious *Handbook of Grounded Theory* appeared in 2007 with Bryant, a British professor of informatics, as coeditor with sociologist Charmaz, and contributions from Australia, Canada, Germany, the United Kingdom, the United States, and New Zealand.[59] Additional GT texts have appeared as well (e.g., Birks & Mills 2011; Corbin & Strauss 2008, 2014; Dey 1999). Charmaz (2005, 2011) also thoughtfully extended GT as a social justice methodology. Many of the theoretical and methodological developments discussed above have also contributed to changes in GT over the nearly five decades of its use and to the recent development of SA, as we shall next see.

SA (Clarke 2003, 2005), an extension of GT, also emerged at this time. It is part of what we term "the (re)turn to the social" or the reconfiguration of relationality taking place across the social sciences and humanities and manifest in both quantitative and qualitative methods. This turn involves heterogeneous and sorely needed reconceptualizations of the social per se. To clarify, historically, research data and analysis were conceptualized as centered on the micro (interpersonal), meso (social/organizational/institutional), and macro (broad historical patterns such as industrialization) levels. Qualitative research was thought to hold sway over the micro (though also pursued at the meso) level, while quantitative survey research targeted micro and meso levels (though aggregations of individuals often qua populations rather than as social grouping of various kinds), and some quantitative research and non- or marginally empirically based theorizing addressed macro levels.[60]

By and large, poststructural theories have abjured this tripartite framework. They argue that this construct is not only outdated and irrelevant but it also does not grasp a fundamental feature—that phenomena are *co-constituted*—produced through the relations of entities at *all* levels of organizational complexity (e.g., Jasanoff 2004). That is, social phenomena are nonfungibly *all of the above*, and analytic focus (both quantitative and qualitative) should instead be on complexities (e.g., Lather 2007; Law 1999, 2004, 2007; Law & Mol 2002; Taylor 2005), relationalities, and ecologies— the study of relations explicitly located in space and time (e.g., Star 1995; Strathern 2002).[61]

This (re)turn toward or reconfiguration of the social largely takes post-structuralisms into account and has coalesced around a number of metaphoric and often overlapping or hybrid approaches, many of which emerged from and/or are lively in science and technology studies, our own area of specialization. In qualitative research, these include:

+ situational analysis, which draws especially but not only on Strauss's ecological social worlds/arenas theory and analysis (e.g., Clarke 2003, 2005; Clarke & Charmaz 2014; Clarke, Friese, & Washburn 2016);
+ Foucauldian discourse analysis (e.g., Foucault 1972, 1973; Keller 2013, 2015; Kendall & Wickham 1999, 2004; Simon 1996);
+ Foucauldian *dispositif* or apparatus as a network of connections among seemingly disparate concepts, discourses, technologies, infrastructures, practices, and institutions (e.g., Bussolini 2010; Foucault 1980:194–228, 1991);
+ actor–network theory (ANT) (e.g., Latour 2005; Law & Hassard 1999) and/or material semiotics (Law 2009);[62]

+ assemblage theory (e.g., Delanda 2006; Deleuze & Guattari 1983; Marcus & Sakka 2006; Ong & Collier 2005; Suchman 2012); and
+ rhizomic analysis (de Freitas 2012; Deleuze & Guattari 1987; Jensen & Rodje 2010).

All have earlier roots but have been varyingly renovated to take recent developments into fuller account.

We find it fascinating that so many approaches to analytically grasping and reconfiguring the social have emerged and are flourishing at this juncture. SA as a relentlessly social approach draws on them as well. For example, from the pragmatist philosophy of Mead (McCarthy 1984; Mead 1972 [1938]) and using the language of ANT, we have adopted and adapted the *nonhuman* (living and not) as wholly worthy of analytic attention, especially in situational maps (see also Braun & Whatmore 2010).[63] Situational maps can themselves be conceptualized as *rhizomic* in Deleuze and Guattari's (1987) sense, drawing on that profound challenge to traditional hierarchical arboreal tree metaphors that pervade our imaginaries. Situational mapping also draws on Foucault's (1978) use of the concept dispositif as a set or network of relations. Social worlds/arenas theory (Becker 1982; Strauss 1978),[64] and Foucaultian concerns with the dispositif are taken up through social worlds/arenas maps. Significantly, Foucaultian attention to discourses is central to positional maps, the third kind of SA map. The SA method explicitly encourages study of narrative, historical, and visual discourses. *All* these maps attend to the *ecology of relations* in the situation in varying ways (Star 1995). (See Chapter 2 for discussion of the centrality of ecological relations in both GT and SA.)

SA draws deeply on Science and Technology Studies, and each of the editors of this volume has a strong STS background, Clarke since 1982. Most of the early roots of STS lie in France and the United Kingdom, and this transdisciplinary field was largely predicated on Foucaultian, Deleuzian, and other poststructural theories from its inception.[65] In fact, Clarke, who initiated SA, read poststructuralist STS work (e.g., Knorr Cetina & Mulkay 1983; Latour & Woolgar 1979) before poststructural theorists. Further, across STS in the 1980s, most scholars had some background in the philosophy of science where, "by the mid-1970s, not one of the defining planks of positivism remained" (Manicas 2007:8). Especially pertinent here, early STS projects routinely elucidated methods issues such as the theory-dependence of what counts as data, boundary construction as part of the creation, and maintenance of disciplines

(Gieryn 1995), the nature of paradigm shifts (going beyond Kuhn) as ongoing displacements of "old truths" (with a small "t"), and the nature and contingency of objectivities (e.g., Daston 1999 [1992]; Daston & Galison 1999).

Over the past several decades, interpretive multi-site or multi-modal case studies have become the most common methodological approaches in STS, typically drawing on interview, ethnographic, archival, and published data sources (e.g., Coleman & von Hellerman 2011; Marcus 1995; Rapp 1999). Precisely because the object of study in STS is, broadly speaking, the production of knowledge, the methods of STS practitioners have themselves always already been under scrutiny—if not by themselves, then by others. Thus, concerns with reflexivity and triangulation of data from different sources are built in rather than added on to the STS methodological tool box. Moreover, STS has been premised on the inseparability of theory and methods (e.g., Jensen 2014), and SA, too, assumes theory–methods packages (Clarke 2005:2–5; Clarke & Star 2008; Star 1989).

STS engagements with methods issues continue to be profound. For example, a 2014 special issue of *Science, Technology and Human Values* 39(2) focused on "The Conceptual and the Empirical—Expanding STS" (Gad & Ribes 2014). And a 2013 special issue of *Social Studies of Science* 43(3) is titled "A Turn to Ontology in Science and Technology Studies?" (Woolgar & Lezaun 2013). Because both methods and poststructuralisms have long been taken-for-granted elements of STS discourse, we bring to the table of qualitative inquiry very different and distinctive sensibilities about aspects of postmodernisms and poststructuralisms, such as seeing these as "always already" part of both methods concerns and an interactionist GT, hence fundamental to SA (Clarke 2005:Chap. 1).

Anselm Strauss was also very much part of the heritage we bring to SA, most directly for Clarke but also for Friese and Washburn. He was an exceptionally gentle man who eschewed confrontation, largely though not always beneficially. His scholarship included developing both the "negotiated order framework" (Clarke In prep.; Strauss 1979, 1982a; Strauss et al. 1963, 1964), which stresses social *processes*, and the social worlds framework (Strauss 1978, 1982a, 1982b, 1984, 1993), which stresses social *structuring*—flip sides of the same theoretical project in his broadly pragmatist/interactionist action-oriented sociology.[66] Theoretically, this combination generated among the most useful concepts in organizations studies—"cooperation without consensus"—that has deep pragmatist roots in Dewey and Mead as well as contemporary manifestations (e.g., Clarke & Star 2008; Star 1993).[67] This interactionist and highly ecological assumption attends to how cooperation can proceed *without* consensus and how individuals and collectivities can "set their differences aside," however temporarily and *contingently*, in the interests of larger shared goals. Thus, it should come as no surprise that, in a classic pluralist cooperative modus operandi that he taught as interactionist, Strauss advocated avoiding "straw man" arguments and prolonged critique, favoring instead doing one's own thing as superbly as possible. "Let the work speak for itself" was one of his adages, and one we share.

While Clarke, Star, and likely others struggled with Strauss about feminism, he collaborated with women across his career and explicitly supported feminist scholars (Clarke 2008a; Clarke & Star 1998; Star 2007; Wiener 2007). Invoking Strauss as a person as well as a scholar, Clarke generated SA and, with this volume, we attempt to sustain GT and SA into the future drawing on heterogeneous theoretical/methodological sources of insight and inspiration and letting the method speak for itself.

In the current qualitative research scene, SA contributes to the overall interpretive project through a broad array of endeavors (e.g., Clarke & Charmaz 2014; Clarke, Friese, & Washburn 2015).[68] These include feminist research (see also Clarke 2006, 2012), postcolonial studies, science and technology studies, critical inquiry, education studies, organizations studies, psychology, health and medicine studies, library and information sciences, ethnic studies, and aging studies. Appendixes B and C list selected exemplary works in each of these areas and selected exemplary works illustrating use of each of the three SA maps.

Issues Confronting Situational Analysis Today

We have deliberately constructed our framework to respect all ways of working because this protects our ability to argue for our own way of working. The alternative, seen too often in the literature, is a vicious circle of contempt between opposing positions. (Carter & Little 2007:1327)

A number of issues currently confront SA. A particularly important one is possible confusion among the different kinds of GT approaches now in circulation. To clarify these alternatives, Jan Morse organized a "grounded theory bash," which led to the book *Developing Grounded Theory: The Second Generation* in 2009. Here, Phyllis Stern represented the Glaserian version of GT, Barbara Bowers dimensional analysis,[69] Juliet Corbin post-positivist/ constructivist basic GT, Kathy Charmaz constructivist interpretive GT, and Adele Clarke interpretive situationist GT (Morse et al. 2009). The volume includes chapters on each emphasis and productive conversations among the contributors aimed at clarifying similarities and persistent differences that demonstrate a generosity of spirit too often missing in such debates, and which Anselm would have appreciated deeply.

Second, as difficult as it is to communicate the profound impact that *Discovery of Grounded Theory* (1967) had at that time, it is equally or more difficult to communicate the profound impact that the poststructural turn and its subsequent schisms have had in qualitative inquiry, especially but not only in the United States and United Kingdom. We would further argue that many of the challenges that have confronted research and researchers since about 1960—including those of feminism, anti-racism, postcolonialism, LGBT and queer studies, indigenous studies, and others—have in the broader domain of qualitative research too often been lumped together with postmodernisms/poststructuralisms. In fact, on reflection, there is relative silence across many of those debates about all of these concerns, perhaps especially sexuality issues. Moreover, as feminists painfully learned, the term must be pluralized as there are many feminisms locally and intersectionally inflected. So, too, are there many forms of racism and anti-racism, and so on. Further, the array of postmodernisms and poststructuralisms seems infinite. A single tarred brush is truly insufficient to the task of dismissing them.

Polarizations such as those manifest in the schisms in qualitative worlds are often simplifications by another name. Leigh Star (1983), in a brilliant article on simplification in science, demonstrates how simplifications can hide the work done, the messy politics of doing it, and often the lower level workers who actually did it. Simplification is often pursued in the interests of easier communication or translation—and academic publication essentially demands (some of) it. However, simplification also not only allows but encourages avoidance of addressing complexities and specificities—hence is highly problematic.

Another issue of concern in qualitative inquiry more broadly is the current proliferation of approaches (e.g., Knoblauch 2014). While some practitioners lament this profusion (e.g., Adler & Adler 2008; Hammersley 2008:181), in contrast, we agree with Yanow and Schwartz Shea (2013 [2006:390]): "If knowledge is power, then methodological pluralism disperses that power, whereas 'one best way' concentrates it. Reembracing interpretive approaches as a legitimate scientific undertaking, then, strengthens both the human sciences and democracy." In researching this brief history of qualitative inquiry, we came across what seems to be a promisingly useful vocabulary with which to continue Gubrium and Holstein's (1997) efforts to create "new languages of qualitative method": the concept of agonistic pluralism. Political theorist Chantal Mouffe (2000:102–103, emphasis in the original) writes:

> *Antagonism* is struggle between enemies, while *agonism* is struggle between adversaries. We can therefore reformulate our problem by saying that envisaged from the perspective of "agonistic pluralism" the aim of democratic politics is to transform *antagonism* into *agonism*. This requires providing channels through which collective passions will be given ways to express themselves over issues which, while allowing enough possibility for identification, will not construct the opponent as an enemy but as an adversary. An important difference with the model of "deliberative democracy" is that for "agonistic pluralism", the prime task of democratic politics is not to eliminate passions from the sphere of the public in order to render a rational consensus possible, but to mobilize those passions towards democratic designs.

Especially important to us is Mouffe's point about *not* eliminating passions, also asserted by Carter and Little (2007:1327) in the epigraph for this section. As Moss (2007:235) emphasizes in his article "Meeting across the Paradigmatic Divide," the concept of agonistic pluralism not only does not give up on or deny profound differences of perspective, but also recognizes and legitimates conflict arising from different interests, values, and perspectives. It promotes engagement *without* requiring domination by one camp or phony consensus, and to us echoes Straussian "cooperation without consensus" (e.g., Clarke & Star 2008; Star 1993; Strauss 1993). We believe *both* engagement without domination and cooperation without consensus are becoming increasingly important as the transnationalization of qualitative inquiry—and most everything else—continues. We will face many challenges of different forms of translation—linguistic, cultural, perspectival, epistemological, and even ontological—wherein cooperation will be of value.

Assuredly, both specific research approaches and innovative theorizing are traveling more widely. There are also more intentionally transnational venues for publication about the research process per se such as the online journal *FQS: Forum: Qualitative Social Research/Sozialforschung*, the *Interna-*

tional Review of Qualitative Research, and the *International Journal of Social Research Methodology*.[70] The free online journal *FQS* innovatively offers abstracts of all articles in English (the new lingua franca of academia) and may also offer them in other languages, while the articles may be in any language(s). This allows much broader access to new developments.

However, countering these expansive moves, major challenges in these times, not only for SA but for all qualitative research and research in general, are the consequences of neoliberalism for the academy (e.g., Lave, Morowski, & Randalls 2012). These include massive structural changes to universities, the essential collapse of public funding of higher education (especially in the United States), tremendous preferences for the "hard" sciences (especially information and computer sciences) over the social sciences and humanities, and the like, brilliantly summarized by David Theo Goldberg.[71] All of these changes have huge implications for how we do our work, who may fund it, what kinds of research are funded, and so on. In short, the constraints discussed above deriving from EBR movements may proliferate in a variety of ways regardless of evidence that is nonetheless deleterious to qualitative inquiry.

The interpretive turn, poststructuralisms, and other intellectual and social justice innovations including epistemological diversity are varyingly salient to qualitative inquiry transnationally today. We assume that it will take many decades and conversations, both easy and challenging, to communicate and translate the range of possibilities these innovations can make thinkable and doable in research and the domains of their possible effects and uses. While the future of qualitative inquiry will involve contestation, there are also calls parallel to ours for methodological pluralism against methodological tribalism from various corners of qualitative worlds (e.g., Carter & Little 2007; Lamont & Swidler 2014; Luker 2010; Yanow & Schwartz-Shea 2013 [2006]).[72] The terrains of qualitative inquiry will also remain uneven as we hope many new and interesting ideas for improving our endeavors will emerge and be negotiated in practice, described by Deleuze and Guattari (1987) as "continuous variation." Like power in Foucauldian analysis and pragmatist philosophy, we see continuing variation as generative.

Overview of the Book

When we began planning this book, we naively thought we could have a tidy table of contents, with each carefully selected article illustrating one or another kind of map and the kinds of work that map can do analytically. Instead, it turned out that the best articles often included two or more kinds of SA maps and illustrated several aspects of the method. Just as the SA method itself was developed to better capture the complexities of social life, we (a bit ironically) have also had to address the complexities of the articles we chose to include.

Part II of this book offers three chapters focused on SA method. The first, by Adele Clarke who developed SA, lives up to its title: "From Grounded Theory to Situational Analysis: What's New? Why? How?" It is very much a "how-to-do-SA" paper, orienting readers to the method to enhance understanding of the rest of the volume. The second chapter, also by Clarke, discusses how both GT and SA were always already feminist approaches as well as ways they had to be tinkered with to enhance their feminist proclivities. A variety of research articles using GT and SA in feminist projects is discussed. The third and last paper here is by Bill Genat and offers an exciting critical interactionist approach to participatory action research that is also highly applicable in many kinds of policy research. It is creatively developed through social worlds/arenas mapping (one of the three SA maps). Genat, who works in Australian Aboriginal communities, draws on the powers of careful listening and representation of the diversity of positions to foreground stakeholders' concerns and enhance epistemic diversity toward creating more effective policy.

Part III includes five chapters that exemplify using SA in diverse empirical projects in feminist women's health, education, science and technology studies, public health nursing, and organizational sociology. We also include reflections by those researchers on their use of SA written for this volume to illuminate how to use the method, what worked best for them, and why. Some of these articles emphasize situational maps, some emphasize social worlds/arenas maps, and some emphasize positional maps. (We introduce these articles in depth in the Introduction to Part III.) It is very gratifying to include such excellent articles, given that the method is relatively new. This is possible because SA builds on GT's advantages and helps strengthen and expand GT, especially by including discourse analyses.

Last, we offer several appendixes, including a list of websites on SA, a list of exemplars of SA by discipline, and a list of exemplars of SA by mapping emphasis. We hope you find the articles and the volume inspirational in learning, using, and teaching SA.

Notes

1. The book won the 2006 Charles Horton Cooley Distinguished Book Award from the Society for the Study of Symbolic Interaction. For an ambitious review, see Mathar (2008).

2. Simplified Chinese translation rights have also been sold, but we have no information on this publication.

3. SA is one of an array of methods seeking to replace former meso-level or middle-range approaches. See discussion of "the (re)turn to the social" in the section on Situating Situational Analysis. On using social worlds arenas maps and assemblage theory together, see Clarke and Friese (2007) and Chen (2011).

4. There is considerable recent attention to the importance of the material. See e.g., Braun & Whatmore (2010) and Puig de la Bellacasa (2011).

5. For the original development of the concept of implicated actors, see Clarke and Montini (1993). See also Clarke (2005:45–51).

6. Erol (2011) similarly takes up issues of women and risk in the social construction of post-menopausal osteoporosis in Turkey as Western patterns of medicalization spread.

7. For discussion of the social justice potentials of GT, which largely pertains to SA as well, see Charmaz (2014 [2006], 2011).

8. See, for example, Harvey (2011), Hess (2001), and Reid (2001).

9. The "democratic" approach of SA, with its origins in American pragmatist philosophy, contrasts sharply with the more "executive" or top-down construction of actor networks in the Latourian actor–network theory tradition (e.g., Latour 1987), also challenging this aspect of Foucault's approach to the analysis of power, which is to follow the powerful. Bowker and Latour (1987) interestingly argue that these differences reflect in part the centralizing tendencies of France versus the pluralizing tendencies of the United States.

10. This is based on a session that generated early versions of these reflections for the 2013 meetings of the International Congress of Qualitative Inquiry in Urbana/Champagne, Illinois. We are delighted to be able to include them here.

11. In writing this section, we are most grateful for the generous assistance of a number of scholars including Reiner Keller, Jorg Strübing, Kathy Charmaz, Monica Casper, Virginia Olesen, and Patti Lather.

12. We have each spent time in other countries teaching SA but make no claims to a fully transnational understanding of trends in qualitative inquiry. On the transnationalization of qualitative inquiry and its consequences, see Knoblauch (2014).

13. Local here references both geopolitical siting and local in Lock's (Lock & Nguyen 2010) sense of "local biologies," asserting that things mean differently at different places and times, including biologies and methods as established and interpreted through local practices. Contra Latour (1987), we do not see "immutable mobiles" but instead "boundary objects" (Star & Griesemer 1989), in which different social worlds always already interpret according to local needs and practices.

14. Other general terms used include life and case history analysis and field research. On the history of qualitative research, see e.g., Manicas (2007), Denzin and Lincoln's "Introductions" (2011 [1994, 2000, 2005]), Vidich and Lyman (1994), Rosaldo (1989), Knoblauch (2014), Atkinson et al. (2001), Seale et al. (2004), and Outhwaite and Turner (2007). The Special Issue on The State of the Art of Qualitative Research in Europe in FQS 6(3):2005 reviews

developments nation by nation, showing how professionalizing varies. See http://www
.qualitative-research.net/index.php/fqs/issue/view/1 (accessed January 27, 2015).

15. We draw lightly here on Denzin and Lincoln's 2011 [1994, 2000, 2005] periodization of
qualitative inquiry, viewing their framing as appropriate until the late 20th century. By that
juncture in the explosion of qualitative research called its revolution, we see both its heterogeneity and hybridity as defying overarching labels. Knoblauch (2014) emphasizes a similar
point, including European complexities.

16. There was, of course, a Department of Anthropology at the University of Chicago, led
by Robert Redfield whose research and that of many of his students focused on Mexico and
Latin America. Lindner (2007) discusses the roots of sociological ethnography in Robert E.
Parks's experiences as a journalist prior to his engagement with the Department of Sociology
in Chicago.

17. Later areas of focus at Chicago included Blumer's work on the movies and conduct, collective behavior and public discourse, and Thomas's interview-based work on unadjusted or
delinquent girls. See, for example, Fine (1995), Bulmer (1997), and Abbott (1999). Moreover,
some would not agree that Chicago School ethnography wholly became part of symbolic
interactionism, asserting instead that a large part of Robert Parks's work has stronger ties
to the human ecology approach further developed by Everett Hughes. In the United States,
Hughes (e.g., 1971) is seen as a symbolic interactionist and human ecology as dwelling there as
well. Again, the local matters.

18. In the United States (and perhaps elsewhere), Simmel's *The Stranger* (1921 [1908]) might
be included, as he was considered inspirational to the Chicago theoretical heritage. However,
in Germany, he is usually considered outside the range of Chicago symbolic interactionism.
He wrote this in Germany, without pursuing empirical work. Both Everett Hughes and Nils
Anderson spent time in Germany post-WWII doing and advising research and discussing
symbolic interaction and the Chicago School.

19. About 1960, the dean of the University of California San Francisco School of Nursing,
Helen Nahm, hired Anselm Strauss to initiate research training for nursing faculty (then
usually not doctorally prepared) in hopes of further professionalization of nursing. Strauss
then hired several other sociologists, including Barney Glaser, Virginia Olesen, Leonard
Schatzman, and Fred Davis. Eventually, doctoral programs in nursing (DNS c1968 and PhD
in 1982) and sociology (PhD in 1968) were established, and the doctoral sociology program
was housed in the Department of Social and Behavioral Sciences (1972), where it remains
today. Glaser left UCSF in the late 1970s. Clarke, Friese, and Washburn all received their
PhDs from this program (in 1985, 2007, and 2007, respectively). Pertinent to this volume,
Strauss was Clarke's advisor. She was hired into his slot in 1989 on his retirement, and later
advised both Friese and Washburn. See Friese (2009, 2010, 2013) and Washburn (2013, 2014)
for their work using SA.

20. A Google search (April 22, 2014) yielded 4,430,000 results—though most are likely
duplicates. While many GT works are excellent, many are not, merely using the term GT
but not the actual analytic practices, not uncommon for any successful method. For example,
Lynch (2012:452), former editor of *Social Studies of Science*, recently commented, "[O]ver the
past decade, I have been led to the sad conclusion that the volume of BADANT (Banal and
Derivative Actor Network Theory) greatly exceeds the well-researched and broadly informa-
tive written work that rides under the ANT banner." Success breeds its own new problems.

21. In a GT ethnography, the researcher focuses less on thick description overall and more on analysis of a particular social process or processes in the site being studied (Charmaz, personal communication).

22. See also Rabinow and Sullivan (1987) and Keller (2012a). T. P. Wilson (1970) was an originator of this term, pointing to the methodological consequences of various theoretical approaches advocating interpretive perspectives.

23. Special thanks to Jürg Strübing for telling me of this development and Wilson's (1970) highly significant paper. A number of later well-known German scholars of interpretive methods, such as Fritz Schütze (2008), translated the texts. See also Strübing (2004).

24. We quote from the original English article. Reiner Keller titled his 2012 book *Das Interpretative Paradigma* following from Thomas's 1970 intervention; Keller's book won the 2014 German Sociological Association prize for the best sociology book of the past two years. Keller and Strübing also note that the German situation vis-à-vis qualitative research was complex in ways that go far beyond the purview of this brief historical overview.

25. Hans-Georg Soeffner invited Strauss to be visiting professor to the University of Konstanz and also contributed to Strauss's festschrift (Maines 1991). See also in English, Soeffner (2004), Charmaz (2008), and Schütze (2008). For exact dates, see the Strauss website: http://sbs.ucsf.edu/medsoc/anselmstrauss/index.html (accessed January 10, 2015).

26. Lye is a website. See: www.brocku.ca/english/jlye/interpturn.php (accessed January 10, 2015). On the interpretive turn, see also Outhwaite & Turner (2007:359–457).

27. We draw here especially from Denzin and Lincoln (2011 [1994:13, 99–104, 2000, 2005]), but have tried to describe the terms as they are more broadly used in the general discourse of qualitative inquiry today—as "sensitizing concepts" in Blumer's (1969) sense of the term (see Clarke 2005:Ch. 1).

28. In that book, Habermas discussed, among others, Mead, Garfinkel, Cicourel, Strauss, and Goffman. After the return of Thomas Luckmann to Germany from the United States in the late 1960s, Alfred Schütz, Mead, and symbolic interaction received greater attention there as well.

29. In sociology, the Society for the Study of Social Problems, founded in 1951, became and remains a congenial venue for critical perspectives.

30. Dorothy Smith trained a cadre of students who generated such studies and helped develop the method (e.g., Campbell & Monicom 1995). Smith's sociology of knowledge approach seeks to grasp what she (1990) calls "the conceptual politics of power" dwelling in discourses particularly oppressive to females.

31. Of course, there were early contributions to this direction of thinking including work by Alice Walker and Audrey Lorde. Of note, *Signs: A Journal of Women in Culture and Society* recently had a special issue on "Intersectionality: Theorizing Power, Empowering Theory" (Summer 2013, vol. 38, no. 4).

32. Mary Louise Pratt was the only woman to contribute a chapter.

33. Institutionally in the United States, this reflects the success both of women's and gender studies and of their doctoral "special emphases" in feminist research, which enroll students from many disciplines on campuses where they are offered. Such special emphases legitimate scholars in terms of future teaching in women's and gender studies, as well as their home disciplines.

34. See Yanow and Schwartz-Shea (2013 [2006:xii]). They (pp. 389–390) also note that "human sciences" is often considered a better translation of a common German term for interpretive work—*Geisteswissenschaften*—in contrast with *Naturwissenschaften* or natural sciences. Of course, this reenacts the Renaissance/Enlightenment split between man and nature that Latour (esp. 1993) and others have taken great pains to challenge.

35. To some, giving up the term "social" could be seen as a major pitfall for qualitative inquiry and interpretive methods, as we are centered around the notion of "the social" (also discussed below regarding SA). There are similar debates about use of the term "science," with some asserting that term pertains primarily to prediction. We advocate retaining understandings of the social as bringing attention to material and organizational aspects of interaction and use both terms.

36. Mead (1972 [1938:98]), a philosopher by training, brilliantly wrote: "[F]acts are not there to be picked up. They have to be dissected out, and the data are the most difficult of abstractions in any field. More particularly, their very form is dependent upon the problem within which they lie."

37. These debates and rifts have occurred both in symbolic interactionism and in other qualitative research worlds. For examples, see Denzin and Lincoln (2011:10 [1994, 2000, 2005]), Snow and Morrill (1995), Denzin (1995), Atkinson and Delamont (2006), Hammersley (2008), and Adler and Adler (2008).

38. The contestation seems especially strong in English-speaking qualitative domains. Parallel arguments regarding "going too far" appear in STS as well, another transdisciplinary specialty that has had enormous success over the past few decades. See, for example, Jensen (2014) and works he cites. Lynch (2012:452) (referencing ANT) discusses how, when approaching travel, there is "drift and slippage from one node to another, with relatively weak and decentralized policing."

39. See, for example, http://humweb.ucsc.edu/foucaultacrossthedisciplines/foucault.htm (accessed January 12, 2015). See also Koopman 2009.

40. The others were naturalism, ethnography, and emotionalism.

41. Silverman and Marvasti (2008:18) deliberately misrepresent the moderate position taken by Gubrium and Holstein, asserting that their critique, taken wholly out of context, is best represented by "ominous words."

42. Robert Adcock, current editor of the section's Newsletter, noted: There was also some question during the opening years of the section as to how broad its understanding of "qualitative" was and whether that understanding incorporated "interpretive" perspectives or not. That issue was resolved over time in favor of a broad, pluralistic section that includes, but is far from limited to, a self-consciously "interpretive" subgroup (personal communication). See http://www1.maxwell.syr.edu/moynihan/cqrm/APSA_s_Qualitative_and_Multi-Method _Research_Section/ (accessed January 10, 2015).

43. For their methods articles see, for example, Glaser (1965, 1969, 1992, 2002) and Strauss (1970, 1978, 1982a, 1982b, 1984, 1991, 1995).

44. Glaser's (1965) early publication on GT was titled "The Constant Comparative Method of Qualitative Analysis." He cited both Merton and Lazarsfeld and thanked them for commenting on drafts. It was later reprinted (Glaser 1969).

45. See Strauss's website for a list of his many publications on Chicago sociology/interactionism: http://sbs.ucsf.edu/medsoc/anselmstrauss/index.html (accessed January 10, 2015).

46. Knoblauch, Flick, and Maeder (2005) also discuss the hegemonic position of Anglo–American research and researchers not only in terms of English becoming the transnational language, but also in terms of the wide distribution of English-language books and journals.

47. Steinmetz (2005) offers analyses of the legacies of positivism across a number of disciplines.

48. See also Verran (2001) and Watson-Verran and Turnbull (1995).

49. Thanks to Kathy Charmaz for helping expand this extraordinary list.

50. For Europe, see, for example, the Special Issue on The State of the Art of Qualitative Research in Europe in FQS 6(3):2005. http://www.qualitative-research.net/index.php/fqs/issue/view/1 (accessed January 10, 2015).

51. However unwittingly, and we believe due in part to efforts to teach the method more clearly, the Strauss and Corbin (1998 [1990]) *Basics* books made it seem like GT could and should be routinized and standardized. A similar situation of success and its many costs and contentions pertains in social studies of science today as well (see, e.g., Jensen 2014). There has been considerable interest in standardization and its problems in the last decade or so. See Bowker and Star (1999), Lampland and Star (2009), Timmermans and Epstein (2010), and Busch (2011). See also the discussion here about evidence-based work.

52. Nursing seeks "evidence-based practices" in the often contested domains of nursing and medicine. One website offers a menu of other sites, each offering different standards. See http://www.nursingworld.org/research-toolkit/appraising-the-evidence (accessed January 27, 2015).

53. See also Patton (2000) and Denzin and Lincoln (2011:2, 716 [1994, 2000, 2005]); compare Morse and Niehaus (2009).

54. See http://www.qualitatives.ca/past-programs (accessed January 12, 2015).

55. See http://www.iiqi.org/ (accessed January 12, 2015).

56. Ethnomethodologists often (but not always) dwell apart from other qualitative communities of practice. See, for example, Pascale (2011:105–138) and Lynch (1998).

57. For a review especially of European discourse analysis, see Keller (2013). On the new *Journal of Discourse Research*, see Matzner and Schmidt (2014).

58. Local is meant in Lock's sense of local biologies. See endnote 14.

59. Like Susan Leigh Star (2007), Antony Bryant was initially trained as a sociologist (he by Giddens, she by Strauss) and later went into informatics.

60. See Seale et al. (2004:3) for elucidation of the Parsonian version of these hierarchical tiers.

61. Gubrium and Holstein (1997:77) note that "postmodern sociologists allow for the possibility of relational patterning." See also related arguments by Burawoy (1998, 2000) and Law (2004, 2007).

62. "Material semiotics" is Law's version of ANT. Like SA, Law emphasizes relationality. See https://www.google.de/#q=material+semiotics+law (accessed January 12, 2015). On ANT in education, see Fenwick and Edwards (2012). On network theory and complexity see Crossley (2010).

63. Special thanks to Cefaï (Forthcoming) for drawing attention to Mead's lovely work on the farmer, the fig tree, and the wasp.

64. Social worlds/arenas (Strauss 1978, 1982a, 1982b, 1984, 1993:209–263; Strauss et al. 1964) and field theories (Bourdieu 1975) emerged at about the same time. In fact, Strauss spent

Spring, 1974, at the University of Paris at Bourdieu's invitation, though Strauss (personal communication) said they actually rarely met. On the history of social worlds concepts in interactionist works, see Cefaï (Forthcoming).

65. We use the term "science and technology studies" (STS) in sharp contrast to the (usually Mertonian) "sociology of science." STS is highly inter/transdisciplinary and transnational and can be dated to the publication of Latour and Woolgar's (1979) classic book *Laboratory Life: The Construction of Scientific Facts* and the founding of the Society for Social Studies of Science as an autonomous organization about the same time. Merton is generally credited with initiating the sociology of science in the 1940s as an American functionalist sociology project based especially at Columbia. Zuckerman (1989) ably reviews Mertonian work and glibly dismisses then emerging STS work. On STS history, see Jasanoff et al. (1995), Hess (1997, 2001), Hackett et al. (2008), and Sismondo (2009).

66. Cooperation without consensus is part of the Straussian negotiated order framework (Clarke In prep.). We use the term "social structuring" to emphasize that, in the interactionist tradition, structures are processual, generated in an on-going fashion through interactions over time, and are not established "once and for all."

67. Clarke and Star (2008) review many studies wherein cooperation without consensus was a major analytic. Leigh Star was a founding coeditor of the journal *Computer Supported Cooperative Work: The Journal of Collaborative Computing* in 1992, which provides an interdisciplinary forum for work linked to cooperation and activity theory.

68. The German translation of the SA text (Clarke 2012) was sponsored by a major figure in European interpretive research, Reiner Keller, whose own work similarly relies not only on the social constructionism of Berger and Luckman (1966), but also on the sociology of knowledge so central to STS, and to SA (e.g., McCarthy 1996).

69. Dimensional analysis was originally developed by Leonard Schatzman, a former student and colleague of Anselm Strauss and faculty member of the doctoral sociology program at UCSF (now deceased). It can be viewed as a variant of GT. See Schatzman (1991), Kools et al. (1996), and Bowers (2009).

70. Knoblauch (2014:para. 11) laments that the increasing transnational requirement to publish in English is, in fact, contributing to the standardization of qualitative methods, an anxiety we share. We believe FQS's approach offers a counterbalancing strategy.

71. For an extraordinary summary of the effects of neoliberalism on the academy, especially but not only in California, see Goldberg's work on "The Afterlife of the Humanities," which goes far far beyond the humanities, at http://humafterlife.uchri.org/ (accessed January 12, 2015). Goldberg also shows what the digital humanities can do—not only the sciences.

72. We do find it notable that the pluralist calls of which we are aware are largely being made by female scholars some of whom are very senior, while it is largely (though far from solely) men on "the battlefield" described by Atkinson and Delamont (2006).

References

Abbott, A. 1999. *Department and Discipline: Chicago Sociology at One Hundred.* Chicago: University of Chicago Press.

Adams, V. 2012. *Markets of Sorrow, Labors of Faith: New Orleans in the Wake of Katrina.* Durham, NC: Duke University Press.

Adler, P. & P. Adler. 2005. Review Essay: Lost in Translation? Review of Wacquant's *Body and Soul*. *Symbolic Interaction* 28(3):433–435.

Adler, P. A. & P. Adler. 2008. The Four Faces of Ethnography. *Sociological Quarterly* 49(4):1–30.

Alvesson, M. 2002. *Postmodernism and Social Research*. Buckingham, UK: Open University Press.

Anderson, E. 2002. The Ideologically-Driven Critique. *American Journal of Sociology* 107(6):1533–1550.

Appadurai, A. & I. Kopytoff (Eds.). 1986. *The Social Life of Things: Commodities in Cultural Perspective*. New York: Cambridge University Press.

Arbeitsgruppe Bielefelder Soziologen. 1973. *Alltagswissen, Interaktion und Gesellschaftliche Wirklichkeit*. Hamburg: Reinbek b. Hamburg.

Atkinson, P., A. Coffey, & S. Delamont. 2003. *Key Themes in Qualitative Research: Continuities and Change*. Walnut Creek, CA: AltaMira.

Atkinson, P., A. Coffey, S. Delamont, J. Lofland, & L. Lofland (Eds.). 2001. *Handbook of Ethnography*. London: Sage.

Atkinson, P. & S. Delamont. 2006. The Roiling Smoke: Qualitative Inquiry and Contested Fields. *International Journal of Qualitative Studies in Education* 19(6):747–755.

Bainbridge, R., M. Whiteside, & J. McCalman. 2013. Being, Knowing and Doing: A Phronetic Approach to Constructing Grounded Theory with Aboriginal Australian Partners. *Qualitative Health Research* 23(2):275–288.

Baiocchi, G., D. Graizbord, & M. Rodríguez-Muñiz. 2013. Actor–Network Theory and the Ethnographic Imagination: An Exercise in Translation. *Qualitative Sociology* 36: 323–341.

Barry, A. & G. Born (Eds.). 2013. *Interdisciplinarity: Reconfigurations of the Social and Natural Sciences*. London: Routledge.

Battiste, M. 2007. Research Ethics for Protecting Indigenous Knowledge and Heritage: Institutional and Researcher Responsibilities. In N. K. Denzin & M. D. Giardina (Eds.), *Ethical Futures in Qualitative Research: Decolonizing the Politics of Knowledge* (pp. 111–132). Walnut Creek, CA: Left Coast Press, Inc.

Becker, H. S. 1982. *Art Worlds*. Berkeley: University of California Press.

Becker, H. S. 2010. How to Find out how to Do Qualitative Research [comment on the National Science Foundation Report on Qualitative Research]. http://home.earthlink.net/~hsbecker/articles/NSF.html (accessed January 27, 2015).

Becker, H., B. Geer, E. C. Hughes, & A. L. Strauss. 1961. *Boys in White: Student Culture in Medical School*. Chicago: University of Chicago Press.

Behar, R. & D. A. Gordon (Eds.). 1995. *Women Writing Culture*. Berkeley: University of California Press.

Berger, P. & T. Luckmann. 1966. *The Social Construction of Realty: A Treatise in the Sociology of Knowledge*. Garden City, NY: Doubleday.

Birks, M. & J. Mills. 2011. *Grounded Theory: A Practical Guide*. London: Sage.

Blumer, H. 1969. *Symbolic Interactionism: Perspective and Method*. Englewood Cliffs, NJ: Prentice Hall.

Bogdan, R. & S. J. Taylor. 1975. *Introduction to Qualitative Research Methods: A Phenomenological Approach to the Social Sciences*. New York: John Wiley.

Bourdieu, P. 1975. The Specificity of the Scientific Field and the Social Conditions of the Progress of Reason. *Social Science Information* 14(6):19–47.

Bourdieu, P. 1977 [1972]. *Outline of a Theory of Practice.* Cambridge, UK: Cambridge University Press.

Bourdieu, P. with L. Waquant. 1992. *An Invitation to Reflexive Sociology.* Chicago: University of Chicago Press.

Bowden, G. & J. Low. 2013. The Chicago School as Symbol and Enactment. In J. Low & G. Bowden (Eds.), *The Chicago School Diaspora: Epistemology and Substance* (pp. 3–28). Montreal: McGill-Queen's University Press.

Bowers, B. 2009. Leonard Schatzman and Dimensional Analysis. In J. M. Morse, P. N. Stern, J. M. Corbin, K. C. Charmaz, B. Bowers, & A. E. Clarke (Eds.), *Developing Grounded Theory: The Second Generation* (pp. 86–126). Walnut Creek, CA: Left Coast Press, Inc.

Bowker, G. & B. Latour. 1987. A Blooming Discipline Short of Discipline: (Social) Studies of Science in France. *Social Studies of Science* 17:715–748.

Bowker, G. & S. L. Star. 1999. *Sorting Things Out: Classification and Its Consequences.* Cambridge, MA: MIT Press.

Boylorn, R. M. & M. P. Orbe (Eds.). 2013. *Critical Autoethnography: Intersecting Cultural Identities in Everyday Lives.* Walnut Creek, CA: Left Coast Press, Inc.

Bulmer, M. 1997. Quantification and Chicago Social Science in the 1920s. A Neglected Tradition. In K. Plummer (Ed.), *The Chicago School: Critical Assessments.* Volume 4: *Methodology and Experience* (pp. 5–31). London, New York: Routledge.

Braun, B. & S. J. Whatmore (Eds.). 2010. *Political Matter: Technoscience, Democracy, and Public Life.* Minneapolis: University of Minnesota Press.

Bryant, A. 2002. Re-grounding Grounded Theory. *Journal of Information Technology Theory and Application* 4(1):25–42.

Bryant, A. & K. Charmaz (Eds.). 2007. *Handbook of Grounded Theory.* London: Sage.

Bulmer, M. 1984. *The Chicago School of Sociology: Institutionalization, Diversity and the Rise of Sociological Research.* Chicago: University of Chicago Press.

Bulmer, M. 1997. Quantification and Chicago Social Science in the 1920s: A Neglected Tradition. In K. Plummer (Ed.), *The Chicago School: Critical Assessments.* Volume 4: *Methodology and Experience* (pp. 5–31). London: Routledge.

Burawoy, M. 1998. The Extended Case Method. *Sociological Theory* 16(1):4–33.

Burawoy, M. 2000. Introduction. In M. Burawoy, J. A. Blum, S. George, Z. Gille, T. Gowan, L. Haney, M. Klawitter, S. H. Lopez, S. O'Riain, & M. Thayer (Eds.), *Global Ethnography: Forces, Connections and Imaginations in a Postmodern World* (pp. 1–40). Berkeley: University of California Press.

Busch, L. 2011. *Standards: Recipes for Reality.* Cambridge, MA: MIT Press.

Bussolini, J. 2010. What Is a Dispositif? *Foucault Studies* 10:85–107.

Campbell, M. L. 1998. Institutional Ethnography and Experience as Data. *Qualitative Sociology* 21(1):55–73.

Campbell, M. L. & F. Gregor. 2002. *Mapping Social Relations: A Primer in Doing Institutional Ethnography.* Aurora, Canada: Garamond.

Campbell, M. L. & A. Monicom (Eds.). 1995. *Knowledge, Experience and Ruling: Studies in the Social Organization of Knowledge.* Toronto: University of Toronto Press.

Cannella, G. & Y. A. Lincoln. 2009. Deploying Qualitative Methods for Critical Social Purposes. In N. K. Denzin & M. D. Giardina (Eds.), *Qualitative Inquiry and Social Justice* (pp. 53–72). Walnut Creek, CA: Left Coast Press, Inc.

Cannella, G., M. S. Pérez, & P. A. Pasque (Eds.). 2015. *Critical Qualitative Inquiry: Foundations and Futures.* Walnut Creek, CA: Left Coast Press, Inc.

Carder, P. C. 2008. Managing Medication Management in Assisted Living: A Situational Analysis. *Journal of Ethnographic and Qualitative Research* 3:1–12.

Carter, S. M. & M. Little. 2007. Justifying Knowledge, Justifying Method, Taking Action: Epistemologies, Methodologies, and Methods in Qualitative Research. *Qualitative Health Research* 17(10):1316–1328.

Cefaï, D. Forthcoming. Social Worlds: The Legacy of Mead's Social Ecology in Chicago Sociology. In H. Joas & D. Huebner (Eds.), *The Timeliness of G. H. Mead*. Chicago: University of Chicago Press.

Charmaz, K. 1995. Between Positivism and Postmodernism: Implications for Methods. In N. K. Denzin (Ed.), *Studies in Symbolic Interaction* 17:43–72.

Charmaz, K. 2000. Grounded Theory: Objectivist and Constructivist Methods. In N. K. Denzin & Y. S Lincoln (Eds.), *Handbook of Qualitative Research* (2nd ed., pp. 509–536). Thousand Oaks, CA: Sage.

Charmaz, K. 2005. Grounded Theory in the 21st Century: A Qualitative Method for Advancing Social Justice Research. In N. K. Denzin & Y. S. Lincoln (Eds.), *Handbook of Qualitative Research* (3rd ed., pp. 507–536). Thousand Oaks, CA: Sage.

Charmaz, K. 2008. The Legacy of Anselm Strauss in Constructivist Grounded Theory. In N. K. Denzin (Ed.), *Studies in Symbolic Interaction* 32:127–142.

Charmaz, K. 2011. Grounded Theory Methods in Social Justice Research. In N. K. Denzin & Y. S. Lincoln (Eds.), *The Sage Handbook of Qualitative Research* (4th ed., pp. 359–380). Thousand Oaks, CA: Sage.

Charmaz, K. 2014 [2006]. *Constructing Grounded Theory: A Practical Guide through Qualitative Analysis*. London: Sage.

Charmaz, K. & R. Mitchell. 2001. Grounded Theory in Ethnography. In P. Atkinson, A. Coffey, S. Delamont, J. Lofland, & L. Lofland (Eds.), *Handbook of Ethnography* (pp. 160–174). London: Sage.

Chen, J. 2011. Studying Up Harm Reduction Policy: The Office as Assemblage. *International Journal of Drug Policy* 22:471–477.

Christians, C. G. 2011. Ethics and Politics in Qualitative Research. In N. K. Denzin & Y. S Lincoln (Eds.), *Handbook of Qualitative Research* (4th ed., pp. 61–80). Thousand Oaks, CA: Sage.

Clarke, A. E. 1991. Social Worlds Theory as Organization Theory. In D. Maines (Ed.), *Social Organization and Social Process: Essays in Honor of Anselm Strauss* (pp. 119–158). Hawthorne, NY: Aldine de Gruyter.

Clarke, A. E. 2003. Situational Analyses: Grounded Theory Mapping after the Postmodern Turn. *Symbolic Interaction* 26(4):553–576.

Clarke, A. E. 2005. *Situational Analysis: Grounded Theory after the Postmodern Turn*. Thousand Oaks, CA: Sage.

Clarke, A. E. 2006. Feminisms, Grounded Theory and Situational Analysis. In S. Hesse-Biber (Ed.), *Handbook of Feminist Research: Theory and Praxis* (pp. 345–370). Thousand Oaks, CA: Sage.

Clarke, A. E. 2007. Grounded Theory: Conflicts, Debates and Situational Analysis. In W. Outhwaite and S. P. Turner (Eds.), *Handbook of Social Science Methodology* (pp. 423–442). Thousand Oaks, CA: Sage.

Clarke, A. E. 2008a. Sex/Gender and Race/Ethnicity in the Legacy of Anselm Strauss. In Special Section: Celebrating Anselm Strauss and Forty Years of Grounded Theory. In N. K. Denzin (Ed.), *Studies in Symbolic Interaction* 32:161–176.

Clarke, A. E. 2008b. Introduction to Special Section: Celebrating Anselm Strauss and Forty Years of Grounded Theory. In N. K. Denzin (Ed.), *Studies in Symbolic Interaction* 32:61–69.

Clarke, A. E. 2009. From Grounded Theory to Situational Analysis: What's New? Why? How? In J. M. Morse, P. N. Stern, J. M. Corbin, K. C. Charmaz, B. Bowers, & A. E. Clarke (Eds.), *Developing Grounded Theory: The Second Generation* (pp. 194–233). Walnut Creek, CA: Left Coast Press, Inc.

Clarke, A. E. 2011. Von der Grounded-Theory-Methodologie zur Situationsanalyse. In G. Mey and K. Mruck (Hrsg.), *Grounded Theory Reader* (pp. 207–232, 2. überarb. u. erweierte Auflage). Wiesbaden, Germany: VS Verlag für Sozialwissenschaften.

Clarke, A. E. 2012. *Situationsanalyse. Grounded Theory nach dem Postmodern Turn*. Hrsg. und mit einer Einleitung von R. Keller. Wiesbaden, Germany: VS-Verlag für Sozialwissenschaften. German Translation.

Clarke, A. E. In prep. "Everyone Was Negotiating about Something": Forty Years of Straussian Negotiated Order Research. To be submitted to *Studies in Symbolic Interaction*.

Clarke, A. E. & K. Charmaz (Eds.). 2014. *Grounded Theory & Situational Analysis*. Sage Benchmarks in Social Research Series, 4 vols. London: Sage.

Clarke, A. E. & C. Friese. 2007. Situational Analysis: Going beyond Traditional Grounded Theory. In K. Charmaz and A. Bryant (Eds.), *Handbook of Grounded Theory* (pp. 694–743). London: Sage.

Clarke, A. E., C. Friese, & R. Washburn. Forthcoming, 2016. *Situational Analysis: Grounded Theory after the Interpretive Turn* (2nd ed.). Thousand Oaks, CA: Sage.

Clarke, A. E. im Gesbrach mit R. Keller. 2011. Fur mich ist die Darstellung der Komplexitat der entscheidende Punkt Zur Begrundung der Situationsanalyse. In G. Mey and K. Mruck (Hrsg.) *Grounded Theory Reader* (pp. 109–133, 2. überarb. u. erweiterte Auflage). Wiesbaden, Germany: VS Verlag für Sozialwissenschaften.

Clarke, A. E. & R. Keller. 2014. Engaging Complexities: Working against Simplification as an Agenda for Qualitative Research Today. *Forum Qualitative Sozialforschung* 15(2). http://www.qualitative-research.net/index.php/fqs/article/view/2186/3668 (accessed January 12, 2015).

Clarke, A. E. & T. Montini. 1993. The Many Faces of RU486: Tales of Situated Knowledges and Technological Contestations. *Science, Technology & Human Values* 18(1):42–78.

Clarke, A. E. & S. L. Star. 1998. On Coming Home and Intellectual Generosity. *Symbolic Interaction* 21(4):341–352.

Clarke, A. E. & S. L. Star. 2008. The Social Worlds/Arenas Framework as a Theory–Methods Package. In E. Hackett, O. Amsterdamska, M. Lynch, & J. Wacjman (Eds.), *Handbook of Science and Technology Studies* (pp. 113–137). Cambridge, MA: MIT Press.

Clifford, J. & G. Marcus. 1986. *Writing Culture: The Poetics and Politics of Ethnography*. Berkeley: University of California Press.

Clough, P. 1992. *The End(s) of Ethnography: From Realism to Social Criticism*. Newbury Park, CA: Sage.

Coleman, S. & P. von Hellerman (Eds.). 2011. *Multi-sited Ethnography: Problems and Possibilities in the Translocation of Research Methods*. New York: Routledge.

Collier, D. & C. Elman. 2008. Qualitative and Multi-method Research: Organizations, Publication, and Reflections on Integration. In *The Oxford Handbook of Political Methodology* (pp. 779–795). Oxford, UK: Oxford University Press.

Collins, P. H. 1990. *Black Feminist Thought: Knowledge, Consciousness, and the Politics of Empowerment*. Boston: Unwin Hyman.

Corbin, J. & A. L. Strauss. 2014 [2008]. *Basics of Qualitative Research: Grounded Theory Procedures and Techniques* (3rd ed.). Thousand Oaks, CA: Sage.

Crenshaw, K. 1989. Demarginalizing the Intersection of Race and Sex: A Black Feminist Critique of Antidiscrimination Doctrine, Feminist Theory and Antiracist Politics. *University of Chicago Legal Forum* 139:139–167.

Crenshaw, K. 1991. Mapping the Margins: Intersectionality, Identity Politics, and Violence against Women of Color. *Stanford Law Review* 43(6):1241–1299.

Crenshaw, K., N. Gotanda, G. Peller, & K. Thomas (Eds.). 1996. *Critical Race Theory: The Key Writings that Formed the Movement.* New York: The New Press.

Cresswell, J. W. 2007. *Qualitative Inquiry and Research Design: Choosing among Five Approaches.* London: Sage.

Crossley, N. 2010. Networks and Complexity: Directions for Interactionist Research? *Symbolic Interaction* 33(3):341–363.

Dahlgren, L., M. Emmelin, & A. Winkvist. 2007. *Qualitative Methodology for International Public Health.* Umea, Sweden: International School of Public Health, Umea University.

Daly, J. 2005. *Evidence-based Medicine and the Search for a Science of Clinical Care.* Berkeley: University of California Press.

Daston, L. 1999 [1992]. Objectivity and the Escape from Perspective. In M. Biagioli (Ed.), *The Science Studies Reader* (pp. 110–123). New York: Routledge.

Daston, L. & P. Galison. 1992. The Image of Objectivity. *Representations* 40:81–128.

de Freitas, E. 2012. The Classroom as Rhizome: New Strategies for Diagramming Knotted Interactions. *Qualitative Inquiry* 18(7):588–601.

de Freitas, E. & N. Sinclair. 2014. *Mathematics and the Body: Material Entanglements in the Classroom.* Cambridge: Cambridge University Press.

Delanda, M. 2006. *A New Philosophy of Society: Assemblage Theory and Social Complexity.* London: Continuum.

Deleuze, G. & F. Guattari. 1983. *Anti-Oedipus: Capitalism and Schizophrenia I.* Minneapolis: University of Minnesota Press.

Deleuze, G. & F. Guattari. 1987. Introduction: Rhizome. In *A Thousand Plateaus: Capitalism and Schizophrenia II* (pp. 3–25). Minneapolis: University of Minnesota Press.

Denzin, N. K. 1991. *Images of Postmodern Society: Social Theory and Contemporary Cinema.* Newbury Park, CA: Sage.

Denzin, N. K. 1995. The Poststructural Crisis in the Social Sciences: Learning from James Joyce. In R. H. Brown (Ed.), *Postmodern Representations: Truth, Power and Memesis in the Human Sciences and Public Culture* (pp. 38–59). Urbana: University of Illinois Press.

Denzin, N. K. 1996. Post-pragmatism. *Symbolic Interaction* 19(1):61–75.

Denzin, N. K. 2001. *Interpretive Interactionism*(2nd ed.). Thousand Oaks, CA: Sage.

Denzin, N. K. 2009a. Apocalypse Now: Overcoming Resistances to Qualitative Research. *International Review of Qualitative Research* (2ne ed.). Thousand Oaks, CA: Sage.

Denzin, N. K. 2009b [1970, 1989]. *The Research Act: A Theoretical Introduction to Sociological Methods.* Chicago: Aldine; Aldine Transaction.

Denzin, N. K. & M. D. Giardina (Eds.). 2009. *Qualitative Inquiry and Social Justice.* Walnut Creek, CA: Left Coast Press, Inc.

Denzin, N. K. & Y. S. Lincoln (Eds.). 2011 [1994, 2000, 2005]. *Handbook of Qualitative Research.* Thousand Oaks, CA: Sage.

Denzin, N. K., Y. S. Lincoln, & M. D. Giardina. 2006. Disciplining Qualitative Research. *International Journal of Qualitative Studies in Education* 19(6):769–782.

Denzin, N. K., Y. S. Lincoln, & L. Tuhiwai Smith (Eds.). 2008. *Handbook of Critical and Indigenous Methodologies*. Thousand Oaks, CA: Sage.

Derrida, J. 1978. Structure, Sign and Play in the Discourse of the Human Sciences. In *Writing and Difference* (A. Bass, Trans.) (pp. 278–293). Chicago: University of Chicago Press.

Devault, M. L. 1999. *Liberating Method: Feminism and Social Research*. Philadelphia: Temple University Press.

Dey, I. 1999. *Grounding Grounded Theory*. San Diego, CA: Academic Press.

Dillard, C. B. 2008. When the Ground Is Black the Ground Is Fertile: Exploring Endarkened Feminist Epistemology and Healing Methodologies of the Spirit. In N. K. Denzin, Y. S. Lincoln, & L. Tuhiwai Smith (Eds.), *Handbook of Critical and Indigenous Methodologies* (pp. 277–293). Thousand Oaks, CA: Sage.

Dunier, M. 2002. What Kind of Combat Sport Is Sociology? *American Journal of Sociology* 107(6):1551–1576.

Erol, M. 2011. Melting Bones: The Social Construction of Postmenopausal Osteoporosis in Turkey. *Social Science & Medicine* 73:1490–1497.

Fassinger, R. E. 2005. Paradigms, Practices, Problems and Promise: Grounded Theory in Counseling Psychology. *Journal of Counseling Psychology* 52(2):156–166.

Fenwick, T. & R. Edwards (Eds.). 2012. *Researching Education through Actor–Network Theory*. Oxford, UK: Wiley Blackwell.

Ferguson, R., M. Gever, T. T. Minh-ha, & C. West (Eds.). 1990. *Out There: Marginalization and Contemporary Culture*. Cambridge, MA: MIT Press.

Fine, G. A. (Ed.). 1995. *A Second Chicago School?: The Development of a Postwar American Sociology*. Chicago: University of Chicago Press.

Fine, M. 1994. Working the Hyphens: Reinventing Self and Other in Qualitative Research. In N. K. Denzin & Y. S. Lincoln (Eds.), *Handbook of Qualitative Research* (pp. 70–82). Thousand Oaks, CA: Sage.

Flick, U. 2005. Qualitative Research in Sociology in Germany and the US—State of the Art, Differences and Developments. *FQS Forum: Qualitative Social Research* 6(3):Art. 23 http://www.qualitative-research.net/index.php/fqs/article/view/17/38 (accessed January 27, 2015).

Flyvberg, B. 2001. *Making Social Science Matter: Why Social Inquiry Fails and How It Can Succeed Again*. Cambridge, UK: Cambridge University Press.

Fonow, M. M. & J. A. Cook. 2005. Feminist Methodology: New Applications in the Academy and Public Policy. *Signs: Journal of Women in Culture and Society* 30(4):211–236.

Fosket, J. 2004. Constructing "High Risk" Women: The Development and Standardization of a Breast Cancer Risk Assessment Tool. *Science, Technology, and Human Values* 29(3):291–323.

Foucault, M. 1972. *The Archeology of Knowledge and the Discourse on Language*. New York: Harper.

Foucault, M. 1973. *The Order of Things: An Archeology of the Human Sciences*. New York: Vintage/Random House.

Foucault, M. 1975. *The Birth of the Clinic: An Archeology of Medical Perception*. New York: Vintage/Random House.

Foucault, M. 1978. *The History of Sexuality*. Volume 1: *An Introduction*. New York: Vintage.

Foucault, M. 1980. *Power/Knowledge: Selected Interviews and Other Writings 1972–1977*. New York: Pantheon.

Foucault, M. 1991. Questions of Method. In G. Burchell, C. Gordon, & P. Miller (Eds.), *The Foucault Effect: Studies in Governmentality* (pp. 73–86). Chicago: University of Chicago Press.

French, M. & F. A. Miller. 2012. Leveraging the "Living Laboratory": On the Emergence of the Entrepreneurial Hospital. *Social Science & Medicine* 75:717–724.

Friese, C. 2009. Models of Cloning, Models for the Zoo: Rethinking the Sociological Significance of Cloned Animals. *BioSocieties* 4:367–390.

Friese, C. 2010. Classification Conundrums: Classifying Chimeras and Enacting Species Preservation. *Theory and Society* 39(2):145–172.

Friese, C. 2013. *Cloning Wild Life: Zoos, Captivity and the Future of Endangered Animals.* New York: NYU Press.

Gad, C. & D. Ribes. 2014. The Conceptual and Empirical in Science and Technology Studies. *Science, Technology & Human Values* 39(2):183–191.

Gagnon, M., J. D. Jacob, & D. Holmes. 2010. Governing through (In)Security: A Critical Analysis of a Fear-based Public Health Campaign. *Critical Public Health* 20(2):245–256.

Gandhi, L. 1998. *Postcolonial Theory: A Critical Introduction.* New York: Columbia University Press.

Garfinkle, H. 1967. *Studies in Ethnomethodology.* Englewood Cliffs, NJ: Prentice-Hall.

Geertz, C. 1973. Thick Description: Toward an Interpretive Theory of Culture. In *The Interpretation of Cultures: Selected Essays* (pp. 3–31). New York: Basic Books.

Gelder, K. & S. Thornton. 2005. *The Subcultures Reader* (2nd ed.). London: Routledge.

Genat, B. 2009. Building Emergent Situated Knowledges in Participatory Action Research. *Action Research* 7:101–115.

Gieryn, T. F. 1995. Boundaries of Science. In S. Jasanoff, G. E. Markle, J. Petersen, & T. Pinch (Eds.), *Handbook of Science and Technology Studies* (pp. 393–445). Thousand Oaks, CA: Sage.

Gitelman, L. (Ed.). 2013. *"Raw Data" Is an Oxymoron.* Cambridge, MA: MIT Press.

Glaser, B. G. 1965. The Constant Comparative Method of Qualitative Analysis. *Social Problems* 12(4):436–445.

Glaser, B. G. 1969. The Constant Comparative Method of Qualitative Analysis. In G. J. McCall & J. L. Simmons (Eds.), *Issues in Participant Observation* (pp. 216–228). Reading, MA: Addison-Wesley.

Glaser, B. G. 1978. *Theoretical Sensitivity: Advances in the Methodology of Grounded Theory.* Mill Valley, CA: Sociology Press.

Glaser, B. G. 1992. *Emergence versus Forcing: Basics of Grounded Theory Analysis.* Mill Valley, CA: Sociology Press.

Glaser, B. G. 2002. Constructivist Grounded Theory? *FQS Forum: Qualitative Social Research* 3(3). http://www.qualitative-research.net/fqs (accessed January 21, 2015).

Glaser, B. G. 2006. *Doing Formal Grounded Theory: A Proposal.* Mill Valley, CA: Sociology Press.

Glaser, B. G. with J. Holton. 2004. Remodeling Grounded Theory. *Forum for Qualitative Social Research*, 5(2). www.qualitative-research .net/fqs-texte/2-04 (accessed January 27, 2015).

Glaser, B. G. & A. L. Strauss. 1967. *The Discovery of Grounded Theory: Strategies for Qualitative Research.* Hawthorne, NY: Aldine [Transaction Pub.].

Gobo, G. 2005. The Renaissance of Qualitative Methods. *FQS Forum: Qualitative Social Research* 6(3). http://www.qualitative-research.net/index.php/fqs/article/view/5 (accessed January 27, 2015).

Greenwood, D. J. & M. Levin. 1998. *Introduction to Action Research: Social Research for Social Change*. Thousand Oaks, CA: Sage.

Grossberg, L., C. Nelson, & P. Treichler (Eds.). 1992. *Cultural Studies*. New York: Routledge.

Gubrium, J. & J. A. Holstein. 1997. *The New Language of Qualitative Method*. London: Oxford University Press.

Gubrium, J. & J. A. Holstein (Eds.). 2002. *Handbook of Interview Research: Context and Method*. New York: Oxford University Press.

Gunaratnam, Y. 2003. *Researching "Race" and Ethnicity: Methods, Knowledge, and Power*. Thousand Oaks, CA: Sage.

Habermas, J. 1967. *Logics of the Social Sciences*. Cambridge, MA: MIT Press.

Hackett, E., O. Amsterdamska, M. Lynch, & J. Wacjman (Eds.). 2008. *Handbook of Science and Technology Studies*. Cambridge, MA: MIT Press.

Hacking, I. 1983. *Representing and Intervening: Introductory Topics in the Philosophy of Natural Science*. Cambridge, UK: Cambridge University Press.

Hammersley, M. 2008. *Questioning Qualitative Inquiry: Critical Essays*. London: Sage.

Haraway, D. 1991. Situated Knowledges: The Science Question in Feminism and the Privilege of Partial Perspective. In D. Haraway (Ed.), *Simians, Cyborgs, and Women: The Reinvention of Nature* (pp. 183–202). New York: Routledge.

Haraway, D. J. 1999. The Virtual Speculum in the New World Order. In A. E. Clarke & V. L. Olesen (Eds.), *Revisioning Women, Health, and Healing: Feminist, Cultural, and Technoscience Perspectives* (pp. 49–96). New York: Routledge.

Harding, S. (Ed.). 1987. *Feminism and Methodology: Social Science Issues*. Bloomington: Indiana University Press.

Harvey, W. S. 2011. Strategies for Conducting Elite Interviews. *Qualitative Research* 11(4): 431–441.

Hekman, S. 2007. Feminist Methodology. In W. Outhwaite and S. P. Turner (Eds.), *Handbook of Social Science Methodology* (pp. 534–546). Thousand Oaks, CA: Sage.

Henwood, K. & I. Lang. 2005. Qualitative Social Science in the UK: Commentary of the "State of the Art." *FQS: Forum: Qualitative Social Research/Sozialforschung* 6(2):Art. 48.

Hess, D. J. 1997. *Science Studies: An Advanced Introduction*. New York: NYU Press.

Hess, D. J. 2001. Ethnography and the Development of Science and Technology Studies. In P. Atkinson, A. Coffey, S. Delamont, J. Lofland, & L. Lofland (Eds.), *Handbook of Ethnography* (pp. 234–245). London: Sage.

Hesse-Biber, S. N. (Ed.). 2013a [2006a]. *Handbook of Feminist Research: Theory and Praxis*. Thousand Oaks, CA: Sage.

Hesse-Biber, S. N. (Ed.). 2013b [2006b]. *Feminist Research Practice: A Primer*. Thousand Oaks, CA: Sage.

Hilgartner, S. 1997. The Sokal Affair in Context. *Science Technology Human Values* 22(4):506–522.

Holstein, J. A. & J. F. Gubrium (Eds.). 2007. *Handbook of Constructionist Research*. Thousand Oaks, CA: Sage.

Holstein, J. A. & J. F. Gubrium (Eds.). 2012. *Varieties of Narrative Analysis*. Thousand Oaks, CA: Sage.

Hughes, E. C. 1971. *The Sociological Eye*. Chicago: Aldine Atherton.

Jackson, A. Y. & L. A. Mazzei. 2012. *Thinking with Theory in Qualitative Research: Viewing Data across Multiple Perspectives*. New York: Routledge.

Jasanoff, S. (Ed.). 2004. *States of Knowledge: The Co-production of Science and Social Order.* London: Routledge.

Jasanoff, S., G. E. Markle, J. C. Peterson, & T. J. Pinch (Eds.). 1995. *Handbook of Science & Technology Studies.* Thousand Oaks, CA: Sage.

Jensen, C. B. 2014. Continuous Variations: The Conceptual and Empirical in STS. *Science, Technology & Human Values* 39(2):192–213.

Jensen, C. B. & K. Rodje (Eds.). 2010. *Deleuzian Intersections: Science, Technology, Anthropology.* New York: Berghahn Books.

Keller, R. 2011. The Sociology of Knowledge Approach to Discourse (SKAD). *Human Studies* 34:43–65.

Keller, R. 2012a. *Das Interpretative Paradigma. Eine Einführung.* Wiesbaden, Germany: VS.

Keller, R. 2012b. Entering Discourses: A New Agenda for Qualitative Research and Sociology of Knowledge. *Qualitative Sociology Review* 8(2):46–75.

Keller, R. 2013. *Doing Discourse Research: An Introduction for Social Scientists.* Translated by B. Jenner. Thousand Oaks, CA: Sage.

Keller, R. Forthcoming, 2015. *The Sociology of Knowledge Approach to Discourse (SKAD).* New York: Springer (translation of 4th German ed.).

Kendall, G. & G. Wickham. 1999. *Using Foucault's Methods.* London: Sage.

Kendall, G. & G. Wickham. 2004. The Foucaultian Framework. In C. Seale, G. Gobo, J. F. Gubrium, & D. Silverman (Eds.), *Qualitative Research Practice* (pp. 141–150). London: Sage.

Khaw, L. 2012. Mapping the Process: An Exemplar of Using Situational Analysis in a Grounded Theory Study. *Journal of Family Theory and Review* 4:138–147.

Kincheloe, J. & P. McLaren. 1994. Rethinking Critical Theory and Qualitative Research. In N. K. Denzin & Y. S. Lincoln (Eds.), *Handbook of Qualitative Research* (pp. 138–157). Thousand Oaks, CA: Sage.

Kincheloe, J. L., P. McLaren, & S. R. Steinberg. 2011. Critical Pedagogy and Qualitative Research: Moving to the Bricolage. In N. K. Denzin & Y. S. Lincoln (Eds.), *Handbook of Qualitative Research* (4th ed., pp. 163–178). Thousand Oaks, CA: Sage.

Kitzinger, C. 2004. Feminist Approaches. In C. Seale, G. Gobo, J. F. Gubrium, & D. Silverman (Eds.), *Qualitative Research Practice* (pp. 125–140). London: Sage.

Klein, N. 2007. *The Shock Doctrine: The Rise of Disaster Capitalism.* New York: Metropolitan Books.

Knaapen, L. 2013. Being "Evidence-based" in the Absence of Evidence: The Management of Non-evidence in Guideline Development. *Social Studies of Science* 43(5):681–706.

Knoblauch, H. 2014. Qualitative Methods at the Crossroads: Recent Developments in Interpretive Social Research. *Forum Qualitative Sozialforschung / Forum: Qualitative Social Research 14*(3):Art. 12. http://nbn-resolving.de/urn:nbn:de:0114-fqs1303128 (accessed January 22, 2015).

Knoblauch, H., U. Flick, & C. Maeder. 2005. Qualitative Methods in Europe: The Variety of Social Research. *FQS Forum: Qualitative Social Research* 6(3):Art. 34. www.qualitative-research.net/index.php/fqs/article/view/3/8 (accessed January 22, 2015).

Knorr Cetina, K. 1999. *Epistemic Cultures: How the Sciences Make Knowledge.* Cambridge, MA: Harvard University Press.

Knorr Cetina, K. & M. Mulkay (Eds.). 1983. *Science Observed: Perspectives on the Social Study of Science.* London: Sage.

Kools, S., M. McCarthy, R. Durham, & L. Robrecht. 1996. Dimensional Analysis: Broadening the Conception of Grounded Theory. *Qualitative Health Research* 6(3):312–330.

Koopman, C. 2009. *Pragmatism as Transition: Historicity and Hope in James, Dewey, and Rorty.* New York: Columbia University Press.

Koopman, C. 2011a. Foucault and Pragmatism: Introductory Notes on Metaphilosophical Methodology. *Foucault Studies* 11:3–10.

Koopman, C. 2011b. Foucault across the Disciplines: Introductory Notes on Contingency in Critical Inquiry. *History of the Human Science* 24(4):1–12.

Krieger, N. 2005. *Embodying Inequality: Epidemiologic Perspectives.* Amityville, NY: Baywood.

Lamont, M. & A. Swidler. 2014. Methodological Pluralism and the Possibilities and Limits of Interviewing. *Qualitative Sociology* 37:153–171.

Lamont, M. & P. White. 2005. *Workshop on Interdisciplinary Standards for Systematic Qualitative Research.* Washington, DC: National Science Foundation.

Lampland, M. & S. L. Star (Eds.). 2009. *Standards and Their Stories: How Quantifying, Classifying and Formalizing Practices Shape Everyday Life.* Ithaca, NY: Cornell University Press.

Lather, P. 1991. *Getting Smart: Feminist Research and Pedagogy with/in the Postmodern.* New York: Routledge.

Lather, P. 1993. Fertile Obsession: Validity after Poststructuralism. *Sociological Quarterly* 34(4):673–693.

Lather, P. 1995. The Validity of Angels: Interpretive and Textual Strategies in Researching the Lives of Women with HIV/AIDS. *Qualitative Inquiry* 1(1):41–68.

Lather, P. 2006. Foucauldian Scientificity: Rethinking the Nexus of Qualitative Research and Educational Policy Analysis. *International Journal of Qualitative Studies in Education* 19(6):783–791.

Lather, P. 2007. *Getting Lost: Feminist Efforts toward a Double(D) Science.* Albany: SUNY Press.

Lather, P. 2010. *Engaging Science Policy: From the Side of the Messy.* New York: Peter Lang.

Lather, P. 2013. Methodology-21: What Do We Do in the Afterward? *International Journal of Qualitative Studies in Education* 26(6):634–645.

Latour, B. 1987. *Science in Action: How to Follow Scientists and Engineers through Society.* Cambridge, MA: Harvard University Press.

Latour, B. 1993. *We Have Never Been Modern.* Cambridge, MA: Harvard University Press.

Latour, B. 2005. *Reassembling the Social: An Introduction to Actor-Network-Theory.* Oxford, UK: Oxford University Press.

Latour, B. & S. Woolgar. 1979. *Laboratory Life: The Social Construction of Scientific Facts.* Beverley Hills, CA: Sage.

Lave, R., P. Morowski, & S. Randalls. 2012. STS [Science and Technology Studies] and Neoliberal Science. *Social Studies of Science* 40(5):659–675.

Law, J. 1999. After ANT: Complexity, Naming and Topology. In J. Law & J. Hassard (Eds.), *Actor Network Theory and after* (1–14). Oxford, UK: Blackwell.

Law, J. 2004. *After Method: Mess in Social Science Research.* London: Routledge.

Law, J. 2007. Making a Mess with Method. In W. Outhwaite & S. P. Turner (Eds.), *Handbook of Social Science Methodology* (pp. 595–606). Thousand Oaks, CA: Sage.

Law, J. 2009. Actor Network Theory and Material Semiotics. In B. S. Turner (Ed.), *The New Blackwell Companion to Social Theory* (pp. 141–158). Oxford, UK: Blackwell Publishing Ltd.

Law, J. & J. Hassard (Eds.). 1999. *Actor Network Theory and After*. Oxford, UK: Blackwell.

Law, J. & A. Mol (Eds.). 2002. *Complexities: Social Studies of Knowledge Practices*. Durham, NC: Duke University Press.

Lempert, L. B. 1996. Women's Strategies for Survival: Developing Agency in Abusive Relationships. *Journal of Family Violence* 11(3):269–289.

Lincoln, Y. S. & E. G. Guba. 2013. *The Constructivist Credo*. Walnut Creek, CA: Left Coast Press, Inc.

Lindner, R. 2007. *Die Entdeckung der Stadtkultur. Soziologie aus der Erfahrung der Reportage* (2nd ed.). Frankfurt: Campus.

Lock, M. & V. K. Nguyen. 2010. *An Anthropology of Biomedicine*. Oxford, UK : Wiley-Blackwell.

Locke, K. 2001. *Grounded Theory in Management Research*. Thousand Oaks, CA: Sage.

Locke, K., K. Golden-Biddle, & M. S. Feldman. 2008. Making Doubt Generative: Rethinking the Role of Doubt in the Research Process. *Organization Science* 19(6):907–918.

Lofland, J. & L. Lofland. 1984. *Analyzing Social Settings* (2nd ed.). Belmont, CA: Wadsworth.

Luker, K. 2010. *Salsa Dancing into the Social Sciences: Research in an Age of Info-glut*. Cambridge, MA: Harvard University Press.

Lury, C. & N. Wakeford (Eds.). 2012. *Inventive Methods: The Happening of the Social*. London: Routledge.

Lynch, M. 1998. Towards a Constructivist Genealogy of Social Constructivism. In I. Velody & R. Williams (Eds.), *The Politics of Constructionism* (pp. 13–32). London: Sage.

Lynch, M. 2012. Self-exemplifying Revolutions: Notes on Kuhn and Latour. *Social Studies of Science* 42(3):449–455.

Maines, D. (Ed.). 1991. *Social Organization and Social Process: Essays in Honor of Anselm Strauss* (pp. 119–158). Hawthorne, NY: Aldine de Gruyter.

Manicas, P. 2007. The Social Sciences since WWII: The Rise and Fall of Scientism. In W. Outhwaite & S. P. Turner (Eds.), *Handbook of Social Science Methodology* (pp. 7–31). Thousand Oaks, CA: Sage.

Marcus, G. E. 1995. Ethnography in/of the World System: The Emergence of Multi-sited Ethnography. *Annual Review of Anthropology* 24:95–117.

Marcus, G. E. 1998. *Ethnography through Thick and Thin*. Princeton, NJ: Princeton University Press.

Marcus, G. E. & M. M. J. Fischer. 1986. The Crisis of Representation in the Human Sciences. In *Anthropology as Cultural Critique* (pp. 7–16). Chicago: University of Chicago Press.

Marcus, G. E. & E. Saka. 2006. Assemblage. *Theory, Culture and Society* 23(2–3):101–109.

Martin, V. & A. Gylnnild (Eds.). 2011. *Grounded Theory: The Philosophy, Method, and Work of Barney Glaser*. Boca Raton, FL: Brown Walker Press.

Martinez, A. 2013. Reconsidering Acculturation in Dietary Change Research among Latino Immigrants: Challenging the Preconditions of US Migration. *Ethnicity & Health* 18(2):115–135.

Mathar, T. 2008. Making a Mess with Situational Analysis? Review Essay: Adele Clarke 2005. Situational Analysis—Grounded Theory after the Postmodern Turn. *Forum Qualitative Sozialforschung / Forum: Qualitative Social Research* 9(2):Art. 4. http://nbn-resolving.de/urn:nbn:de:0114-fqs080244 (accessed January 27, 2015).

Matzner, N. & L. M. Schmidt. 2014. Conference Report: Project Journal of Discourse Research and the Prospects of Disciplinary, Interdisciplinary and Transdisciplinary Cooperation. *Forum Qualitative Social Research/ Sozialforschung* 15(3). http://www.qualitative-research.net/index.php/fqs/article/view/2219 (accessed January 27, 2015).

McCarthy, D. 1984. Towards a Sociology of the Physical World: George Herbert Mead on Physical Objects. In N. K. Denzin (Ed.), *Studies in Symbolic Interaction* 5:105–121.

McCarthy, D. 1996. *Knowledge as Culture: The New Sociology of Knowledge.* New York: Routledge.

Mead, G. H. 1964 [1927]. The Objective Reality of Perspectives. In A. J. Reck (Ed.), *Selected Writings of George Herbert Mead* (pp. 306–319). Chicago: University of Chicago Press.

Mead, G. H. 1962 [1934]. *Mind, Self and Society.* (C. W. Morris, Ed.). Chicago: University of Chicago Press.

Mead, G. H. 1972 [1938]. *The Philosophy of the Act.* Chicago: University of Chicago Press.

Mertens, D. M., F. Cram, & B. Chilia (Eds.). 2014. *Indigenous Pathways into Social Research: Voices of a New Generation.* Walnut Creek, CA: Left Coast Press, Inc.

Meyer, M. A. 2008. Indigenous and Authentic: Hawaiian Epistemology and the Triangulation of Meaning. In N. K. Denzin, Y. S. Lincoln, & L. Tuhiwai Smith (Eds.), *Handbook of Critical and Indigenous Methodologies* (pp. 217–233). Thousand Oaks, CA: Sage.

Mills, C. W. 1940. Situated Actions and Vocabularies of Motive. *American Sociological Review* 6:904–913.

Mills, C. W. 1959. *The Sociological Imagination.* New York: Oxford University Press.

Minkler, M. (Ed.). 2012. *Community Organizing and Community Building for Health and Welfare* (3rd ed.). New Brunswick, NJ: Rutgers University Press.

Minkler, M. & N. Wallerstein (Eds.). 2008. *Community-based Participatory Research for Health: From Process to Outcomes* (2nd ed.). San Francisco: Jossey-Bass.

Morse, J. M. 1989. *Qualitative Nursing Research: A Contemporary Dialogue.* Newbury Park, CA: Sage.

Morse, J. M. & L. Niehaus. 2009. *Mixed Method Design: Principles and Procedures.* Walnut Creek, CA: Left Coast Press, Inc.

Morse, J. M., P. N. Stern, J. Corbin, B. Bowers, K. Charmaz, & A. E. Clarke. 2009. *Developing Grounded Theory: The Second Generation.* Walnut Creek, CA: Left Coast Press, Inc.

Moss, P. 2007. Meetings across the Paradigmatic Divide. *Educational Philosophy and Theory* 39(3):229–245.

Mouffe, C. 2000. *The Democratic Paradox.* London: Verso.

Mykhalovskiy, E. & L. Weir. 2004. The Problem of Evidence-based Medicine: Directions for Social Science. *Social Science and Medicine* 59:1059–1069.

Naples, N. A. 2003. *Feminism and Method: Ethnography, Discourse Analysis and Activist Research.* New York: Routledge.

Newbury, J. 2011. Situational Analysis: Centerless Systems and Human Service Practices. *Child & Youth Services* 32(2):88–107.

Newman, K. 2002. No Shame: The View from the Left Bank. *American Journal of Sociology* 107(6):1577–1599.

Noffke, S. E. & B. Somekh (Eds.). 2009. *The Sage Handbook of Educational Action Research.* London: Sage.

Olesen, V. L. 1994. Feminisms and Models of Qualitative Research. In N. K. Denzin & Y. S. Lincoln (Eds.), *Handbook of Qualitative Research* (pp. 158–174). Thousand Oaks, CA: Sage.

Olesen, V. L. 2000. Feminisms and Qualitative Research at and into the Millennium. In N. K. Denzin & Y. S. Lincoln (Eds.), *Handbook of Qualitative Research* (2nd ed., pp. 215–256). Thousand Oaks, CA: Sage.

Olesen, V. L. 2005. Early Millennial Feminist Qualitative Research: Challenges and Contours. In N. K. Denzin & Y. S. Lincoln (Eds.), *Handbook of Qualitative Research* (3rd ed., pp. 235–278). Thousand Oaks, CA: Sage.

Olesen, V. L. 2011. Feminist Qualitative Research in the Millennium's First Decade: Developments, Challenges, Prospects. In N. K. Denzin & Y. S. Lincoln (Eds.), *Handbook of Qualitative Research* (4th ed., pp. 129–146). Thousand Oaks, CA: Sage.

Oliver, C. 2012. Critical Realist Grounded Theory: A New Approach for Social Work. *British Journal of Social Work* 42(2):371–387.

Ong, A. & S. J. Collier (Eds.). 2005. *Global Assemblages: Technology, Politics and Ethics as Anthropological Problems*. Malden, MA: Blackwell.

Outhwaite, W. & S. P. Turner (Eds.). 2007. *Handbook of Social Science Methodology*. Thousand Oaks, CA: Sage.

Pascale, C. M. 2008. Talking about Race: Shifting the Analytical Paradigm. *Qualitative Inquiry* 14(5):723–741.

Pascale, C. M. 2011. *Cartographies of Knowledge: Exploring Qualitative Epistemologies*. Los Angeles: Sage.

Patton, C. 2000. Introduction: Helping Ourselves: Research after (the) Enlightenment. *Health* 4(3):267–287.

Pérez, M. S. & G. S. Cannella. 2011. Using Situational Analysis for Critical Qualitative Research Purposes. In N. K. Denzin & M. D. Giardina (Eds.), *Qualitative Inquiry and Global Crisis* (pp. 97–117). Walnut Creek, CA: Left Coast Press, Inc.

Pérez, M. S. & G. S. Cannella. 2013. Situational Analysis as an Avenue for Critical Qualitative Research: Mapping Post-Katrina New Orleans. *Qualitative Inquiry* 19(7):1–13.

Phellas, C. N. (Ed.). 2012. *Researching Non-heterosexual Sexualities*. Farnham, UK: Ashgate.

Pilcher, J. 2012. *Planet Taco: A Global History of Mexican Food*. London: Oxford University Press.

Plummer, K. 2005. Critical Humanism and Queer Theory: Living with the Tensions. In N. K. Denzin & Y. S. Lincoln (Eds.), *Handbook of Qualitative Research* (3rd ed., pp. 357–373). Thousand Oaks, CA: Sage.

Pratt, M. L. 1992. *Imperial Eyes: Travel Writing and Transculturation*. London: Routledge.

Puddephatt, A., W. Shaffir, & S. W. Kleinecht (Eds.). 2009. *Ethnographies Revisited: Constructing Theory in the Field*. New York: Routledge.

Puig de la Bellacasa, M. 2011. Matters of Care in Technoscience: Assembling Neglected Things. *Social Studies of Science* 41(1):85–106.

Rabinow, P. & W. M. Sullivan (Eds.). 1987. The Interpretive Turn: A Second Look. In P. Rabinow & W. M. Sullivan (Eds.), *Interpretive Social Science: A Second Look* (2nd ed., pp. 1–30). Berkeley: University of California Press.

Ragin, C. C., J. Nahgel, & P. White. 2004. *Workshop on Scientific Foundations of Qualitative Research*. Washington, DC: National Science Foundation. See http://www.nsf.gov/pubs/2004/nsf04219/nsf04219.pdf (accessed January 27, 2015).

Rapp, R. 1999. *Testing Women/Testing the Fetus: The Social Impact of Amniocentesis in America*. New York: Routledge.

Reason, P. 1994. Three Approaches to Participative Inquiry. In N. K. Denzin & Y. S. Lincoln (Eds.), *Handbook of Qualitative Research* (pp. 324–339). Thousand Oaks, CA: Sage.

Reason, P. & H. Bradbury-Huang (Eds.). 2008 [2001]. *The Sage Handbook of Action Research: Participative Inquiry and Practice*. Thousand Oaks, CA: Sage.

Reid, R. 2001. Researcher or Smoker? Or, When the Other Isn't Other Enough in Studying "Across" Tobacco Control. In R. Reid and S. Traweek (Eds.), *Doing Science and Culture* (pp. 119–150). New York: Routledge.

Reid, R. 2005. *Globalizing Tobacco Control: Anti-smoking Campaigns in California, France, and Japan.* Bloomington: Indiana University Press.

Reynolds, L. & N. Herman-Kinney (Eds.). 2003. *Handbook of Symbolic Interactionism.* Walnut Creek, CA: AltaMira.

Riessman, C. K. 1993. *Narrative Analysis.* Newbury Park, CA: Sage.

Rorty, R. 1967. *The Linguistic Turn: Recent Essays in Philosophical Method.* Chicago: University of Chicago Press.

Rorty, R. 1979. *Philosophy and the Mirror of Nature.* Princeton, NJ: Princeton University Press.

Rorty, R. 1982. *Consequences of Pragmatism: Essays, 1972–1980.* Minneapolis: University of Minnesota Press.

Rosaldo, R. 1989. Culture and Truth: The Remaking of Social Analysis. Boston: Beacon Press.

Ross, D. 1990. *The Origins of American Social Science.* Cambridge, UK: Cambridge University Press.

Said, E. 1978. *Orientalism.* New York: Random House.

Samik-Ibrahim, R. M. 2000. Grounded Theory Methodology as the Research Strategy for a Developing Country. *FQS Forum: Qualitative Social Research* 1(1). http://www.qualitative-research.net/index.php/fqs/article/view/1129) (accessed January 5, 2015).

Savage, M. & R. Burrows. 2007. The Coming Crisis of Empirical Sociology. *Sociology* 41(5): 885–899.

Schatzki, T. R., K. Knorr Cetina, & E. von Savigny (Eds.). 2001. *The Practice Turn in Contemporary Theory.* London: Routledge.

Schatzman, L. 1991. Dimensional Analysis: Notes on an Alternative Approach to the Grounding of Theory in Qualitative Research. In D. Maines (Ed.), *Social Organization and Social Process: Essays in Honor of Anselm Strauss* (pp. 303–314). Hawthorne, NY: Aldine de Gruyter.

Schatzman, L. & A. L. Strauss. 1973. *Field Research: Strategies for a Natural Sociology.* Englewood Cliffs, NJ: Prentice Hall.

Schreiber, R. S. & P. N. Stem (Eds.). 2001. *Using Grounded Theory in Nursing.* New York: Springer.

Schulz, A. J. & L. Mullings. (Eds.). 2006. *Gender, Race, Class, and Health: Intersectional Approaches.* San Francisco: Jossey-Bass.

Schütze, F. 2008. The Legacy in Germany Today of Anselm Strauss's Vision and Practice in Sociology. In N. K. Denzin (Ed.) *Studies in Symbolic Interaction* 31:103–126.

Schwalbe, M. L. 2008. *Rigging the Game: How Inequality Is Reproduced in Everyday Life.* New York: Oxford University Press.

Schwanen, T. & M. P. Kwan. 2009. Doing Critical Geographies with Numbers. *The Professional Geographer* 61(4):459–464.

Seale, C., G. Gobo, J. F. Gubrium, & D. Silverman (Eds.). 2004. *Qualitative Research Practice.* London: Sage.

Seboni, N. 1997. Young People's Health Needs in Botswana: A Challenge for Nursing. *International Nursing Review* 44(4):110–114.

Seloilwe, E. S. 1998. Family Caregiving of the Mentally Ill in Botswana: Experiences and Perceptions. *Mosenodi* 6(1):17–25.

Shaibu, S. 2002. Access to Health Care: Perspectives of Family Caregivers of the Elderly. *Mosenodi* 10(2):44–52.

Shim, J. K. 2010. Cultural Health Capital: A Theoretical Approach to Understanding Health Care Interactions and the Dynamics of Unequal Treatment. *Journal of Health and Social Behavior* 51(1):1–15.

Silverman, D. & A. Marvasti. 2008. *Doing Qualitative Research: A Comprehensive Guide.* London: Sage.

Simmel, G. 1921 [1908]. The Sociological Significance of the "Stranger." In R. E. Park & E. W. Burgess (Eds.), *Introduction to the Science of Sociology* (pp. 322–327). Chicago: University of Chicago Press.

Simon, J. 1996. Discipline and Punish: The Birth of a Middle-range Research Strategy. *Contemporary Sociology—A Journal of Reviews* 25:316–319.

Sismondo, S. 2009. *An Introduction to Science and Technology Studies.* Malden, MA: Wiley Blackwell.

Smith, D. E. 1987. *The Everyday World as Problematic: A Feminist Sociology.* Boston: Northeastern University Press.

Smith, D. E. 1990. *The Conceptual Politics of Power.* Boston: Northeastern University Press.

Smith, D. E. 2005. *Institutional Ethnography: A Sociology for People.* Lanham, MD: Rowman & Littlefield.

Snow, D. A. & C. Morrill. 1995. A Revolutionary Handbook or a Handbook for Revolution? *Journal of Contemporary Ethnography* 24(3):341–362.

Soeffner, H. G. 2004 [1983]. Social Science Hermeneutics. In U. Flick, E. Kardoff, & I. Steinke (Eds.), *A Companion to Qualitative Research* (pp. 95–100). London: Sage.

Spencer, J. 2001. Ethnography after Post-modernism. In P. Atkinson, A. Coffey, S. Delamont, J. Lofland & L. Lofland (Eds.), *Handbook of Ethnography* (pp. 443–452). London: Sage.

Spradley, J. R. 1979. *The Ethnographic Interview.* New York: Holt, Rinehart & Winston.

Sprague, J. 2005. *Feminist Methodologies for Critical Researchers: Bridging Differences.* Lanham, MD: Rowman & Littlefield.

Springer, K.W., J. M. Stellman, & R. Jordan-Young. 2012. Beyond a Catalogue of Differences: A Theoretical Frame and Good Practice Guidelines for Researching Sex/Gender in Human Health. *Social Science & Medicine* 74(11):1817–1824.

Stanley, L. (Ed.). 1990. *Feminist Praxis: Research, Theory and Epistemology in Feminist Sociology.* London: Routledge.

Star, S. L. 1983. Simplification in Scientific Work: An Example from Neuroscience Research. *Social Studies of Science* 13:208–226.

Star, S. L. 1989. *Regions of the Mind: Brain Research and the Quest for Scientific Certainty.* Stanford, CA: Stanford University Press.

Star, S. L. 1993. Cooperation without Consensus in Scientific Problem Solving: Dynamics of Closure in Open Systems. In S. Easterbrook (Ed.), *Computer-supported Cooperative Work: Cooperation or Conflict?* (pp. 93–105). London: Springer-Verlag.

Star, S. L. (Ed.). 1995. *Ecologies of Knowledge: Work and Politics in Science and Technology.* Albany: SUNY Press.

Star, S. L. 2007. Living Grounded Theory: Cognitive and Emotional Forms of Pragmatism. In A. Bryant & K. Charmaz (Eds.), *Handbook of Grounded Theory* (pp. 75–94). Thousand Oaks, CA: Sage.

Star, S. L. & G. Bowker. 2007. Enacting Silence—Residual Categories as a Challenge for Ethics, Information Systems, and Communication Technology. *Ethics and Information Technology* 9:273–280.

Star, S. L., & J. Griesemer. 1989. Institutional Ecology, "Translations" and Boundary Objects: Amateurs and Professionals in Berkeley's Museum of Vertebrate Zoology, 1907–1939. *Social Studies of Science* 19:387–420.

St. Pierre, E. & W. Pillow (Eds.). 2000. *Working the Ruins: Feminist Poststructural Theory and Methods in Education.* New York: Routledge.

Steinberg, S. R. 2012. Preface: What's Critical about Qualitative Research? In G. S. Canella and S. R. Steinberg (Eds.), *Critical Qualitative Research Reader* (pp. ix–x). New York: Peter Lang Publishers.

Steinberg, S. R. & G. S. Cannella (Eds.). 2012. *Critical Qualitative Research Reader.* New York: Peter Lang Publishers.

Steinmetz, G. (Ed.). 2005. *The Politics of Method in the Human Sciences: Positivism and Its Epistemological Others.* Durham, NC: Duke University Press.

Stonequist, E. V. 1961 [1937]. *The Marginal Man: A Study in Personality and Culture.* New York: Russell & Russell.

Strathern, M. 2002. On Space and Depth. In J. Law & A. Mol (Eds.), *Complexities: Social Studies of Knowledge Practices.* Durham, NC: Duke University Press.

Strauss, A. L. 1970. Discovering New Theory from Previous Theory. In T. Shibutani (Ed.), *Human Nature and Collective Behavior: Papers in Honor of Herbert Blumer* (pp. 46–53). Englewood Cliffs, NJ: Prentice-Hall.

Strauss, A. L. 1978. A Social Worlds Perspective. In N. K. Denzin (Ed.), *Studies in Symbolic Interaction* 1:119–128.

Strauss, A. L. 1979. *Negotiations: Varieties, Contexts, Processes and Social Order.* San Francisco: Jossey-Bass.

Strauss, A. L. 1982a. Interorganizational Negotiation. *Urban Life* 11(3):350–367.

Strauss, A. L. 1982b. Social Worlds and Legitimation Processes. In N. K. Denzin (Ed.), *Studies in Symbolic Interaction* 4:171–190.

Strauss, A. L. 1984. Social Worlds and Their Segmentation Processes. In N. K. Denzin (Ed.), *Studies in Symbolic Interaction* 5:123–139.

Strauss, A. L. 1987. *Qualitative Analysis for Social Scientists.* Cambridge, UK: Cambridge University Press.

Strauss, A. L. 1991. *Creating Sociological Awareness: Collective Images and Symbolic Representation.* New Brunswick, NJ: Transaction Publications.

Strauss, A. L. 1993. *Continual Permutations of Action.* New York: Aldine de Gruyter.

Strauss, A. L. 1995. Notes on the Nature and Development of General Theories. *Qualitative Inquiry* 1(1):7–18.

Strauss, A. L. & J. Corbin. 1994. Grounded Theory Methodology: An Overview. In N. K. Denzin & Y. S. Lincoln (Eds.), *Handbook of Qualitative Research* (pp. 273–285). Thousand Oaks, CA: Sage.

Strauss, A. L. and J. Corbin (Eds.). 1997. *Grounded Theory in Practice.* Thousand Oaks, CA: Sage.

Strauss, A. L., & J. Corbin. 1998 [1990]. *The Basics of Qualitative Analysis: Grounded Theory Procedures and Techniques.* Newbury Park, CA: Sage.

Strauss, A. L., L. Schatzman, R. Bucher, D. Erlich, R. Bucher, & M. Sabshin. 1964. *Psychiatric Ideologies and Institutions.* Glencoe, IL: Free Press.

Strauss, A. L., L. Schatzman, D. Erlich, R. Bucher, & M. Sabshin. 1963. The Hospital and Its Negotiated Order. In E. Freidson (Ed.), *The Hospital in Modern Society* (pp. 147–168). New York: The Free Press.

Strong, T., J. Gaete, I. N. Sametband, J. French, & J. Eeson. 2012. Counsellors Respond to the DSM-IV-TR. *Canadian Journal of Counseling and Psychotherapy* 46(2):85–106.

Strübing, J. 2004. *Anselm Strauss*. Konstanz, Germany: UVK Verlagsgesellschaft mbH.

Strübing, J. 2007. Research as Pragmatic Problem-solving: The Pragmatist Roots of Empirically-grounded Theorizing. In A. Bryant & K. Charmaz (Eds.), *Handbook of Grounded Theory* (pp. 580–602). London: Sage.

Suchman, L. 2012. Configuration. In C. Lury & N. Wakeford (Eds.), *Inventive Methods: The Happening of the Social* (pp. 49–60). London: Routledge.

Taylor, P. J. 2005. *Unruly Complexity: Ecology, Interpretation, Engagement*. Chicago: University of Chicago Press.

Thomas, W. I. 1978 [1923]. The Definition of the Situation. In R. Farrell & V. Swigert (Eds.), *Social Deviance* (pp. 54–57). Philadelphia: Lippincott.

Thomas, W. I. & D. S. Thomas. 1970 [1928]. Situations Defined as Real Are Real in Their Consequences. In G. P. Stone & H. A. Farberman (Eds.), *Social Psychology through Symbolic Interaction* (pp. 154–155). Waltham, MA: Xerox College Publishing.

Timmermans, S. & M. Berg. 2003. *The Gold Standard: The Challenge of Evidence-based Medicine and Standardization in Health Care*. Philadelphia: Temple University Press.

Timmermans, S. & S. Epstein. 2010. A World of Standards but Not a Standard World: Toward a Sociology and Standards and Standardization. *Annual Review of Sociology* 36: 69–89.

Timmermans, S. & A. Mauck. 2005. *The Promises and Pitfalls of Evidence-based Medicine*. *Health Affairs* 24(1):18–28.

Tuhiwai Smith, L. 2012 [1999]. *Decolonizing Methodologies: Research and Indigenous People*. London: Zed.

Urquhart, C. 2007. The Evolving Nature of Grounded Theory Method: The Case of the Information Systems Discipline. In A. Bryant & K. Charmaz (Eds.), *Handbook of Grounded Theory* (pp. 339–360). London: Sage.

Van Maanen, J. 1995. An End to Innocence: The Ethnography of Ethnography. In J. Van Maanen (Ed.), *Representation in Ethnography* (pp. 1–35). Thousand Oaks, CA: Sage.

Velody, I. & R. Williams (Eds.). 1998. *The Politics of Constructionism*. London: Sage.

Verran, H. 2001. *Science and African Logic*. Chicago: University of Chicago Press.

Vidich, A. J. & S. M. Lyman. 1994. Qualitative Methods: Their History in Sociology and Anthropology. In N. K. Denzin & Y. S. Lincoln (Eds.), *Handbook of Qualitative Research* (pp. 23–59). Thousand Oaks, CA: Sage.

Visweswaran, K. 1994. *Fictions of Feminist Ethnography*. Minneapolis: University of Minnesota Press.

Wacquant, L. 2002. Scrutinizing the Street: Poverty, Morality, and the Pitfalls of Urban Ethnography. *American Journal of Sociology*, 107, 1468-1532.

Walter, M. & C. Anderson. 2013. *Indigenous Statistics: A Quantitative Methodology*. Walnut Creek, CA: Left Coast Press, Inc.

Washburn, R. 2013. The Social Significance of Human Biomonitoring. *Sociology Compass* 7(2):162–179.

Washburn, R. 2014. Measuring Personal Chemical Exposures through Biomonitoring: The Experiences of Research Participants. *Qualitative Health Research* 24(3):329–344.

Watson-Verran, H. & D. Turnbull. 1995. Science and Other Indigenous Knowledge Systems. In S. Jasanoff, G. Markle, J. Petersen, & T. Pinch (Eds.), *Handbook of Sciences and Technology Studies* (pp. 115–139). Thousand Oaks, CA: Sage.

Wertz, F. J. 2011. The Qualitative Revolution and Psychology: Science, Politics and Ethics. *The Humanistic Psychologist* 39(2):77–104.

Wiener, C. 2007. Making Teams Work in Conducting Grounded Theory. In A. Bryant & K. Charmaz (Eds.), *Handbook of Grounded Theory* (pp. 293–310). London: Sage.

Wilson, T. P. 1970. Conceptions of Interaction and Forms of Sociological Explanation. *American Sociological Review* 35(4):697–710.

Wolf, D. (Ed.). 1996. *Feminist Dilemmas in Fieldwork*. Boulder, CO: Westview Press.

Woolgar, S. & J. Lezaun. 2013. The Wrong Bin Bag: A Turn to Ontology in Science and Technology Studies? *Social Studies of Science* 43(3):321–340.

Wyly, E. 2009. Strategic Positivism. *The Professional Geographer* 61(3):310–322.

Yanow, D. & P. Schwartz-Shea. 2013 [2006]. *Interpretation and Method: Empirical Research Methods and the Interpretive Turn*. New York: Routledge.

Zuckerman, H. 1989. The Sociology of Science. In N. Smelser (Ed.), *Handbook of Sociology* (pp. 511–574). Newbury Park, CA: Sage.

PART II

ON SITUATIONAL ANALYSIS AS AN INTERPRETIVE QUALITATIVE METHOD

INTRODUCTION

PART II INTRODUCES the method of Situational Analysis (SA) in some depth. It offers two articles about SA by its originator, Adele Clarke, and one by Bill Genat on his approach to participatory action research (PAR) based on social worlds/arenas maps from SA.

Clarke was a student of Anselm Strauss. She later became a faculty member in his department upon his retirement and taught the qualitative research sequence of courses there for over twenty years. The courses emphasize grounded theory (GT), phenomenology and field research approaches, and more recently SA. Clarke first published on SA in 2003 in a Special Issue on Theory and Method of the journal *Symbolic Interaction*, but soon realized a book was needed to properly frame and launch this new method (Clarke 2005). SA both relies on *and* radically extends GT by pushing that method around the postmodern/poststructural/interpretive turn and taking into account other theoretical and methodological developments since the introduction of GT by Glaser and Strauss in 1967.

The first article in this section, "From Grounded Theory to Situational Analysis: What's New? Why? How?" by Adele Clarke (2009), answers those questions, providing an excellent overview of SA. This article was written for an exceptional edited book that brought together all the major second-generation contributors to GT method (discussed above in Chapter One). Starting in about 1990, scholars in this second generation began publishing their own versions of GT, featuring different facets. Jan Morse, a nurse researcher who specializes in qualitative inquiry and edits *Qualitative Health Research*, organized a "grounded theory bash," which generated *Developing Grounded Theory: The Second Generation* (Morse et al. 2009). In that book, Phyllis Stern represents Glaserian classic GT, Barbara Bowers dimensional analysis,[1] Juliet Corbin post-positivist basic GT, Kathy Charmaz construc-tionist interpretive GT, and Adele Clarke interpretive situationist GT. Adele Clarke's chapter on situationist GT is included here.

Clarke begins her *Second Generation* paper with a bit of intellectual biography—how she came to learn, use, and teach GT, and eventually develop SA to address what she saw as problematic about GT. She then discusses the roots of SA in both GT and symbolic interactionism as a "theory–methods package." That is, theories and methods are mutually dependent—each implicates the other in engaging epistemological and ontological questions. In short, epistemology concerns *how*—by what means—we can learn and know. Ontology is concerned with *what can be known*—the nature and boundaries of knowledge and knowing (see also Carter & Little 2007). Both differ across paradigms such as positivism/realism, constructivism/interpre-tation, and so on.

Next, Clarke turns to the specific new roots of SA, especially Straussian social worlds/arenas theory on which one of the three kinds of SA maps is based. While Strauss had developed this theory over some years, he had never integrated it with GT, which Clarke did. Another new root is Foucault's emphasis on studying discourses, which led Clarke to develop positional maps based on analyzing the array of positions taken on different issues in the dis-courses in the situation. The SA method is particularly strong at analyzing narrative, visual, and historical discourses (see Clarke 2005:Chs. 4–7).

Based on her own and others' work in science and technology studies, Clarke explicitly integrated nonhuman elements into the situation to be analyzed, including discourses. Latour and Woolgar (1979) had pioneered in grasping the importance of "things" in the laboratory. Clarke (1987) contrib-uted to this stream of work, focusing on the procurement and organization of living and specimen materials for research in the reproductive sciences (see also Clarke & Fujimura 1992). Nonhuman things can be central in an analysis.

The roots of situational maps lie in Clarke's engagement with things, her teaching of GT, and in Deleuze and Guattari's (1987) concept of rhizomes, a plant-based metaphor for multiple emergent shoots emerging from a plane with widespread horizontal, entwined networks of underground roots. Rhi-zomes contrast with and resist tree metaphors, which are vertical, have local-ized roots, and an original source (such as acorns and oak trees). In contrast, rhizomes invoke multiplicities of connections, relationality, linkages across people and nonhuman objects and beings, nomadic propagation, and growth. They are complex, contingent, and ultimately indeterminate—messy like life itself! One version of the situational map is actually called a "messy map." SA explicitly engages such complexities (e.g., Clarke with Keller 2014).

Clarke then provides an overview of SA method and focuses on doing one of the three kinds of SA maps—situational maps. Such maps are especially useful at the earliest design stages of research projects as they help make visible the kinds and range of data necessary to address the research questions. Clarke's paper also introduces the concept of implicated actors, important in analyzing power in situations (see also Clarke 2005:46–48). The particular capacity of SA to help researchers pursue increasingly popular multi-sited projects (including, for example, interview, observational, and discourse data) is noted.

Some of the key inspirations for SA came from feminism, especially its poststructural versions (e.g., Haraway 1991; Lather 2007). Hence, the second article in this section is Adele Clarke's (2012) "Feminisms, Grounded Theory and Situational Analysis Revisited," which appeared in the *Handbook of Feminist Research: Theory and Praxis* (2nd ed.; see also Clarke 2007). Clarke begins by describing GT and how it has always already been *implicitly* feminist in its pragmatist assumptions. Turning to recent feminist GT literature, Clarke then demonstrates how scholars have made GT more *explicitly* feminist through using it in feminist projects. This allows us to see how SA, as a method, both relies on and emerges from GT.

Next Clarke discusses the SA method, how it, too, is always already implicitly feminist through similar avenues as GT and through some of its own innovations. Here Clarke uses examples of feminist research to illustrate SA. Certain challenges have been posed by Glaser's and Strauss's own largely agnostic positions vis-à-vis gender, race, and class, which were not given the primacy that they now often receive in the academy. Clarke discusses resulting constraints and explores opportunities (see also Clarke 2006, 2008). In conclusion, Clarke frames her hopes for feminist futures of both GT and SA so these methods can be used in ways that further emphasize their feminist and social justice tendencies and capacities. (We include current citations on feminist approaches to methods in the references at the end of this section. See also Charmaz 2005, 2011.)

The third paper in this section on SA method moves us into exciting new territory. Bill Genat (2009) is an Australian qualitative researcher who works in Aboriginal communities on health issues. He deployed SA social worlds/ arenas maps and theory in developing a particularly interactionist approach to participatory action research (PAR) that is also broadly relevant for all kinds of policy research. Drawing deeply on symbolic interactionism (e.g., Denzin 2001 [1989]), feminist standpoint epistemologies (e.g., Naples 2003; Sprague 2005), and situated knowledges (e.g., Haraway 1991), Genat aligns his approach with postcolonial theory (e.g., Gandhi 1998) and decolonizing methodologies (e.g., Denzin, Lincoln, & Tuhiwai Smith 2008; Mertens, Cram, & Chilia 2014; Tuhiwai Smith 2012 [1999]).

Genat (2009:102) "describes the social arena of the research act as an interacting system of social worlds of specific stakeholders, each defined by discourse and with particular understandings and investments in a particular framing of phenomena in this social arena and beyond." That is, he makes a social worlds/arenas map of the PAR project itself—and carefully lays out all the worlds that should be involved, studied and analyzed. (See also Clarke & Montini 1993; Clarke & Star 2008.)

In the introductions to both Parts I and II of this book we discuss how careful and thorough representation of *all* the actors (human and nonhuman), organizations, institutions, and so forth in the situation is both a radical act and crucial for SA. Genat places this democratizing representational practice at the heart of his version of PAR. He then pushes on this practice to generate "meaningful theory at the local level thereby enabling researchers, researcher-participants and their local partners to foreground local understandings to critique more dominant discourses and policy positions regarding their circumstances" (Genat 2009:101). Instead of the usual epistemological subjugation of those being researched, their own understandings are explicitly sought out over time, creating enhanced *epistemological diversity and equity* and a better chance that policy interventions will address the lived needs and goals of the local community per se.

As a method, SA intentionally seeks to "turn up the volume" on *all* the "lesser but still present discourses" in a situation (Clarke 2005:175). Genat utilizes this capacity brilliantly to *structure and organize* his approach to PAR to accomplish a deeper collaboration rather than merely gesture toward it (Minkler & Wallerstein 2003). Significantly, Genat's model has much broader possibilities for use across social policy research of all kinds (e.g., health, education). Here, the policy arena should be constructed to include research strategies that seek to understand the needs and goals of *all* those both *directly* involved *and* those who are *implicated* in the research. The more ambitiously inclusive the design, the greater the likelihood that: (1) the diversity of needs and goals can be understood in advance and reasonably addressed, and (2) the kinds of problems likely to ensue can be anticipated

and engaged. Two words that policy developers hate to hear are "unanticipated consequences." A broad arena design and ambitious inclusiveness
reduces such risks.

We do have one minor criticism of Genat's map in Figure 4.1. The map
or diagram is excellent, but the outer circle framing the research arena should
be a dotted or broken line rather than a solid one. This symbolizes how the
arena itself is open to change—people, things, technologies, ideas, and so
forth flow into and out of arenas over time and circumstance. In fact, making
maps of different historical moments and comparing them gives SA a particular capacity to "hold" history and to be able to represent it comparatively.
This is especially true of social worlds/arenas maps but also of the others.

As qualitative researchers, many of us share the hope that our research
might "make the world a better place." Genat (2009:108) notes:

> Now that many of us are over the idea that "Truth" is somehow waiting
> to be discovered, we realize that to exist well on the planet we need to live
> easefully alongside the many truths in play. In this context, the search for
> abstract theories that add to the "body of knowledge" seem far less urgent
> in comparison to generating greater understanding of how people can
> transform their particular life situation for the better.

The radical inclusiveness of Genat's version of PAR can be extended
across policy arenas to the benefit of many. We are deeply gratified that SA
can be useful in such endeavors.

Note

1. Dimensional analysis was originally developed by Leonard Schatzman, a colleague of
Anselm Strauss and a founding faculty member of the doctoral sociology program at UCSF.
It can be viewed as a variant of GT. See Schatzman (1991), Kools et al. (1996), and Bowers
(2009).

References

Bowers, B. 2009. Leonard Schatzman and Dimensional Analysis. In J. M. Morse, P. N. Stern,
    J. M. Corbin, K. C. Charmaz, B. Bowers, & A. E. Clarke (Eds.), *Developing Grounded
    Theory: The Second Generation* (pp. 86–126). Walnut Creek, CA: Left Coast Press, Inc.
Carter, S. M. & M. Little. 2007. Justifying Knowledge, Justifying Method, Taking Action:
    Epistemologies, Methodologies, and Methods in Qualitative Research. *Qualitative Health
    Research* 17(10):1316–1328.

Charmaz, K. 2005. Grounded Theory in the 21st Century: A Qualitative Method for Advancing Social Justice Research. In N. K. Denzin & Y. S. Lincoln (Eds.), *Handbook of Qualitative Research* (3rd ed., pp. 507–536). Thousand Oaks, CA: Sage.

Charmaz, K. 2011. Grounded Theory Methods in Social Justice Research. In N. K. Denzin & Y. S. Lincoln (Eds.), *The Sage Handbook of Qualitative Research* (4th ed., pp. 359–380). Thousand Oaks, CA: Sage.

Clarke, A. E. 1987. Research Materials and Reproductive Science in the United States, 1910–1940. In G. L. Geison (Ed.), *Physiology in the American Context, 1850–1940* (pp. 323–350). Bethesda, MD: American Physiological Society. Reprinted with an Epilogue in S. L. Star (Ed.), *Ecologies of Knowledge: New Directions in Sociology of Science and Technology* (pp. 183–219). Albany: State University of New York Press, 1995.

Clarke, A. E. 2003. Situational Analyses: Grounded Theory Mapping after the Postmodern Turn. *Symbolic Interaction* 26(4):553–576.

Clarke, A. E. 2005. *Situational Analysis: Grounded Theory after the Postmodern Turn.* Thousand Oaks, CA: Sage.

Clarke, A. E. 2006. Feminisms, Grounded Theory and Situational Analysis. In S. Hesse-Biber (Ed.), *Handbook of Feminist Research: Theory and Praxis* (pp. 345–370). Thousand Oaks, CA: Sage.

Clarke, A. E. 2007. Grounded Theory: Conflicts, Debates and Situational Analysis. In W. Outhwaite and S. P. Turner (Eds.), *Handbook of Social Science Methodology* (pp. 423–442). Thousand Oaks, CA: Sage.

Clarke, A. E. 2008. Sex/Gender and Race/Ethnicity in the Legacy of Anselm Strauss. Special Section: Celebrating Anselm Strauss and Forty Years of Grounded Theory. In N. K. Denzin (Ed.), *Studies in Symbolic Interaction* 32:161–176.

Clarke, A. E. 2009. From Grounded Theory to Situational Analysis: What's New? Why? How? In J. M. Morse, P. N. Stern, J. M. Corbin, K. C. Charmaz, B. Bowers, & A. E. Clarke (Eds.), *Developing Grounded Theory: The Second Generation* (pp. 194–233). Walnut Creek, CA: Left Coast Press, Inc.

Clarke, A. E., & J. Fujimura. 1992. Introduction: What Tools? Which Jobs? Why Right? In *The Right Tools for the Job: At Work in Twentieth Century Life Sciences* (pp. 3–44). Princeton, NJ: Princeton University. French translation: *La Materialite des Sciences: Savoir-faire et Instruments dans les Sciences de la Vie.* Paris: Synthelabo Groupe, 1996.

Clarke, A. E. in conversation with R. Keller. 2014. Engaging Complexities: Working against Simplification as an Agenda for Qualitative Research Today. *FQS Forum: Qualitative Social Research* 15(2). http://www.qualitative-research.net/index.php/fqs/article/view/2186 (accessed January 22, 2015).

Clarke, A. E. & T. Montini. 1993. The Many Faces of RU486: Tales of Situated Knowledges and Technological Contestations. *Science, Technology & Human Values* 18(1):42–78.

Clarke, A. E. & S. L. Star. 2008. The Social Worlds/Arenas Framework as a Theory–Methods Package. In E. Hackett, O. Amsterdamska, M. Lynch, & J. Wacjman (Eds.), *Handbook of Science and Technology Studies* (pp. 113–137). Cambridge, MA: MIT Press.

Deleuze, G. & F. Guattari. 1987. Introduction: Rhizome. In *A Thousand Plateaus: Capitalism and Schizophrenia II* (pp. 3–25). Minneapolis: University of Minnesota Press.

Denzin, N. K. 2001 [1989]. *Interpretive Interactionism.* Newbury Park, CA: Sage.

Denzin, N. K., Y. S. Lincoln, & L. Tuhiwai Smith (Eds.). 2008. *Handbook of Critical and Indigenous Methodologies.* Thousand Oaks, CA: Sage.

Gandhi, L. 1998. *Postcolonial Theory: A Critical Introduction*. New York: Columbia University Press.

Genat, B. 2009. Building Emergent Situated Knowledges in Participatory Action Research. *Action Research* 7:101–115.

Glaser, B. G. & A. L. Strauss. 1967. *The Discovery of Grounded Theory: Strategies for Qualitative Research*. Chicago: Aldine.

Haraway, D. 1991. Situated Knowledges: The Science Question in Feminism and the Privilege of Partial Perspective. In D. Haraway (Ed.), *Simians, Cyborgs, and Women: The Reinvention of Nature* (pp. 183–202). New York: Routledge.

Kools, S., M. McCarthy, R. Durham, & L. Robrecht. 1996. Dimensional Analysis: Broadening the Conception of Grounded Theory. *Qualitative Health Research* 6(3):312–330.

Lather, P. 2007. *Getting Lost: Feminist Efforts toward a Double(D) Science*. Albany: State University of New York Press.

Latour, B. & S. Woolgar. 1979. *Laboratory Life: The Social Construction of Scientific Facts*. Beverley Hills, CA: Sage.

Mertens, D. M., F. Cram, & B. Chilia (Eds.). 2014. *Indigenous Pathways into Social Research: Voices of a New Generation*. Walnut Creek, CA: Left Coast Press, Inc.

Minkler, M. & N. Wallerstein (Eds.). 2003. *Community-based Participatory Research for Health: From Process to Outcomes* (2nd ed.). San Francisco: Jossey-Bass.

Morse, J., P. N. Stern, J. Corbin, B. Bowers, K. Charmaz, & A. E. Clarke. 2009. *Developing Grounded Theory: The Second Generation*. Walnut Creek, CA: Left Coast Press, Inc.

Naples, N. A. 2003. *Feminism and Method: Ethnography, Discourse Analysis and Activist Research*. New York: Routledge.

Schatzman, L. 1991. Dimensional Analysis: Notes on an Alternative Approach to the Grounding of Theory in Qualitative Research. In D. Maines (Ed.), *Social Organization and Social Process: Essays in Honor of Anselm Strauss* (pp. 303–314). Hawthorne, NY: Aldine de Gruyter.

Sprague, J. 2005. *Feminist Methodologies for Critical Researchers: Bridging Differences*. Lanham, MD: Rowman & Littlefield.

Tuhiwai Smith, L. 2012 [1999]. *Decolonizing Methodologies: Research and Indigenous People*. London: Zed Books.

CHAPTER 2

FROM GROUNDED THEORY TO SITUATIONAL ANALYSIS
WHAT'S NEW? WHY? HOW?

Adele E. Clarke

Introduction[1]

One of the subtitles I considered for this event was, drawing on Simone de Beauvoir ([1959] 2005), "From 'Great Men' to 'Dutiful Daughters.'" We are some but not all of the major players of the second generation of grounded theorists.[2] And it is interesting that all of us here are women and we all studied with the two "great men" of grounded theory (hereafter GTM)—Anselm Strauss and Barney Glaser—the first generation. The world—including academia—has changed a lot over the past forty years since they published *The Discovery of Grounded Theory* (Glaser & Strauss, 1967). The contributors to this volume demonstrate the shift from the then predominant "chilly climate in the classroom" for women (if not people of color) to what might be described as "political global warming" fueled by feminism, civil-rights/anti-racism, anti-ageism, anti-war, disability rights, postcolonial theory, and so on. And these changes also inform some of our scholarship.

When Jan Morse extended the invitation to this "GT Bash," I was initially quite anxious. I for one have not enjoyed in the least the tenor of much of the Glaserian/Straussian debate. For some years, Leigh Star (another student of Anselm's) and I took the position of hoping it would "just go away" and intentionally tried not to feed into it. We explicitly did not want to promote the "disciplining" of this or that version of GTM. My anxiety about a GT bash was that it would encourage "bash*ing*" along just such lines. Well, fifteen years after "Round 1" (Glaser, 1992), the debates have clearly not gone away, but happily have instead turned into more productive scholarly conversations and have generated clarifications and extensions of grounded theory, including

From Morse, Janice M, et al. 2009. *Developing Grounded Theory*, 194–233. © Taylor & Francis. Republished in *Situational Analysis in Practice*, by Adele E. Clarke, Carrie Friese, and Rachel Washburn, 84–118. (Taylor & Francis, 2015). All rights reserved.

my own.[3] So, instead of aiding and abetting "bash*ing*," this GTM bash is a big gala—a fete. I was reminded of Anselm's comment that symbolic interactionism is a banquet—people come and take what they want and leave the rest (Strauss & Fischer, 1979). So, too, are grounded theory and situational analysis (hereafter SA) (e.g., Clarke, 2003, 2005). I will return to this banquet metaphor.

Continuing to think with Simone de Beauvoir, one is not born a grounded theorist but may, with good fortune, become one. So I will start, a la Strauss, with a bit of intellectual autobiography in terms of how I came to be one and came to be here today. The roots of situational analysis go deep. I was first a sociology student in the scientistic 1960s, at Barnard College of Columbia University (yes where Glaser was, too, though we did not meet then). My exposure to qualitative research there was minimal. But one of my teachers was the esteemed medical sociologist Renee Fox, who was an amazing ethnographer. Another was Mira Komarovsky who, like de Beauvoir, studied gender in the 1950s.

At NYU, where I received a Master's degree in sociology, we were trained only in statistics and survey methods, although many of the faculty did interview-based ethnographic research on the professions. However, Eliot Freidson brought Howie Becker in to give a talk, and we read Goffman, Garfinkle, and other "great men." When I then worked in survey research (for a Columbia University doctoral student), I noticed that some of the most interesting data were left in the file cabinets—answers to "open-ended" questions—because no one knew what to do with them. I had done the interviews and was quite haunted by our failure to include these materials.

A decade later, I sought a doctoral program in sociology that would allow me to specialize in qualitative research, medical sociology, and women's health. I was then teaching in the Women's Studies Program at Sonoma State University, and Kathy Charmaz both directed me to the University of California, San Francisco (UCSF) and wrote me a letter of recommendation. Her exceptional generosity to me continues to this day.

At UCSF in 1980, I finally "came home" intellectually in all three sites of my desire (Clarke & Star, 1998). As sociology students, we pursued our own hands-on "do-it-yourself" qualitative research projects from design and human subjects approval (yes—even in 1980) to final presentations with superb faculty: Ginnie Olesen and Lenny Schatzman taught field research,[4] while Anselm followed with qualitative analysis organized as a small working group. We were welcome to sit in on his ongoing analysis group as long as we desired. We desired! My cohort also met with Barney Glaser for analysis groups, probably the last to do so as he was no longer at UCSF.

Conceiving Situational Analysis

Significantly for situational analysis, during my graduate studies I fell in love not only with Strauss's grounded theory but also with his social worlds/ arenas theory, which he had worked on (individually and collaboratively) at about the same time during the heart of his career. He pursued these as separate projects, more often on his own than with his research team,[5] and his publications rarely engaged both at the same time.[6] But I soon did. Almost all of my own work from the early eighties onward relied on and then began to elaborate social worlds and arenas theory.[7] I was particularly riveted by the idea of social worlds as universes of discourse, bounded by how far they reached in terms of space, time, and meaning-making. Discourse as an analytic concept was just emerging, and I was truly thrilled at having a way to think about and study what we are awash in. I distinctly remember yearning for such a concept in the 1960s.

In the mid-1990s, I began to think about writing about qualitative methods. I was at the time a research fellow at the UC Humanities Research Institute at Irvine in a group focused on "Feminist Epistemologies and Methodologies." Patti Lather (e.g., 1991, 2007; Clarke, 2009), who became my major interlocutor about methods, was there, too. And this is really where what I later called situational analysis began—from my attempt to reground grounded theory in Straussian social worlds and arenas suffused with the assumptions of feminism that had been part of my life since the early seventies (Clarke, 2006b; Olesen, 2007), and the poststructuralisms that had been part of my life since the early nineties (especially Foucault). After I returned to San Francisco in 1996, Anselm and Fran Strauss came to dinner at the end of August, and I told Anselm about my idea. He was excited about this fusion of GTM and social worlds/arenas, and we were to discuss it further. Very very sadly he died on September 6.

What's New in Situational Analysis?

So, drawing deeply but not only on Strauss, SA both extends and goes beyond grounded theory. What is SA about? Why create a new approach? How are Anselm's contributions both preserved and reconfigured for the new millennium? I answer these questions elaborately in my book (Clarke, 2005, pp. xvii-81). I argue for a grounded theory grounded in symbolic interactionist sociology, very much à la Strauss, to be understood as a "theory/methods package." This concept of theory/methods packages focuses on the integral—and ultimately nonfungible—aspects of ontology and epistemology. What can be known and how we can know are inseparable. Such packages thus include epistemological and ontological assumptions, along with concrete practices through which social scientists go about their work, including relating to/with one another and with the various nonhuman entities involved in the situation.

A symbolic interactionist grounded theory/situational analysis theory/methods package, then, is about the "goodness of fit" between the fundamentals of symbolic interactionist theory (e.g., Blumer, [1969] 1993; Reynolds & Herman, 2003; Strauss, 1993), constructionist grounded theory (Charmaz, 2000, 2006; Strauss, 1987), and situational analysis including Foucautian discursive formations (Clarke, 2003, 2005) as methodological approaches in terms of questions of ontology and epistemology. The theory/methods package concept does *not* mean that one can opt for two items from column A and two from column B to "tailor" a package. Nor does it mean that one element automatically "comes with" the other as a prefabricated package. Using a "package" takes all the work involved in learning the theory *and* the practices and how to articulate them across time and circumstance (see Clarke 1991, 2005, pp. 2-5, 2006b, 2007; Star, 1989, 1991a, 1991b, 1999, 2007; Star & Strauss, 1998; Strauss & Corbin, 1997). It becomes a way of knowing and doing *together*. The very idea of theory/methods packages assumes that "method, then, is not the servant of theory: method actually grounds theory" (Jenks, 1995, p. 12).

There are a number of ways in which Strauss's interactionist grounded theory/methods package was always already around the postmodern turn and ways that grounded theory was recalcitrant against that turn—the lurking scientisms, positivisms, and realisms that Kathy Charmaz (2000, 2006) has ably detailed. I won't reiterate those here (Clarke, 2005, pp. 11-19, 2007).

I want to focus instead on what is new in situational analysis. What new possibilities does it bring to the grounded theory banquet table—on offer to all? I will discuss four facets: First are the Chicago social ecologies from the early twentieth century that served as the deep tap roots for social worlds/arenas/discourses theory. Second, I take up Foucault, discourse studies, and moving beyond the knowing subject. The third issue takes the nonhuman

elements in a situation explicitly into account. Last are the concepts of implicated actors and actants in situations. I then frame the shift from the conditional matrix to the situational matrix and describe the three kinds of maps
that constitute SA. I conclude with some peeks at possible futures of SA.

From Chicago Social Ecologies to
Social Worlds/Arenas/Discourses Theory

Early Chicago School sociology focused on communities of different types
(e.g., ethnic communities, elite neighborhoods, impoverished slums), distinctive locales (e.g., taxi dancehalls, the stockyards), and signal events of varying
temporal durations (e.g., a strike). The sociological task was "to make *the group*
the focal center and to build up from its discoveries *in concrete situations,* a
knowledge of the whole" (Eubank in Meltzer, Petras, & Reynold, 1975, p. 42,
emphases added). But, as Baszanger and Dodier (1997, p. 16) have asserted:

> Compared with the anthropological tradition, the originality of the first
> works in the Chicago tradition was that they did not necessarily integrate
> the data collected around a collective whole in terms of a common cul-
> ture, but *in terms of territory or geographic space.* The problem with which
> these sociologists were concerned was based on human ecology: interac-
> tions of human groups with the natural environment and interactions of
> human groups in a given geographic milieu. . . . The main point here was
> to make an *inventory of a space* by studying the different communities and
> activities of which it is composed, that is, which encounter and confront
> each other in that space.

These "inventories of space" often took the form of maps (e.g., Fine, 1995;
Kurtz, 1984).

Traditional Chicago School studies were undergirded by an areal field
model—a "map" of some kind done from "above" such as a city map (e.g.,
Blumer, 1958; Hughes, 1971, esp. pp. 267, 270; Park, 1952). Most important
here, the communities, organizations, kinds of sites, and collectivities represented on such maps were to be explicitly viewed *in relation to the sitings or
situations of one another, and within their larger contexts.* Thus, relationality
was a featured concern. "The power of the ecological model underlying the
traditional Chicago approach lies in the ability to focus now on the niche and

now on the ecosystem which defined it" (Dingwall, 1999, p. 217). Leigh Star (1995) has called this "the figure/ground gestalt switch," and analytically it is fundamentally important.

In the 1950s and 1960s, researchers in this tradition continued the study of "social wholes" in new ways, shifting to studies of work, occupations, and professions, moving from local to national and international groups. Geographic boundaries were dropped as necessarily salient, replaced by *shared discourses* as boundary-making and marking. Perhaps most significantly, they increasingly attended to the relationships of those groups to other "social wholes," the *interactions* of collective actors and discourses. (In today's methodological vernacular, many such studies would be termed "multi-sited."[8])

In SA, the root metaphor for grounded theorizing shifts from social process/action to social ecology/situation—grounding the analysis deeply and explicitly in the broader situation of inquiry of the research project. Social worlds theory assumes multiple collective actors—social worlds—in all kinds of negotiations in a broad and often contentious substantive arena. Arenas are focused on matters about which all the involved social worlds and actors care enough to be (1) committed to act, and (2) to produce discourses about arena concerns. Thus, arenas are sites of action *and* discourse. They are discursive sites in often complicated ways. Particular social worlds are constructed in other world's discourses as well as producing their own. But arenas usually endure for some time, and longstanding arenas are typically characterized by multiple, complex, and layered discourses that interpolate and combine old(er) and new(er) elements in on-going, contingent, and inflected practices. Further, because perspectives and commitments differ, arenas are usually sites of contestation and controversy. As such, they are especially good for analyzing heterogeneous perspectives or positions and for analyzing power in action (a lesson from technoscience studies) (e.g., Nelkin, 1995).

Arenas are also especially amenable conceptual frames through which to work at a more meso/organizational level, analyzing *collective* actors (social worlds), their work, and discourses in those arenas. For example, Peter Hall (1997, p. 397) noted: "A view of social organization is offered that emphasizes relations among situations, linkages between consequences and conditions, and networks of collective activity across space and time." Significantly, it is through such frames that symbolic interactionist studies can address more global elements, increasingly important today.[9] But, like the basic social process/action frameworks fundamental to traditional grounded theory, social worlds/arenas/discourses analyses also cannot do everything we want to do analytically, hence my expansion of them into the several forms of situational analysis.

Foucault: Discourse Studies and Moving beyond the "Knowing Subject"

Interactionism, if it is to thrive and grow, must incorporate elements of post-structural and postmodern theory (e.g., the works of Barthes, Derrida, Foucault, Baudrillard, etc.) into its underlying views of history, culture, and politics. (Denzin, 1992, p. xvii)

Let us turn now to the first new root of situational analysis: Foucault's work on discourse and the importance of moving beyond "the knowing subject." Simon (1996, p. 319) has asserted that the work of Foucault "might be called a postmodern version of middle range theory." Foucault challenged the social sciences by decentering the "knowing subject" (the individual human as agentic social actor) to focus instead on "the social" as constituted through discursive practices and on discourses as constitutive of subjectivities. Foucault (1972) began with the concept of "the order of discourse," asserting that ways of framing and representing linguistic conventions of meanings and habits of usage together constitute specific discursive fields or terrains. Conceptually, discourses are analytic modes of ordering the chaos of the world. His concept of "discursive practices" described ways of being in the world that could, when historicized, be understood to produce distinctive "discursive formations"—dominant discourses that bind together social injunctions about particular practices (Dreyfus & Rabinow, 1983, p. 59). Dominant discourses are reinforced through extant institutional systems of law, media, medicine, education, and so on—often operating in conjunction. A discourse is effected in disciplining practices, which produce subjects/subjectivities through surveillance, examination, and various technologies of the self—ways of producing ourselves as properly disciplined subjects (e.g., Foucault, 1973, 1975, 1978, 1988). For example, the various institutions of medicine (from hospitals to pharmaceutical companies) and the media (from newspapers to TV and the Internet) together produce "healthscapes"—extensive narrative and visual discourses on health and the responsibilities of citizens to pursue it. We constitute ourselves and are constituted by and through them—the focus of my own current work (Clarke, 2010a).

SA goes beyond "the knowing subject" as centered knower and decision-maker to *also* address and analyze salient discourses dwelling within the situation of inquiry. We are all, like it or not, constantly awash in seas of discourses that are constitutive of life itself. SA enrolls Foucault's poststructural approaches to help push grounded theory around the postmodern turn to take these into account. Specifically, situational analysis follows "Foucault's footsteps" (Prior, 1997) into sites of his serious theorizing—historical, narrative/textual, and visual discourses. Grounded theory aided and abetted by situational analysis facilitates such moves.

Taking the Nonhuman Explicitly into Account

In the postmodern, studying action—the analytic center of GTM—is not enough. So, having begun down the discursive path, it quickly becomes obvious that if the human subject is decentered—no longer the analytic everything—"the object is also and always decentered" (Dugdale, 1999, p. 16). Humans are not enough. Fresh methodological attention needs to be paid to *nonhuman objects* in situations—things of all kinds. These may include cultural objects, technologies, animals, media, nonhuman animate and inanimate pieces of material culture, and the lively discourses that also constitute the situations we study—from cups and saucers to lab animals to TV programs. Some are products of human action (and we can study the production processes); others are construed as "natural" (and we can study how they have been constructed as such).

Many of us actually using grounded theory have taken the nonhuman into account in our substantive research for decades (Clarke & Star, 2003), but we did so without the methodological reflexivity that would make these innovations explicit—adequately visible to others seeking to use grounded theory in such postmodern ways. Things have also had an important place in interactionist history (e.g., McCarthy, 1984, pp. 108-109; Park & Burgess, [1921] 1970). Blumer, drawing deeply on Mead, offered a specific framework on the:

Nature of Objects. The position of symbolic interactionism is that the "worlds" that exist for human beings and for their groups are composed of "objects" and that these *objects are the product of symbolic interaction*. An object is anything that can be indicated, anything that is pointed to or

referred to—a cloud, a book, a legislature, a banker, a religious doctrine, a
ghost, and so forth. ([1969] 1993, pp. 10-11, emphasis added)

This explicit constructionist *and* materialist view of the nonhuman has tacitly informed the research of a number of us (Clarke & Star, 2003, 2007).

Let me further clarify and situate the term nonhuman. Over the past several decades, the theoretical importance of things—materialities—has been
retheorized in a number of ways through poststructural lenses. Certainly
Foucault's (1973) *The Order of Things* raised fresh ways of conceptualizing
how "things" order the world. It was through actor-network theory, developed since c1975 especially by Bruno Latour, Michel Callon, John Law, and
Madeleine Akrich in the transdisciplinary field of science and technology
studies that I first encountered this move (e.g., Latour, 1987, 2005; Law &
Hassard, 1999; Law & Mol, 1995). Actor-network theory initiated a much
more explicit and full(er) theoretical and methodological status for the nonhuman and explicitly uses that term.[10]

"Nonhuman actants" are not only present as nodes in the actor network
in this approach, but also have agency. In science and technology studies,
such conceptions exploded dualistic notions of a technical core and social
superstructure—the separability of humans and machines. Instead, the
social and technical together become a "seamless web," co-constructed and
mutually embedded (Bijker, Pinch, & Hughes, 1987; Latour, 1987). Woolgar
(1991) captured this vividly in research on "how computers configure their
users," featuring the agency of the nonhuman in making us do things differently. With laptops or cell phones in place, we become "cyborgs"—cybernetic
organisms (Haraway, [1985] 1991a).

This reconceptualization of the nonhuman as not only important but
also agentic is deeply provocative and productive. *Adequate analyses of situations being researched must include the nonhuman explicitly and in considerable
detail.* "Seeing" the agency of the nonhuman elements present in the situation
disrupts the taken-for-granted, creating Meadian (e.g., [1927] 1964) moments
of conceptual rupture through which we can see the world afresh. For
example, "Magazines exist to sell readers to advertisers" ruptures the taken-
for-granted and offers a different perspective. The agency of magazines per se
in the distribution of advertising discourses, normally invisible or at least not
the lead point, is here rendered explicit and primary.

Significantly, including the nonhuman as agentic actors/actants in
research takes up the postmodern challenge of posthumanism—the idea

that only humans "really" matter or "matter most." "By acknowledging non-humans as components and determinants of the arrangements that encompass people, this line of research *problematizes the social and challenges traditional renderings of it as relations between people*" (Schatzki, Cetina, & von Savigny, 2001, p. 11, emphasis added). A key argument in science and technology studies has been that the nonhuman and the human are co-constitutive—together constitute the world *and each other*. Similar arguments have also been made in material culture studies: "Material forms were often of significance precisely because being disregarded as trivial, they were often a key unchallenged mechanism for social reproduction and ideological dominance .... [S]ocial worlds were as much constituted by materiality as the other way around" (Miller, 1998, p. 3; see also Hodder, 2000). Consumption studies—focused on relations between humans and things—is another site where taking the nonhuman seriously has occurred (e.g., Applbaum, 2004; Hearn & Roseneil, 1999).

Such processes of co-construction and co-constitution can be studied through using the situation as the locus of analysis, explicitly including all analytically pertinent nonhuman (including technical) elements along with the human in situational maps. This is one of the key ways in which a GTM rooted in symbolic interactionism offers a distinctively *materialist* constructionism through SA. Nonhuman actants structurally condition the interactions within the situation through their specific material properties and requirements.[11] Their agency is everywhere. SA explicitly takes the nonhuman elements in the situation of inquiry into account both materially and discursively.

Implicated Actors and Actants

There can also be *implicated actors and/or actants* in social worlds and arenas (Clarke, 2005, pp. 46-48; Clarke & Montini, 1993). This concept provides a means of analyzing the situatedness of less powerful actors and the consequences of others' actions for them and raises issues of discursive constructions of actors and of nonhuman actants. There are at least two kinds of implicated actors. First are those implicated actors who are physically present but generally silenced/ignored/invisibled by those in power in the social world or arena. Second are those implicated actors *not* physically present in a given social world but solely discursively constructed by others in the situation. They are conceived, represented, and perhaps targeted by the work of those others, hence they are *discursively* present.

Neither category of implicated actors is actively involved in the actual negotiations of self-representation in the social world or arena, nor are their thoughts or opinions or identities explored or sought out by other actors through any openly empirical mode of inquiry (such as by asking them questions). They are neither invited by those in greater power to participate nor to represent themselves on their own terms. If physically present, their perceptions are largely ignored and/or silenced. The difference between the two types turns on the issue of their physical presence.

Let me give examples. First, those actors present but silenced/invisible in the situation of inquiry can be exemplified by women scholars and scholars of color in traditional histories of academic disciplines and professions. They were there in those worlds, doing many things, but their presence and contributions have been largely ignored and/or erased, requiring usually feminist and anti-racist archaeologies to excavate, resurrect, and resituate them (e.g., Deegan, 1990; DuBois, 1993). Second, an example of actors solely discursively constructed are women users of most contraceptives by the reproductive scientists who designed them (Clarke, 1998, 2000), who were rather surprised at women's objections and rejections of the technologies (e.g., Bruce, 1987).

There can, of course, also be *implicated actants*—implicated nonhuman actors—in situations of concern.[12] Like humans, implicated actants can be physically *and/or* discursively present in the situation of inquiry. That is, human actors (individually and/or collectively as social worlds) routinely discursively construct nonhuman actants from those human actors' own perspectives. The analytic question here is who is discursively constructing what, and how and why are they doing so? For example, a heterogeneously constructed implicated actant is the male (birth control) pill. Most people, if they have heard of it at all, will have done so in the question: "Whatever happened to the male pill?" Nelly Oudshoorn's (2003) *The Male Pill: A Biography of a Technology in the Making* answers that question. Though technically feasible since the 1970s, the very intensity of the discursive constructions of the male pill and of men as consumers of it has delayed its release for decades.

The concept of implicated actors and actants can be particularly useful in the explicit analysis of power in social worlds and arenas. Such analyses are both complicated and enhanced by the fact that there are generally *multiple* discursive constructions circulating of both the human and nonhuman actors in any given situation. Analyzing power involves analyzing whose constructions of whom/what exist? Which are taken as "the real" constructions—or the ones that "matter" most in the situation by the various participants? Which are contested? Whose are ignored? By whom? What happens when heretofore silent/silenced implicated actors suddenly open their mouths and speak? Through understanding the discursive constructions of implicated actors and actants, analysts can grasp a lot about the social worlds and the arena in which they are active and some of the consequences of those actions for the less powerful.

In sum, the tap roots of SA lie in Chicago School ethnographies and pragmatist philosophy. The new roots include Foucauldian discourse studies going beyond "the knowing subject," taking the nonhuman explicitly into account, and analyzing implicated actors and actants. These come together in the shift to situations per se as focal—as units of analysis—to which we next turn.

From the Conditional Matrix to Situational Maps

In his later work, Strauss was relentlessly sociological in seeking to incorporate and integrate analyses of structural process in new ways. The term "structural process" was used in *The Discovery of Grounded Theory*:

> One of the central issues in sociological theory is the relationship of structure to process. . . . Sociological theory ordinarily does not join structure and process so tightly as our notion of "structural process" does. . . . A major implication of our book is that structure and process are related more complexly (and more interestingly) than is commonly conceived. (Glaser & Strauss, 1967, pp. 239-242)

Thus, from the outset, grounded theory was aimed at what today might be called "deconstructing" and complicating this age-old, tired if not exhausted, binary (e.g., Hildenbrand, 2007).

Strauss pursued this through the methodological framework of the conditional matrix developed with Julie Corbin. And it was most especially through dealing with the matrices, through my own teaching of qualitative research methods, and through my own engagement with science and technology studies that I ended up developing situational analysis.

Through the conditional matrix, Strauss sought to develop ways to do grounded theory analysis that included *specifying structural conditions*— literally making them visible in the analysis. Strauss's interactionist sociology was already rooted in process—classic GTM "basic social processes." He was interested most of all in understanding *action as situated activity* (see Figure 2.1 (Strauss & Corbin, 1990, p. 163)). Note that action is in the center of the diagram—the GTM basic social process.

The several versions of the conditional and conditional/consequential matrices that Strauss and Corbin produced were intended to provide systematic paths for grounded theorists to follow in order to facilitate specifying the salient structural conditions that obtained for the phenomenon under study. These conditional matrices frame a number of concerns that are to be considered by the analyst, generally organized into "levels": international (economic, cultural, religious, scientific, and environmental issues); national (political, governmental, cultural, economic, gender, age, ethnicity, race, particular national issues, etc.); and, depending on where the research is undertaken, community, organizational, institutional, or local group and individual/(inter)actional setting. At the core for Strauss is action—both strategic and routine (see also Clarke, 2008a, 2010b; Strauss, 1993).

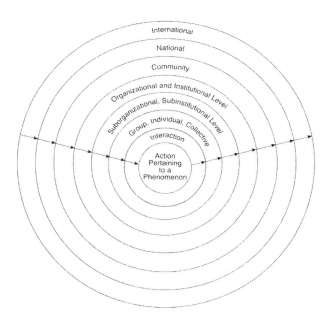

Figure 2.1: Strauss and Corbin's 1990 Conditional Matrix (From Strauss and Corbin [1990] *Basics of Qualitative Research.* Copyright 1990 by Sage Publications, Inc. Reprinted with permission of the publisher.)

Looking at the 1998 *Basics* matrix in Figure 2.2 (Strauss & Corbin, 1998, p. 184), we can see that the concentric circles apparently represent the more structural conditions *within* which the focus of analysis dwells. The structural conditions are portrayed as *context,* arrayed *around* the central focus from local to global (from near the center/core to far away places on the periphery). In Corbin's revisions after Strauss's death, the individual replaces action as the central analytic. All in all, especially given the primacy of the nation state, it remains a very modernist vision. Peter Hall's (1997) critique on this point, which I share, is that "the imagery of the conditional matrix as a set of concentric circles, while perhaps simply a heuristic device, conveys an erroneous vision of social topography, *one that I would rather leave to empirical examination*" (p. 401, emphasis added).

To me, the conditional matrices do not do the conceptual analytic work Strauss wanted done in terms of grounded theory method. Strauss was gesturing too abstractly toward the possible salience of the structural elements of situations rather than insisting on their concrete and detailed *empirical*

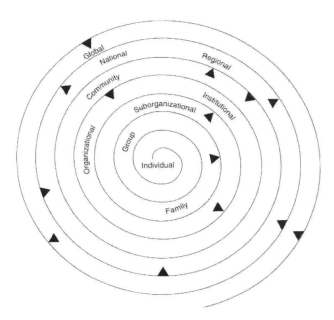

Figure 2.2: Strauss and Corbin's 1998 Conditional Matrix (From Strauss and Corbin [1998] *Basics of Qualitative Research.* Copyright 1998 by Sage Publications, Inc. Reprinted with permission of the publisher.)

Figure 2.3: Clarke's Situational Matrix (From Clarke [2005] *Situational Analysis: Grounded Theory after the Postmodern Turn.* Copyright 2005 by Sage Publications, Inc. Reprinted with permission of the publisher.)

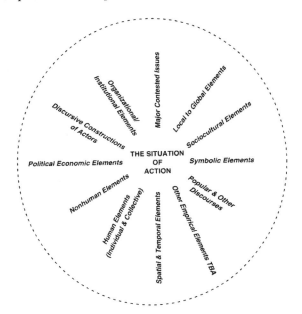

specification and clear explication as a requisite part of grounded theory *analysis.* Figure 2.3 is my alternative—the situational matrix.

Here *the conditions of the situation are in the situation.* There is no such thing as "context." The conditional elements of the situation need to be specified in the analysis of the situation itself as *they are constitutive of it,* not merely surrounding it or framing it or contributing to it. They *are* it. Regardless of whether some actors might construe them as local or global, internal or external, close-in or far away, or whatever, the fundamental question is: *"How do these conditions appear—make themselves felt as consequential—as integral parts of the empirical situation under examination?"* At least some answers to that question can be found through doing situational analyses.

This matrix, like those of Strauss and Corbin, is an abstract version. The diagram as a whole *is* the situation of inquiry. Many kinds or genres of people and things can be in that situation, and the labels are intended as generic. The fundamental assumptions are that everything *in* the situation *both constitutes and affects* most everything else in the situation in some way(s). Everything actually in the situation or understood to be so "conditions the possibilities" (yes, Foucault) of interpretation and action. People and things, humans and nonhumans, fields of practice, discourses, disciplinary and other regimes/ formations, symbols, technologies, controversies, organizations and institutions—each and all can be present and mutually consequential.

The concept of situation is key. I was inspired by several scholars here. First, the Thomas's theorem from the 1920s that "if situations are perceived as real, they are real in their consequences," a theorem at the heart of social constructionism and symbolic interactionism, is foundational for SA as well (Thomas & Thomas, [1928] 1970). Second, I was inspired by C. Wright Mills's (1940) work on situated motives, third by Norm Denzin's ([1970] 1989) early efforts at situating research in his book *The Research Act.* And last, a major resource on the concept of situation is Donna Haraway's (1991b) classic feminist theory paper on "situated knowledges." The key point is that in SA, *the situation itself becomes the fundamental unit of analysis* (Clarke, 2005, esp. pp. 21-23, 71-73).

Mapping Situations

The situation of inquiry is to be *empirically* constructed through the making of three kinds of maps and following through with analytic work and memos of various kinds.
   1. **situational maps** lay out the major human, nonhuman, discursive, and other elements in the research situation of inquiry and provoke analysis of relations among them;
   2. **social worlds/arenas maps** lay out the collective actors and the arena(s) of commitment and discourse within which they are engaged in ongoing negotiations—mesolevel interpretations of the situation; and
   3. **positional maps** lay out the major positions taken, and *not* taken, in the data vis-à-vis particular axes of difference, concern, and controversy around issues in the situation of inquiry.

All three kinds of maps are intended as analytic exercises, fresh ways into social science data that are especially well suited to contemporary studies from solely interview-based to multi-sited research projects. They are intended as supplemental to traditional grounded theory analyses that center on action. Instead, these maps center on elucidating the key elements, discourses, structures, and conditions of possibility that characterize the situation of inquiry. Thus, situational analysis can deeply situate research projects individually, collectively, social organizationally/ institutionally, temporally, geographically, materially, discursively, culturally, symbolically, visually, and historically.

Abstract Situational Maps

In this chapter, I will only introduce situational maps. The initial maps done in SA—situational maps—lay out the major human, nonhuman, discursive, historical, symbolic, cultural, political, and other elements in the research situation of concern and provoke analysis of relations among them. These maps are intended to capture the messy complexities of the situation in their dense relations and permutations. They intentionally work *against* the usual simplifications so characteristic of scientific work (Star 1983) in particularly postmodern ways. See Figure 2.4.

Here I am also going to emphasize something I did not fully realize until I had finished the book—that situational maps are excellent research design

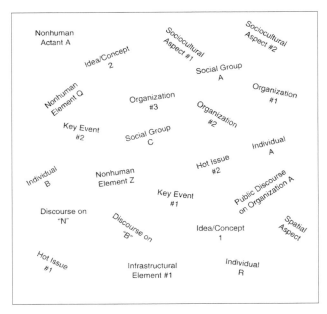

Figure 2.4: Abstract Situational Map: Messy/Working Version (From Clarke [2005] *Situational Analysis: Grounded Theory after the Postmodern Turn.* Copyright 2005 by Sage Publications, Inc. Reprinted with permission of the publisher.)

tools. Because they are intended to be done and redone multiple times across the life of a research project, there is no one "right" map. If you put something on it that turns out not to be important, you can delete it later or just ignore it. But if it was there in the first place, or got there during the research, at least you integrated it into the research design and sought some data about it systematically and have some sense of its relative importance.

So you can do a situational map to plan a research project. This can be very helpful today in that one typically has to discuss such things even in seeking dissertation grants. The goal for the researcher in doing a situational map for design purposes is to get everything you think might be worth a peek in terms of data gathering onto the map, and then plan what data to gather about it and include these plans in your preliminary research design. Over time, one adds and deletes from the situational map as your research directions and interests clarify and intensify. If an element falls away, that's fine. Research is *empirical* after all. The map also changes downstream as you pursue what is known in GTM as "theoretical sampling" —seeking fresh data sources pertinent to a particular *theoretical* point you are exploring. Always keep copies of old maps (with dates on them!).

I actually formulated my first situational maps in teaching qualitative research to grad students—usually their pilot dissertation projects. Over the years, I developed the habit of getting one piece of paper going for each student and adding to it during the months of working together on their projects in small groups. As the teacher, I needed a way to remember what they had done already and what we might want to come back to. These messy pieces of paper with notes, tentative analytic diagrams, etc., became inspirational. I realized that it was *not only me* who needed help remembering and holding all the odd pieces together![13]

See Figure 2.5 for the Abstract Situational Map—Ordered Version. Here you can see the categories a bit more clearly. The categories derive in part from my own work and from Strauss's (1993, p. 252) "general orders" within his negotiated/processual ordering framework: spatial, temporal, technological, work, sentimental, moral, aesthetic, and so on. In terms of laying out the major elements in situations, these categories seem basic to me.

It is important to note that *there is no absolute need to have all of these categories in any given analysis.* You may also have other categories. Using your own messy map to build this orderly one allows for new and different categories and/or modifications of these. What appears in *your* situational map is based on *your* situation of inquiry—your project. The ordered situational

Figure 2.5: Abstract Situational Map: Ordered/Working Version (From Clarke [2005] *Situational Analysis: Grounded Theory after the Postmodern Turn.* Copyright 2005 by Sage Publications, Inc. Reprinted with permission of the publisher.)

INDIVIDUAL HUMAN ELEMENTS/ACTORS e.g., key individuals and significant (unorganized) people in the situation	**NONHUMAN ELEMENTS/ACTIONS** e.g., technologies; material intfrastructures; specialized information and/or knowledges; material "things"
COLLECTIVE HUMAN ELEMENTS/ACTORS e.g., particular groups; specific organizations	**IMPLICATED/SILENT ACTORS/ACTANTS** As found in the situation
DISCURSIVE CONSTRUCTIONS OF INDIVIDUAL AND/OR COLLECTIVE HUMAN ACTORS As found in the situation	**DISCURSIVE CONSTRUCTION OF NONHUMAN ACTANTS** As found in the situation
POLITICAL/ECONOMIC ELEMENTS e.g., the state; particular industry/ies; local/regional/global orders; political parties; NGOs; politicized issues	**SOCIOCULTURAL/SYMBOLIC ELEMENTS** e.g., religion; race; sexuality; gender; ethnicity; nationality; logos; icons; other visual and/or aural symbols
TEMPORAL ELEMENTS e.g., historical, seasonal, crisis, and/or trajectory aspects	**SPATIAL ELEMENTS** e.g., spaces in the situation, gegraphical aspects, local, regional, national, global spatial issues
MAJOR ISSUES/DEBATES (USUALLY CONTESTED) As found in the situation; and see positional map	**RELATED DISCOURSES (HISTORICAL, NARRATIVE, AND/OR VISUAL)** e.g., normative expectations of actors, actants, and/or other specified elements; moral/ethical elements; mass media and other popular cultural discourses; situation-specific discourses
OTHER KINDS OF ELEMENTS As found in the situation	

maps should also be done and redone across the career of the research project. Things may well move around. And they may well—and usually do—appear in more than one category. You can learn to do both messy and ordered maps in MS Word.

The key key key key point that I cannot stress too much is that you should not slavishly try and fill in blank categories on the ordered map. I worry very seriously about people doing that. I do so because it would violate the fundamental assumptions of both GTM and SA. GTM and SA are both deeply *empirical* approaches to the study of social life. The very term "grounded theory" means data-grounded theorizing. In the words of Atkinson, Coffey, & Delamont (2003, p. 150): "[G]rounded theory is not a description of a kind of theory. Rather, it represents a general way of generating

theory (or, even more generically, a way of having ideas on the basis of empirical research)." The theorizing is generated by tacking back and forth between
the nitty-gritty specificities of empirical data and more abstract ways of
thinking about them. Philosophically, this tacking back and forth is called
"'abductive' reasoning . . . a sort of 'third way' between the Scylla of inductive
reasoning and the Charybdis of hypothetico-deductive logic" (Atkinson,
Coffey, & Delamont, 2003, p. 149). "Abduction is to move from a conception
of something to a different, possibly more developed or deeper conception of
it" (Dey, 2004, p. 91; see also Locke, 2007; Reichertz, 2007; Richardson &
Kramer, 2006; Strübing, 2007b).

SA wholly shares in these assumptions. So filling in any "blank" categories of the ordered situational map would be disastrous because it would
shift the method from using induction (building from the empirical to the
more abstract/conceptual) and abduction (taking back and forth between
the empirical and the more abstract/conceptual) into deduction (moving
from the abstract/conceptual to the concrete). Yet there is also a tension here
that must be acknowledged. The very *doing* of the maps provokes thinking—
analysis—and may and should help you work through your data more
systematically. So, although blanks should not be "filled in" mechanically or
perfunctorily, nor should one stop thinking and analyzing! If it feels perfunc-
tory, stop.

Note that in doing initial situational maps, the analyst should specify the
nonhuman elements in the situation and how they are constructed in discourses, thus making pertinent materialities and discourses visible from the
outset. Actually, all three kinds of maps are keyed to taking the nonhuman—
including discourses—in the situation of inquiry seriously.

I use both kinds of maps—messy and orderly—returning again and
again to messy versions precisely because they stay "open" more and more
easily. The ordered ones often seem too final too fast. Yet my tired brain
sometimes needs the neatness and orderliness to try and make thinking and
writing more coherent.

Exemplar Situational Maps

Next let me provide exemplar maps. I am using as an exemplar here my project on RU486 (also known as the "French abortion pill") because abortion
politics are so transparent in North America today that I need not explain
much! Approved and used in France since 1982 and in many other European

nations, the contested nature of abortion in the United States considerably delayed and complicated its approval here. I began the project in 1989 as an interview/ethnographic endeavor to follow the FDA approval process "in practice" because it was to have had some local San Francisco components. Several years later, because FDA approval was so delayed and the local element had totally disappeared, my third research assistant on the project and I "ended up" doing a discourse analysis (Clarke & Montini, 1993). RU486 was actually not FDA approved until September 2000, and even then in a highly overregulated fashion (Joffe & Weitz, 2003, p. 2353).

The research was not pursued with explicit use of situational analysis but with an incipient form that relied on social worlds/arenas analysis. Analytically, we examined the discursive constructions of RU486 put forward by most of the key social worlds (and some subworlds) that had committed themselves to action of some kind in the abortion arena regarding this abortion technology. We focused largely but not exclusively on the United States,

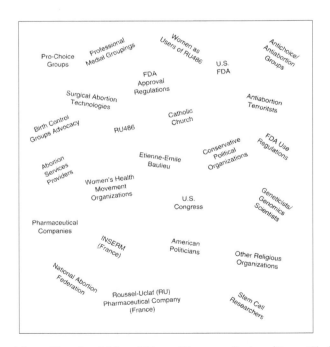

Figure 2.6: Messy Situational Map: RU486 Discourse Project (From Clarke [2005] *Situational Analysis: Grounded Theory after the Postmodern Turn*. Copyright 2005 by Sage Publications, Inc. Reprinted with permission of the publisher.)

and especially on reproductive and other scientists, birth control/population control organizations, pharmaceutical companies, medical groups, anti-abortion groups, pro-choice groups, women's health movement organizations, politicians, the U.S. Congress, and the FDA. We also examined what little research existed on women users or consumers of RU486 as a narrative discourse. I conceptualized these women as "implicated actors" (discussed above).

This was a multi-site study with a nonhuman object—a new abortion technology—at the center. Our data included published materials, interviews with key players, documents produced by involved organizations, and observations of some (but not all) key events. [Today, we would use websites as a means of access to pertinent organizational discourses.]

In Figure 2.6, we can see the elements in the messy RU486 map. I have not entered the specific names of the many different organizations involved here, but categorized them under general rubrics (e.g., feminist organizations; women's health movement organizations) for a simpler and more easily readable "teaching" map for this text. Particular organizations would, of course, be entered in the actual situational map and are discussed in the publication (Clarke & Montini, 1993). In the situational map, then, we can see the varied collective actors concerned about abortion, committed to act *and* to producing discourses in that arena. The main nonhuman actant is RU486. Anyone familiar with U.S. abortion politics will note that "all the usual suspects" are gathered here.

Part of the power of SA compared to most other approaches lies in "helping silences to speak"—noting where there are absences as well as presence. There are two sets of silent scientific collective actors here. Both are concerned with reproductive phenomena and are constituencies for whom abortion is of considerable importance but who seek to keep the proverbial "ten-foot-pole" between their social worlds and the white heat of the current U.S. abortion controversy. First are geneticists and others active in human genomics and/or involved in any and all aspects of prenatal genetic screening. Because there are no therapeutic interventions for most of the conditions current and anticipated screening will find, abortion remains the only therapeutic alternative. Enhanced access to and options for abortion for women who wish to terminate such a pregnancy, such as those provided by RU486, would seemingly be of central concerns for these actors. Yet abortion was and remains largely absent from their public discourse. The second silent set of collective scientific actors is fetal tissue researchers—today called "stem cell

Figure 2.7: Ordered Situational Map: RU486 Discourse Project (From Clarke [2005] *Situational Analysis: Grounded Theory after the Postmodern Turn.* Copyright 2005 by Sage Publications, Inc. Reprinted with permission of the publisher.)

INDIVIDUAL HUMAN ELEMENTS/ACTORS Etienne-Emile Baulieu	NONHUMAN ELEMENTS/ACTORS RU486 Surgical abortion technologies FDA regulations for approval FDA regulations for use
COLLECTIVE HUMAN ELEMENTS/ACTOR U.S. FDA U.S. Congress Pro-choice groups Anti-choice/anti-abortion groups Birth control advocacy groups Women's health movement groups Abortion services providers National Abortion Federation Professional medical groups	IMPLICATED/SILENT ACTORS/ACTANTS Women as users Genetic/genomic scientists Stem cell researchers Anti-abortion terrorists
DISCURSIVE CONSTRUCTION(S) OF HUMAN ACTORS Social world constructions of others Social world constructions of Baulieu Social world construction of FDA	DISCURSIVE CONSTRUCTION OF NONHUMAN ACTANTS Social world constructions of RU486 Social world construction of abortion Construction of approval regulations Construction of use regulations
POLITICAL/ECONOMIC ELEMENTS Access to abortion Costs of abortion Political party concerns re abortion	SOCIOCULTURAL/SYMBOLIC ELEMENTS Morality of abortion Morality of unwanted children Pill for abortion as "magic bullet"
TEMPORAL ELEMENTS Lateness of approval compared to Europe Rise of religious right in U.S. politics since 1970s	SPATIAL ELEMENTS Potential ease of wide geographic availability of RU486 Lack of abortion services in 84% of U.S. counties
MAJOR ISSUES/DEBATES (USUALLY CONTESTED) Safety of RU486 Safety of abortion Morality of abortion Morality of unwanted children	RELATED DISCOURSES (NARRATIVE AND/OR VISUAL) Abortion discourses Birth control discourses Sex/gender/feminism discourses Sexuality discourses

researchers." They have been silent about abortion despite the use of fetal tissue from induced abortions as materials for certain scientific research.

Readers may have noted that I was actually doing situational analyses here. As a feminist researcher, I knew about these silent actors and I put them "on the map"—a map where they would likely rather *not* appear. This illustrates the importance of the analyst's *own* knowledge of the situation in situational analysis as well as the legitimacy of using that knowledge "up front." Specifically, the analyst uses his or her knowledge to help design data collection and does not wait quietly for magically appearing data to speak! That is, the analyst needs to anticipate data that should be gathered in the initial design and/or theoretically sample appropriately downstream with great care and sensitivity (Charmaz, 2006).

Figure 2.7 is the ordered RU486 situational map. There are LOTS of discursive constructions because the data I gathered were that. The ordered map reveals one significant individual, Etienne-Emile Baulieu, the scientist primarily responsible for its development and who also served as a public advocate. There were many significant collective actors organized by and large into recognizable social worlds. But the most important new point to emerge through doing the ordered map concerns attending to spatial elements. A key feature of RU486 as a medical abortion technology is that it potentially could be distributed where there are no abortion clinics. Fully 84% of U.S. counties do not have abortion services (Joffe & Weitz, 2003, p. 2354)! Potentially, RU486 could legally put abortion services in the offices of primary care physicians and gynecologists in all of those counties. This element was and continues to be key in the politics of RU486. But as Joffe and Weitz detail, the regulations governing its distribution have limited access to it.

Using Situational Maps to Map Relationality

Relations among the various elements in the situation are key to its analysis. Once you have your messy map, you can do relational analyses. This is the next phase of analytic work to be done with the messy map. The procedure here is to first make a bunch of photocopies of your best version to date of the situational map. Then you take each element in turn and think about it in relation to each other element on the map. Literally center on one element and draw lines between it and the others and *specify the nature of the relationship by describing the nature of that line.* One does this *systematically,* one at a time, from every element on the map to every other. Use as many maps as seem useful to diagram yourself through this analytic exercise. This to me is the major work one does with the situational map once it is constructed. This is one of those sites where being highly systematic in considering data can flip over into the exciting and creative moments of intellectual work. And sometimes there is no payoff.

Relational maps also help the analyst to decide which stories—which relations—to pursue. This is especially helpful in the early stages of research when we tend to feel a bit mystified about where to go and what to memo. A session should produce several relational analyses with the situational maps and several memos. One would return to elaborate on these memos several times as data are collected. They should also be useful guides for theoretical sampling.

Conclusions

SA offers three kinds of maps as fresh analytic devices for grounded theorists. The importance of Strauss's social worlds and arenas theory; Foucault's emphasis on discourse and going beyond the knowing subject; the analytic centrality of the nonhuman; and the concept of situation are clear. I myself am especially fond of "helping silences speak." For both GTM and SA, the theorizing offered downstream in research reports should comfortably "handle" the data at a conceptual level, offer some integration of the concepts generated, be sufficient to address variation and change, and offer a fresh theoretical grasp of the phenomenon that may also open up sites for practical application (on such pragmatist problem-solving, see Strübing, 2007b).

In concluding, I want to look to the future and talk a bit about the emerging generation using and/or writing about situational analysis. Only a few articles other than my own work have appeared to date. Mills and colleagues (2007, p. 72) supplemented their grounded theory research on Australian rural nurses' experiences of mentoring with situational and social worlds mapping. This generated "increased awareness of how outside actors influenced participants' constructions of mentoring." Positional maps did not work for this project as it focused on action and agency rather than discourses (see also Mills, Francis, & Bonner, 2007, 2008). Polish sociologist Anny Kacperczyk (2007) has published an introduction to SA in Polish. And there are papers in the pipeline of which I am aware. Jennifer Fosket (2004, 2010, 2014) has used GTM and SA in her research on a large-scale clinical trial, and has written on the usefulness of doing situational maps. Sara Shostak (2003, 2005; Clarke, 2005, pp. 137-138) used social worlds/arenas maps to plot the disciplinary emergence of toxicogenomics.

Carrie Friese (2009; Clarke, 2005, pp. 139-140) used situational analysis to map the cloning of endangered species in the United States and has challenged the empirical adequacy of the social worlds/arenas metaphor and maps in important ways (Clarke & Friese, 2007). That is, there exist multiple meso-level analytics/metaphors in circulation, and we now think that the choice of which to draw on in a research project should be driven by empirical (rather than prescriptive) considerations. We are therefore considering writing a paper that compares actor network theory, network theories, assemblages, and social worlds/arenas in terms of their empirical strengths and weaknesses. This would update Clarke's (1991) earlier work comparing social worlds/arenas with other organizational theories.

Last, I return to my theme of being a dutiful daughter. Ans was a brilliant teacher in terms of making you as students do the work of design, data gathering, and analysis yourselves. He was very supportive and asked wonderful questions but would never do the analysis *for* you. As a student, this can be very hard—and disappointing! But the great gift given is that you really learn to do your own research. And that was what he wanted most from his students. I have thought much about being a dutiful daughter, about how to both honor and extend and even go beyond one's revered teacher. Like most of us, I have had much too much academic experience observing those who need to put others down in order to put themselves up. Through working with Ans, I learned that doing one's own work was the best path "up" and that trying to improve tools is a worthy endeavor. I was indeed most fortunate in "finding a creative present in the context of a revered past" (Dunning, 2003, p. 10).

In my efforts to create and sustain SA, I thus felt very reassured by the epigraph from John Dewey on the dedication page of Strauss and Corbin's (1990, 1998) *Basics* books. John Dewey offers a commentary on the importance of change to keeping ideas vital: "If the artist does not perfect new vision in his process of doing, he acts mechanically and repeats some old model fixed like a blueprint in his mind" (Dewey 1934/2005, p. 50). Strauss and Corbin (1994, p. 283) further noted that "no inventor has permanent possession of the invention—certainly not even of its name—and furthermore we would not wish to do so." I hope to eventually become that comfortable about situational analysis!

It *was* a great GTM bash. I hope situational analysis makes useful contributions to the GTM banquet. Please feel free to sample.

Notes

1. Thanks to Kathy Charmaz for ongoing, thoughtful, and useful critique about situational analysis. I have cited lightly here. The complete bibliography for *Situational Analysis* (Clarke,

2005) can be found in downloadable form at http://clarkessituationalanalysis.blogspot.com/ A current listing of my own methods publications is also at that site. The Anselm Strauss website has his complete CV, topical publications lists, and pdfs of a number of papers, along with a number of essays about his work. See appendixes. See also Clarke, 2008b).

2. In the second generation, in addition to those of us represented in this volume, I would also include (based on publication of their own books on GTM) Dahlgren, Emmelin, and Winkvist (2007), Dey (1999, 2004), Kearney (1998, 1999), Konecki (2000), Locke (1996, 2001), and Strübing (2004, 2007a). Leigh Star (e.g., 1995, 1999) and Antony Bryant (2002, 2006) brought GTM into information and computer science. Kris Koniecke also organized the online journal *Qualitative Sociological Review* (http://www.qualitativesociologyreview. org/ENG/index_eng.php) that features GTM. Thousands of others have, of course, published work using GTM, and there are a number of books on GTM in other languages (see listing in Morse et al. 2009).

3. On the diversity of grounded theory, including hollow claims of its use, in addition to this volume, see Bryant and Charmaz (2007, esp. pp. 1-57) and O'Connor, Netting, and Thomas (2008).

4. Their syllabi and reading lists were precious resources and they have been reincarnated annually for the Sociology and Nursing qualitative research courses.

5. Carolyn Wiener (personal communication, January 3, 2008) responded as follows when I asked her about this recently:

> We did not emphasize arenas/social worlds in our publications. I was the only one on the team who was interested in pursuing it, stemming from the timing of my dissertation/ book, *The Politics of Alcoholism*, which coincided with Anselm's working out the usefulness of this formulation. It fit so beautifully with what I had observed in my first exposure to the alcohol arena at a huge meeting in San Francisco which addressed alcohol problems from a myriad of perspectives. I had been given a fellowship that required I choose a research subject related to alcoholism, which I just assumed was a clearly defined entity. I told Anselm about the contentious discussion in the sessions and described the field as a "mess." You will appreciate his glee when he told me, "That's your subject, the mess!"

6. For Strauss's more theoretical publications focused on social worlds/arenas, see Strauss (1978a, 1978b, 1982a, 1982b, 1984, 1991a, 1991b); for his capstone statement, see Strauss (1993, pp. 209-244). The only major published empirical study was *Psychiatric Ideologies and Institutions* (Strauss et al., 1964) through which, I would argue, he and colleagues created the framework rather than used it. Wiener and Strauss also wrote an (unpublished) social worlds/arenas analysis of the early years of HIV/AIDS in the San Francisco Bay Area, available online on the Strauss website noted in the appendixes.

7. See Clarke (1990a, 1990b, 1991, 1998, 2005, pp. 109-117, 2006a), Clarke and Montini (1993), Clarke and Star (2003, 2007), and Clarke and Friese (2007).

8. On multi-sited research, see, for example, Marcus (1998). For examples, see Freidson's (1970, 1975) work on the profession of medicine, and Bucher's (1962, 1988; Bucher & Strauss, 1961) on reform-oriented segments as social movements inside a profession.

9. Other works discussing or using the social worlds/arenas framework include Baszanger (1998a, 1998b), Bucher (1988), Casper (1998a, 1998b), Garrety (1997), Star (1989), Wiener (1981, 1991, 2000), and reviews in Clarke and Star (2003, 2007). Becker (1982) and Shibutani (1955, 1962, 1986, pp. 109-116) also wrote on social worlds, though not using grounded theory methods.

10. For interactionist critiques of actor-network-theory, see Star (1991a, b, 1995), Fujimura (1991), and Clarke and Montini (1993). Especially on nonhuman agency, see Casper (1994), Latour (2005), and Law and Hassard (1999).

11. Monica Casper's (1998b, see also 1994) concept of "work objects" generated through her research on fetal surgery nicely allows the question of whether the focus of work is or is not "human" to be empirically addressed. See Clarke (1995) on the salience of nonhumans in scientific research on reproductive physiology, and Haraway (2007) on the vexed boundary between human and nonhuman.

12. Special thanks to Laura Mamo for discussions on this point.

13. As I began to get serious about situational maps, I remembered that earlier, in *Negotiations*, Strauss (1978b, pp. 98-99) had distinguished between a broader structural context and a narrower and more immediate negotiation context. Later, Strauss and Corbin (1990, p. 100) distinguished among causal, intervening, and contextual conditions. This was provocative for my thinking. Although I would agree that some elements are more important than others, and some are certainly experienced by those in the situation as "closer in" than others, it is precisely such an in principle dualism/determinism that I am struggling against.

References

Applbaum, K. (2004). *The marketing era: From professional practice to global provisioning.* New York: Routledge.

Atkinson, P., Coffey, A., & Delamont, S. (2003). *Key themes in qualitative research: Continuities and change.* Walnut Creek, CA: AltaMira.

Baszanger, I. (1998a). *Inventing pain medicine: From the laboratory to the clinic.* New Brunswick, NJ: Rutgers University Press.

Baszanger, I. (1998b). The work sites of an American interactionist: A. L. Strauss (1917-1996). *Symbolic Interaction*, 21(4), 353–378.

Baszanger, I. & Dodier, N. (1997). Ethnography: Relating the part to the whole. In D. Silverman (Ed.), *Qualitative research: Theory, method, and practice* (pp. 8-23). London: Sage.

Becker, H. S. (1982). *Art worlds.* Berkeley: University of California Press.

Bijker, W., Pinch, T., & Hughes, T. (Eds.). (1987). *The social construction of technical systems: New directions in the sociology and history of technology.* Cambridge, MA: MIT Press.

Blumer, H. (1958). Race prejudice as a sense of group position. *Pacific Sociological Review*, 1(1), 3–8.

Blumer, H. (1969, 1993). *Symbolic interactionism: Perspective and method.* Berkeley: University of California Press.

Bruce, J. (1987). Users' perspectives on contraceptive technology and delivery systems: Highlighting some feminist issues. *Technology in Society*, 9(3–4), 359–383.

Bryant, A. (2002). Re-grounding grounded theory. *Journal of Information Technology, Theory and Application*, 4(1), 25–42.

Bryant, A. (2006). *Thinking informatically: A new understanding of information, communication and technology.* Lampeter, UK: Edwin Mellen.

Bryant, A. & Charmaz, K. (Eds.). (2007). *Handbook of grounded theory.* London: Sage.

Bucher, R. (1962). Pathology: A study of social movements within a profession. *Social Problems*, 10(1), 40–51.

Bucher, R. (1988). On the natural history of health care occupations. *Work and Occupations,*
15(2), 131–147.

Bucher, R. & Strauss, A. (1961). Professions in process. *American Journal of Sociology,* 66(4),
325–334.

Casper, M. J. (1994). Reframing and grounding nonhuman agency: What makes a fetus an
agent? *American Behavioral Scientist,* 37(6), 839–856.

Casper, M. J. (1998a). *The making of the unborn patient: A social anatomy of fetal surgery.* New
Brunswick, NJ: Rutgers University Press.

Casper, M. J. (1998b). Negotiations, work objects and the unborn patient: The interactional
scaffolding of fetal surgery. *Symbolic Interaction,* 21(4), 379–400.

Charmaz, K. (2000). Grounded theory: Objectivist and constructivist methods. In N. K.
Denzin & Y. S. Lincoln (Eds.), *Handbook of qualitative research,* 2nd ed. (pp. 509–536).
Thousand Oaks, CA: Sage.

Charmaz, K. (2006). *Constructing grounded theory.* London: Sage.

Clarke, A. E. (1990a). A social worlds research adventure: The case of reproductive science.
In S. Cozzens & T. Gieryn (Eds.), *Theories of science in society* (pp. 15–42). Bloomington:
Indiana University Press.

Clarke, A. E. (1990b). Controversy and the development of American reproductive sciences.
Social Problems 37(1), 18–37.

Clarke, A. E. (1991). Social worlds theory as organizational theory. In D. Maines (Ed.), *Social
organization and social process: Essays in honor of Anselm Strauss* (pp. 119–158). Hawthorne,
NY: Aldine de Gruyter.

Clarke, A. E. (1995). Research materials and reproductive science in the United States, 1910-
1940. In S. L. Star (Ed.), *Ecologies of knowledge: New directions in sociology of science and
technology* (pp. 183–219). Albany: State University of New York Press.

Clarke, A. E. (1998). *Disciplining reproduction: Modernity, American life sciences and the "problem of sex."* Berkeley: University of California Press.

Clarke, A. E. (2000). Maverick reproductive scientists and the production of contraceptives
c1915-2000. In A. Saetnan, N. Oudshoorn, & M. Kirejczyk (Eds.), *Bodies of technology:
Women's involvement with reproductive medicine* (pp. 37–89). Columbus: Ohio State University Press.

Clarke, A. E. (2003). Situational analyses: Grounded theory mapping after the postmodern
turn. *Symbolic Interaction,* 26(4), 553–576.

Clarke, A. E. (2005). *Situational analysis: Grounded theory after the postmodern turn.* Thousand
Oaks, CA: Sage.

Clarke, A. E. (2006a). Social worlds. In G. Ritzer (Ed.), *The Blackwell encyclopedia of sociology*
(pp. 4547–4549). Malden, MA: Blackwell.

Clarke, A. E. (2006b). Feminisms, grounded theory and situational analysis. In S. Hesse-
Biber (Ed.), *The handbook of feminist research: Theory and praxis* (pp. 345–370). Thousand
Oaks, CA: Sage.

Clarke, A. E. (2007). Grounded theory: Conflicts, debates and situational analysis. In W.
Outhwaite & S. P. Turner (Eds.), *Handbook of social science methodology* (pp. 838–885).
Thousand Oaks, CA: Sage.

Clarke, A. E. (2008a). Sex/gender and race/ethnicity in the legacy of Anselm Strauss. *Studies
in Symbolic Interaction,* 32, 159–176.

Clarke, A. E. (2008b). Anselm L. Strauss. In G. Ritzer (Ed.), *The Blackwell encyclopedia of
sociology.* Malden, MA: Blackwell.

Clarke, A. E. (2009). On Getting Lost and Found and Lost Again with Patti Lather. In Special Issue on Knowledge that Matters, *Frontiers: A Journal of Women's Studies* 30(1):212–222.

Clarke, A. E. (2010a). From the rise of medicine to biomedicalization: U.S. healthscapes and iconography c1890-present. In A. E. Clarke, J. Shim, L. Mamo, J. Fosket, & J. Fishman (Eds.), *Biomedicalization: Technoscience and transformations of health and illness in the U. S.* (pp. 104-146). Durham, NC: Duke University Press.

Clarke, A. E. (2010b). Anselm Strauss en heritage: Sexe/genre et race/ethnicite.In French in D. Chabaud-Rychter, V. Descoutures, A. Devreux, & E. Varikas (Eds.), *Questions de genre aux sciences sociales "normales* (pp. 245–259). Paris: La Decouverte.

Clarke, A. E. & Friese, C. (2007). Situational analysis: Going beyond traditional grounded theory. In A. Bryant & K. Charmaz (Eds.), *Handbook of grounded theory* (pp. 694–743). London: Sage.

Clarke, A. E. & Montini, T. (1993). The many faces of RU486: Tales of situated knowledges and technological contestations. *Science, Technology and Human Values*, 18(1), 42–78.

Clarke, A. E. & Star, S. L. (1998). On coming home and intellectual generosity. Introduction to special issue: New work in the tradition of Anselm L. Strauss. *Symbolic Interaction* 21(4), 341–349.

Clarke, A. E. & Star, S. L. (2003). Symbolic interactionist studies of science, technology and medicine. In L. Reynolds & N. Herman (Eds.), *Handbook of symbolic interactionism* (pp. 539–574). Walnut Creek, CA: AltaMira.

Clarke, A. E. & Star, S. L. (2007). Social worlds/arenas as a theory-methods package. In E. Hackett, O. Amsterdamska, M. Lynch & J. Wacjman (Eds.), *Handbook of science and technology studies* (pp. 113–137). Cambridge, MA: MIT Press, 2nd ed.

Dahlgren, L., Emmelin, M., & Winkvist, A. (2007). *Qualitative methodology for international public health.* Umea, Sweden: International School of Public Health, Umea University.

De Beauvoir, S. ([1959] 2005). *Memoirs of a dutiful daughter.* New York: HarperCollins Publishers.

Deegan, M. J. (1990). *Jane Addams and the men of the Chicago School: 1892-1918.* New Brunswick, NJ: Transaction Publishers.

Denzin, N. K. ([1970] 1989). *The research act: A theoretical introduction to sociological methods.* Chicago: Aldine.

Denzin, N. K. (1992). *Symbolic interactionism and cultural studies: The politics of interpretation.* Oxford: Basil Blackwell.

Dewey, J. ([1934] 2005). *Art as experience.* New York: Perigee Books.

Dey, I. (1999). *Grounding grounded theory: Guidelines for qualitative inquiry.* San Diego, CA: Academic Press.

Dey, I. (2004). Grounded theory. In C. Seale, G. Gobo, J. F. Gubrium, & D. Silverman (Eds.), *Qualitative research practice* (pp. 80-93). London: Sage.

Dingwall, R. (1999). On the nonnegotiable in sociological life. In B. Glassner & R. Hertz (Eds.), *Qualitative sociology and everyday life* (pp. 215–225). Thousand Oaks, CA : Sage.

Dreyfus, H. L. & Rabinow, P. (1983). *Michel Foucault: Beyond structuralism and hermeneutics,* 2nd ed. Chicago: University of Chicago Press.

DuBois, W.E.B. (1993). *WE.B. Dubois reader.* New York: Scribner.

Dugdale, A. (1999). Materiality: Juggling sameness and difference. In J. Law & J. Hassard (Eds.), *Actor-network theory and after* (pp. 113–135). Oxford, UK: Blackwell Publishers.

Dunning, J. (2003). Limon's troupe now bears her signature. *New York Times,* Sunday, April 27:10AR.

Fine, G. A. (1995). *A second Chicago school?: The development of a postwar American sociology.* Chicago: University of Chicago Press.

Fosket, J. R. (2004). Constructing 'high risk" women: The development and standardization of a breast cancer risk assessment tool. *Science, Technology, and Human Values,* 29(3), 291–323.

Fosket, J. R. (2010). Breast cancer risk as disease: Biomedicalizing risk. In A. E. Clarke, J, Shim, L. Mamo, J. Fosket, & J. Fishman (Eds.), *Biomedicalization: Technoscience health and illness in the U.S.* (pp. 331–352). Durham, NC: Duke University Press.

Fosket, J. R. 2014. Situating knowledge. In A. E. Clarke & K. Charmaz (Eds.) *Grounded theory and situational analysis* (pp. 91–110). Sage Benchmarks in Social Research Series, 4 volumes. London: Sage.

Foucault, M. (1972). *The archeology of knowledge and the discourse on language.* New York: Harper.

Foucault, M. (1973). *The order of things: An archeology of the human sciences.* New York: Vintage/Random House.

Foucault, M. (1975). *The birth of the clinic: An archeology of medical perception.* New York: Vintage/Random House.

Foucault, M. (1978). *The history of sexuality.* Vol. 1: *An introduction.* New York: Vintage Books.

Foucault, M. (1988). Technologies of the self. In L. Martin, H. Gutman, & P. Hutton (Eds.), *Technologies of the self: A seminar with Michel Foucault* (pp. 16-49). Amherst: University of Massachusetts Press.

Freidson, E. (1970). *Profession of medicine: A study of the sociology of applied knowledge.* New York: Harper and Row.

Freidson, E. (1975). *Doctoring together: A study of professional social control.* Chicago: University of Chicago Press.

Friese, C. 2009. Models of cloning, models for the zoo: Rethinking the sociological significance of cloned animals. *BioSocieties* 4:367–390

Fujimura, J. H. (1991). On methods, ontologies and representation in the sociology of science: Where do we stand? In D. Maines (Ed.), *Social organization and social process: Essays in honor of Anselm Strauss* (pp. 207-248). Hawthorne, NY: Aldine de Gruyter.

Garrety, K. (1997). Social worlds, actor-networks and controversy: The case of cholesterol, dietary fat and heart disease. *Social Studies of Science,* 27(5), 727–773.

Glaser, B. G. (1992). *Emergence versus forcing: Basics of grounded theory analysis.* Mill Valley, CA: Sociology Press.

Glaser, B. G. & Strauss, A. L. (1967). *The discovery of grounded theory: Strategies for qualitative research.* Chicago: Aldine.

Hall, P. (1997). Meta-power, social organization, and the shaping of social action. *Symbolic Interaction,* 20(4), 39–418.

Haraway, D. ([1985] 1991a). *Simians, cyborgs, and women: The reinvention of nature.* New York: Routledge.

Haraway, D. (1991b). Situated knowledges: The science question in feminism and the privilege of partial perspective. In D. Haraway (Ed.), *Simians, cyborgs, and women: The reinvention of nature* (pp. 183–202). New York: Routledge.

Haraway, D. (2007). *When species meet.* Minneapolis: University of Minnesota Press.

Hearn, J. & Roseneil, S. (Eds.). (1999). *Consuming cultures: Power and resistance.* London: Macmillan.

Hildenbrand, B. (2007). Mediating structure and interaction in grounded theory. In A. Bryant & K. Charmaz (Eds.), *Handbook of grounded theory* (pp. 539–564). London: Sage.

Hodder, I. (2000). The interpretation of documents and material culture. In N. K. Denzin & Y. S. Lincoln (Eds.), *Handbook of qualitative research*, 2nd ed. (pp. 703–715). Thousand Oaks, CA: Sage.

Hughes, E. C. (1971). *The sociological eye*. Chicago: Aldine Atherton.

Jenks, C. (1995). The centrality of the eye in Western culture: An introduction. In C. Jenks (Ed.), *Visual culture* (pp. 1–25). London: Routledge.

Joffe, C. & Weitz, T. A. (2003). Normalizing the exceptional: Incorporating the "abortion pill" into mainstream medicine. *Social Science and Medicine*, 56(12), 2353–2366.

Kacperczyk, A. (2007). Badacz i jego poszukiwania w swietle "Analizy Sytuacyjnej" Adele E. Clarke. Przeglad Socjologii Jakosciowej. *Qualitative Sociology Review* III(2).

Kearney, M. H. (1998). Ready to wear: Discovering grounded formal theory. *Research in Nursing and Health*, 21(2), 179–186.

Kearney, M. H. (1999). *Understanding women's recovery from illness and trauma*. Thousand Oaks, CA: Sage.

Konecki, K. (2000). *Studies in qualitative methodology: Grounded theory* [in Polish]. Warsaw, Poland: PWN.

Kurtz, L. R. (1984). *Evaluating Chicago sociology: A guide to the literature, with an annotated bibliography*. Chicago: University of Chicago Press.

Lather, P. (1991). *Getting smart: Feminist research and pedagogy with/in the postmodern*. New York: Routledge.

Lather, P. (2007). *Getting lost: Feminist efforts toward a double(d) science*. Albany: State University of New York Press.

Latour, B. (1987). *Science in action*. Cambridge, MA: Harvard University Press.

Latour, B. (2005). *Reassembling the social: An introduction to actor-network theory*. Oxford: Oxford University Press.

Law, J. & Hassard, J. (Eds.). (1999). *Actor network theory and after*. Malden, MA: Blackwell.

Law, J. & Mol, A. (1995). Notes on materiality and sociality. *The Sociological Review*, 43(2), 274–294.

Locke, K. (1996). Rewriting the discovery of grounded theory after 25 years? *Journal of Management Inquiry*, 5(1), 239–245.

Locke, K. (2001). *Grounded theory in management research*. Thousand Oaks, CA: Sage.

Locke, K. (2007). Rational control and irrational free-play: Dual-thinking modes as necessary tension in grounded theorizing. In A. Bryant & K. Charmaz (Eds.), *Handbook of grounded theory* (pp. 565–579). London: Sage.

Marcus, G. (1998). *Ethnography through thick and thin*. Princeton, NJ: Princeton University Press.

McCarthy, D. (1984). Towards a sociology of the physical world: George Herbert Mead on physical objects. *Studies in Symbolic Interaction*, 5, 105–121.

Mead, G. H. ([1927] 1964). The objective reality of perspectives. In A. J. Reck (Ed.), *Selected writings of George Herbert Mead* (pp. 306–319). Chicago: University of Chicago Press.

Meltzer, B. N., Petras J. W., & Reynolds, L. T. (1975). *Symbolic interactionism: Genesis, varieties and criticism*. Boston: Routledge and Kegan Paul.

Miller, D. (1998). Why some things matter. In D. Miller (Ed.), *Material cultures: Why some things matter* (pp. 3–21). London: University College of London Press.

Mills, C. W. (1940). Situated actions and vocabularies of motive. *American Sociological Review*, 5(6), 904–913.

Mills, J., Chapman, Y., Bonner, A., & Francis, K. (2007). Grounded theory: A methodological spiral from positivism to postmodernism. *Journal of Advanced Nursing*, 58(1), 72–79.

Mills, J., Francis, K., & Bonner, A. (2007). Live my work: Rural nurses and their multiple perspectives of self. *Journal of Advanced Nursing*, 59(6), 583–590.

Mills, J., Francis, K., & Bonner, A. (2008). Getting to know a stranger—rural nurses' experiences of mentoring: A grounded theory. *International Journal of Nursing Studies*, 45(4), 599–607.

Nelkin, D. (1995). Scientific controversies. In S. Jasanoff, G. E. Markle, J. Petersen, and T. Pinch (Eds.), *Handbook of science & technology studies* (pp. 444–456). Thousand Oaks, CA: Sage.

O'Connor, M. K., Netting, F. E., & Thomas, M. L. (2008). Grounded theory: Managing the challenge for those facing institutional review board oversight. *Qualitative inquiry*, 14(1), 28–45.

Olesen, V. L. (2007). Feminist qualitative research and grounded theory: Complexities, criticisms and opportunities. In A. Bryant & K. Charmaz (Eds.), *Handbook of grounded theory* (pp. 417–435). London: Sage.

Oudshoorn, N. (2003). *The male pill: A biography of a technology in the making*. Durham, NC: Duke University Press.

Park, R. E. (1952). *Human communities*. Glencoe, IL: Free Press.

Park, R. E. & Burgess, E. W. ([1921]1970). *Introduction to the science of sociology*. Chicago: University of Chicago.

Prior, L. (1997). Following in Foucault's footsteps: Text and context in qualitative research. In D. Silverman (Ed.), *Qualitative research: Theory, method, practice* (pp. 63–79). London: Sage.

Reichertz, J. (2007). Abduction: The logic of discovery of grounded theory. In A. Bryant & K. Charmaz (Eds.), *Handbook of grounded theory* (pp. 214–228). London: Sage.

Reynolds, L. & Herman, N. (Eds.). (2003). *Handbook of symbolic interactionism*. Walnut Creek, CA: AltaMira.

Richardson, R. & Kramer, E. H. (2006). Abduction as the type of inference that characterizes the development of a grounded theory. *Qualitative Research*, 6(4), 497–513.

Schatzki, T. R., Cetina, K. K., & von Savigny, E. (Eds.). (2001). *The practice turn in contemporary theory*. London: Routledge.

Shibutani, T. (1955). Reference groups as perspectives. *American Journal of Sociology*, 60(6), 562–569.

Shibutani, T. (1962). Reference groups and social control. In A. Rose (Ed.), *Human behavior and social processes* (pp. 128–145). Boston: Houghton Mifflin.

Shibutani, T. (1986). *Social processes: An introduction to sociology*. Berkeley: University of California Press.

Shostak, S. (2003). Locating gene-environment interaction: At the intersections of genetics and public health. *Social Science and Medicine*, 56(11), 2327–2342.

Shostak, S. (2005). The emergence of toxicogenomics: A case study of molecularization. *Social Studies of Science*, 35(3), 367–404.

Simon, J. (1996). Discipline and punish: The birth of a middle-range research strategy. *Contemporary Sociology*, 25(3), 316–319.

Star, S. L. (1983). Simplification in scientific work: An example from neuroscience research. *Social Studies of Science*, 13(2), 208–226.

Star, S. L. (1989). *Regions of the mind: Brain research and the quest for scientific certainty.* Stanford, CA: Stanford University Press.

Star, S. L. (1991a). Power, technologies and the phenomenology of conventions: On being allergic to onions. In J. Law (Ed.), *A sociology of monsters: Essays on power, technology and domination* (pp. 26–56). Sociological Review Monograph No. 38. New York: Routledge.

Star, S. L. (1991b). The sociology of the invisible: The primacy of work in the writings of Anselm Strauss. In D. Maines (Ed.), *Social organization and social process: Essays in honor of Anselm L. Strauss* (pp. 265–283). Hawthorne, NY: Aldine de Gruyter.

Star, S. L. (1995). The politics of formal representations: Wizards, gurus and organizational complexity. In S. L. Star (Ed.), *Ecologies of knowledge: Work and politics in science and technology* (pp. 88–118). Albany: State University of New York Press.

Star, S. L. (1999). The ethnography of infrastructure. *American Behavioral Scientist*, 43(3), 377–391.

Star, S. L. (2007). Living grounded theory: Cognitive and emotional forms of pragmatism. In A. Bryant & K. Charmaz (Eds.), *Handbook of grounded theory* (pp. 75–94). London: Sage.

Star, S. L. & Strauss, A. L. (1998). Layers of silence, arenas of voice: The ecology of visible and invisible work. *Computer Supported Cooperative Work: The Journal of Collaborative Computing*, 8(1), 9–30.

Strauss, A. L. (1978a). A social worlds perspective. *Studies in Symbolic Interaction*, 1, 119-128.

Strauss, A. L. (1978b). *Negotiations: Varieties, contexts, processes and social order.* San Francisco: Jossey Bass.

Strauss, A. L. (1982a). Interorganizational negotiation. *Urban Life*, 11(3), 350–367.

Strauss, A. L. (1982b). Social worlds and legitimation processes. In N. K. Denzin (Ed.), *Studies in symbolic interaction*, 4th ed. (pp. 171–190). Greenwich, CT: JAI Press.

Strauss, A. L. (1984). Social worlds and their segmentation processes. In N. K. Denzin (Ed.), *Studies in symbolic interaction*, 5th ed. (pp.123–139). Greenwich, CT: JAI Press.

Strauss, A. L. (1987). *Qualitative analysis for social scientists.* Cambridge: Cambridge University Press.

Strauss, A. L. (1991a). *Creating sociological awareness: Collective images and symbolic representation.* New Brunswick, NJ: Transaction Publishers.

Strauss, A. L. (1991b). Social worlds and spatial processes: An analytic perspective. In W. R. Ellis (Ed.), *A person-environment theory series/The Center for Environmental Design Research Working Paper Series.* Berkeley: Department of Architecture, University of California. Online at Anselm Strauss's website (see appendixes).

Strauss, A. L. (1993). *Continual permutation of action.* New York: Aldine de Gruyter.

Strauss, A. L. & Corbin, J. (1990). *The basics of qualitative analysis: Grounded theory procedures and techniques.* Thousand Oaks, CA: Sage.

Strauss, A. L. & Corbin, J. (1994). Grounded theory methodology: An overview. In N. K. Denzin & Y. S. Lincoln (Eds.), *Handbook of qualitative research* (pp. 273–285). Newbury Park, CA: Sage.

Strauss, A. L. & Corbin, J. (Eds.). (1997). *Grounded theory in practice.* Thousand Oaks, CA: Sage.

Strauss, A. L., & Corbin, J. (1998). *The basics of qualitative analysis: Grounded theory procedures and techniques*, 2nd ed. Thousand Oaks, CA: Sage.

Strauss, A. & Fisher, B. (1979). George Herbert Mead and the Chicago tradition of sociology, Part I. *Symbolic Interaction, 2*(1), 9–26.

Strauss, A., Schatzman, L., Bucher, R., Ehrlich, D. and Sabshin, M. (1964). *Psychiatric ideologies and institutions.* Glencoe, IL: The Free Press of Glencoe.

Strübing, J. (2004). *Grounded theory: Zur sozialtheoretischen und epistemologischen Fundierung des Verfahrens der empirisch begrundeten Theoriebildung.* Wiesbaden, Germany: VS Verlag für Sozialwissenschaften.

Strübing, J. (2007a). *Anselm Strauss.* Konstanz, Germany: UVK VerlagsgesellschaftmbH.

Strübing, J. (2007b). Research as pragmatic problem-solving: The pragmatist roots of empirically-grounded theorizing. In A. Bryant & K. Charmaz (Eds.), *Handbook of grounded theory* (pp. 580–602). London: Sage.

Thomas, W. I. & Thomas, D. S. [1928] (1970). Situations defined as real are real in their consequences. In G. P. Stone & H. A. Farberman (Eds.), *Social psychology through symbolic interaction* (pp. 154–155). Waltham, MA: Xerox College Publishing.

Wiener, C. L. (1981). *The politics of alcoholism: A social worlds analysis.* New Brunswick, NJ: Transaction Press.

Wiener, C. L. (1991). Arenas and careers: The complex interweaving of personal and organizational destiny. In D. Maines (Ed.), *Social organization and social process: Essays in honor of Anselm Strauss* (pp. 175–188). New York: Aldine De Gruyter.

Wiener, C. L. (2000). *The elusive quest: Accountability in hospitals.* New York: Aldine de Gruyter.

Wiener, C., Strauss, A., Fagerhaugh, S., & Suczek, B. (1992). The AIDS policy arena: Contingent aspects of social world/arena theory. Unpublished ms. Available online at Strauss's website (see appendixes).

Woolgar, S. (1991). Configuring the user: The case of usability trials. In J. Law (Ed.), *A sociology of monsters: Essays on power, technology and domination* (pp. 57–102). New York: Routledge.

CHAPTER THREE

FEMINISM, GROUNDED THEORY, AND SITUATIONAL ANALYSIS REVISITED

Adele E. Clarke

Simply finding grounded theory was not self-evident. It meant walking a twisted path, full of contingency and accidental proximities. . . . In bringing both contingencies and commitments to explicit, overt analysis, one creates the chance to . . . include the heart of method as a part of lived experience. . . . The growing community of analysts, critics, and students is my ground of reflection, and we give each other the courage to go on.

—Susan Leigh Star (2007, pp. 79, 91)

Grounded theory (hereafter GT), developed by Barney Glaser and Anselm Strauss (1967), has become such a leading method in qualitative research transnationally that it now merits its own hefty *Handbook of Grounded Theory* (Bryant & Charmaz, 2007), a major new text (Charmaz, 2006, 2014), and a four-volume reader in the SAGE Benchmarks in Social Research Methods series, titled *Grounded Theory and Situational Analysis* (Clarke & Charmaz, 2014). Interestingly, in the book devoted to the diversity of approaches within GT generated by the second generation of scholars (Morse et al., 2009), all of those scholars are women, most if not all feminists.

AUTHOR'S NOTE: In sorrow I dedicate this chapter to the memory of a superb feminist grounded theorist, Susan Leigh Star, mentor, colleague, friend (Star, 2007; Clarke, 2010b). For comments on this and related work, I thank Leigh, Monica Casper, Kathy Charmaz, Carrie Friese, and Virginia Olesen. I cite the grounded theory and situational analysis literatures lightly because of space, and I omitted many citations found in my earlier version (Clarke, 2007a). See also bibliographies in Bryant and Charmaz (2007) and at www.situationalanalysis.com.

GT merits such ambitious works especially because of its transnational and transdisciplinary travels (e.g., Morse et al., 2009, pp. 254-256; Schutze, 2008; Tarozzi, 2008). It is renowned today not only in sociology (e.g., Clarke & Charmaz, 2014; Strauss & Corbin, 1997) and nursing (e.g., Keamey, 2007; Plummer & Young, 2010; Schreiber & Stern, 2001; Stern, 2007), where it was originally taught, but also in organization and management studies (e.g., Dougherty, 2005; Locke, 2001; Pearse & Kanyangale, 2009; Suddaby, 2006); education (e.g., Creswell, 2007); library science (e.g., Star & Bowker, 2007); counseling psychology (e.g., Fassinger, 2005); computer and information science (Bryant, 2006; Urquhart, 2007); social work (e.g., Gilgun, 2013; Padgett, 2008); public health (e.g., Dahlgren, Emmelin, & Winkvist, 2007); science, technology, and medicine studies (e.g., Clarke & Star, 2008); and queer studies (e.g., Plummer, 2005). GT has been quite well elaborated over the years by a number of scholars, most especially Charmaz.[1] Situational analysis (hereafter SA), which I developed, is an extension of GT inspired in part by Donna Haraway's (1991) concept of "situated knowledges" and by Norm Denzin's (1970/1989) early efforts at situating research in his book *The Research Act*. It integrates poststructural assumptions with those of GT and strong feminist emphases on elucidating differences, the analysis of power, and including documentary, historical, and visual discourses (Clarke, 2003, 2005; Clarke & Charmaz, 2014).

Feminisms here are approaches fundamentally provoking research toward improving the heterogeneous situations of women and promoting social justice. The feminisms I have been involved in seek to elucidate the dynamics of sexism, racial and ethnic discrimination, classism, homo- and queer-phobias, discrimination against the disabled, looksism, and ageism— and their complex interrelations are often theorized as intersectionality (e.g., Collins, 2004; Dill & Zambrana, 2009; Schulz & Mullings, 2006; Weber, 2010). In addition to this broad research agenda, feminist practices— praxis—matter. Feminisms also affect how we go about research (and other aspects of life). Pushing ourselves and others to be open to new ways of seeing and knowing, to legitimate and promote epistemic diversity (knowledge production by differently situated producers), and to work against epistemic violence that erases or silences minor voices and perspectives are each and all important. In sum, I share with Dorothy Smith (2007) her goal of opening her feminism "from a sociology for women to a sociology for people."

In terms of feminism(s) and GT and SA, there exist vast numbers of citations from multiple disciplines and recent reviews (Olesen, 2007, 2011). My goal here is to examine a range of selected research using GT and SA vis-à-vis their contributions to feminist research and praxis.[2] It is requisite to remember that no one method can do everything that feminists might want to do. Fonow and Cooke (2005), for example, assert that "there has never been one correct feminist epistemology generating one correct feminist methodology" (p. 213), and I would add, there never will be.

I first elucidate what GT is and specify the ways in which GT has always already been implicitly feminist in its pragmatist epistemologic ontology. I then turn to the feminist GT literature and demonstrate how scholars have to date made GT more explicitly feminist through using it in feminist projects. Next I discuss what SA is, how it, too, is also always already implicitly feminist, and some feminist research using it to date. In conclusion, I frame my hopes for the feminist futures of both GT and SA.

What Is Grounded Theory?

Social phenomena are complex. Thus they require complex grounded theory. (Strauss, 1987, p. 1)

GT and SA are both first and foremost modes of analysis of qualitative research data. That is, neither claims to offer a fully elaborated methodology from soup to nuts—from project design to data collection to final write-up. Many elements of a full-blown methodology are offered by both, and situational maps can be especially useful for design stages. But analysis is their core goal. Building on traditional GT, which is usually used with field data or in-depth interviews, SA explicitly extends analysis to discursive data including narrative and historical documents and visual materials. Across many disciplines, there has been a dramatic increase in multi-site or multi-modal research projects that generate many kinds of data. Both GT and SA can be used across heterogeneous data sources and are thus excellent for such projects.

GT and SA are both deeply empirical approaches to the study of social life. The very term *grounded theory* means data-grounded theorizing. In the words of Atkinson, Coffey, and Delamont (2003), "Grounded theory is not a description of a kind of theory. Rather it represents a general way of generating theory (or, even more generically, a way of having ideas on the basis of empirical research)" (p. 150). The theorizing is generated *abductively* by tacking back and forth between the nitty-gritty specificities of empirical data and more abstract ways of thinking about them.[3] In doing SA, too, the analyst relentlessly returns to the crudest of the maps to remind herself of the palpability and heterogeneity of the data and their interconnections.

In using or doing GT, the analyst initially codes the qualitative data (open coding)—word by word, segment by segment—and gives temporary labels (codes) to particular phenomena. Over time, the analyst determines whether codes generated through one data source also appear elsewhere, and elaborates their properties. Related codes that seem robust through the ongoing coding process are then densified into more enduring and analytically ambitious "categories" (Charmaz, 2006). Memos are written about each designated code and category: What does it mean? What are the instances of it? What is the variation within it in the data? What does and doesn't it seem to "take into account" (Lempert, 2007)? Ideally, the categories generated and deemed robust are ultimately integrated into a theoretical analysis of the substantive area of the current research project. Thus, a "grounded theory" of a particular phenomenon is composed of the analytic codes and categories generated abductively in the analysis and explicitly integrated to form a theory of the substantive area. The analyst generates an empirically based "substantive theory" (Strauss, 1987). In traditional GT, over time, after the researchers have generated multiple substantive theories of a particular broad area of interest through an array of empirical research projects, so the argument went, more "formal theory" could be developed (see Glaser, 2007; Keamey, 2001, 2007; Moore, 2007; Strauss, 1995). Formal theory was originally used here in the modernist sense of social theory, aiming at "Truth," and I return to this point later.

What remains relatively unique and very special to this approach is first GT's requiring that analysis begin as soon as there are data. Coding begins immediately, and theorizing based on that coding does as well, however provisionally (Glaser, 1978). Second, there are at least two kinds of sampling involved in doing grounded theory research. First is the usual sampling driven by attempts to be "representative" of some social body or population and its heterogeneities—to examine a full array of persons and sites of the phenomenon. Second is "theoretical sampling" guided explicitly by *theoretical* concerns that have emerged in the provisional analysis. Such "*theoretical sampling*" focuses on finding *new data sources* (persons and/or things—and *not* theories) that are excellent for explicitly addressing specific theoretically interesting facets of the emergent analysis. Theoretical sampling has been integral to GT from the outset, remains a fundamental strength of this analytic approach, and is also crucial for SA.[4]

In fact, it can be argued that precisely what is to be studied *emerges* from the analytic process over time, rather than being designated a priori: "The true legacy of Glaser and Strauss is a collective awareness of the heuristic value of developmental research designs [through doing theoretical sampling] and exploratory data analytic strategies, not a 'system for conducting and analyzing research'" (Atkinson et al., 2003, p. 163). I see this emergence as implicitly feminist in that it tries to build an adequate "database" for a project through expanding the data to be collected "as needed" analytically and also through researchers' mining their own reflexivity. This is a much more modest than arrogant approach to the production of new knowledge—assuming that we learn as we go (Haraway, 1997). Thus it takes "experience" into account in all its densities and complexities (Scott, 1992)—especially the experiences of the researchers with their project and their reflexivity about it (Charmaz, 2006).

Most research using GT has relied on field work to generate interview and/or ethnographic data through which to analyze human action (e.g., Strauss & Corbin, 1997). Conventional GT has focused on generating the "basic social process" occurring in the data concerning the phenomenon of concern—the basic form of human *action*. The key or basic social process is typically articulated in gerund form connoting ongoing action at an abstract level. Studies have been done, for example, on *living with* chronic illness (Charmaz, 2010), *classifying* and its consequences (Lampland & Star, 2009), *producing* accountability in hospitals (Wiener, 2000), *explaining* suspicious deaths at the morgue (Timmermans, 2006), *creating* a new social actor—the unborn patient—via fetal surgery (Casper, 1998), and *disciplining* the scientific study of reproduction (Clarke, 1998).

Around this basic process, the analyst then constellates the particular and distinctive conditions, strategies, actions, and practices engaged in by the human and nonhuman actors involved. For example, the subprocesses of disciplining the scientific study of reproduction include *formalizing* a scientific discipline, *establishing* stable access to research materials, *gleaning* fiscal support for research, *producing* contraceptives and other technoscientific products, and *handling* the social controversies the science provokes, for example, regarding the use of contraceptives (Clarke, 1998). Many excellent projects have been done using basic GT, and this action-centered approach will continue to be fundamentally important analytically (Clarke & Charmaz, 2014).

Grounded Theory as Always Already Implicitly Feminist

There are several ways in which I and others such as Susan Leigh Star[5] have long understood GT to have been always already implicitly feminist: (1) its roots in American symbolic interactionist sociology and pragmatist philosophy emphasizing actual experiences and practices—the lived doingness of social life; (2) its use of George Herbert Mead's concept of perspective that emphasizes partiality, situatedness, and multiplicity; (3) its assumption of a materialist social constructionism; (4) its foregrounding deconstructive analysis and multiple simultaneous readings; and (5) its attention to range of variation as featuring of difference(s) (Clarke, 2005; Star, 2007).

First and foremost here are what I and other feminists see as the roots of GT in symbolic interactionist sociology and pragmatist philosophy.[6] This was not always the case. Historically, Glaser and Strauss (1967), Glaser (1978), and Schatzman and Strauss (1973) argued that GT as a methodological approach could be effectively used by people from a variety of theoretical as well as disciplinary perspectives. That is, they initially took a "mix and match" approach. Their challenge—which they ably met—was to articulate a new qualitative methodology in the belly of the haute positivist quantitative sociological beast of the 1960s (Bryant & Charmaz, 2007; Olesen, 2007). They sought to do so through a systematic approach to analyzing qualitative research data.[7] Their emphases in the early works cited were on taking a *naturalistic* approach to research, having initially *modest* (read, substantively focused) theoretical goals, and being *systematic* in what we might today call the interrogation of qualitative research data in order to work against what they and others then saw as the *distorting subjectivities* of the researcher in the concrete processes of interpretive analysis (discussed further below).[8]

In considerable contrast, it can be argued that GT is rooted in American pragmatist philosophy and the approach to sociology generated through it—symbolic interactionism (e.g., Blumer, 1969; Strübing, 2007). That is, grounded theory/symbolic interactionism can be seen as constituting a theory/methods package that is implicitly feminist. Star framed such theory/methods packages as including a set of epistemological and ontological assumptions along with concrete practices through which a set of practitioners go about their work, including relating to and with one another and the various nonhuman entities involved in the situation. This concept of a theory/methods package focuses on the ultimately nonfungible aspects of ontology and epistemology—viewing these as co-constitutive (Star, 2007; Clarke & Star, 2008). Vis-à-vis symbolic interactionism, this features researching the meanings held by the actors themselves—an implicitly feminist stance (Clarke, 2005).

Specifically, I and others have argued that GT is a methodology inherently predicated on various forms of symbolic interactionist theoretical and philosophical ontology (e.g., Charmaz, 2006; Locke, 2001; Olesen, 2007). "Method, then, is not the servant of theory: method actually grounds theory" (Jenks, 1995, p. 12). Historically, as GT grew in stature and began to be used more and more widely, and as the implications of Berger and Luckmann's (1966) *The Social Construction of Reality* began to be taken up more explicitly, more and more practitioners of GT began tugging GT in constructionist and postmodernist directions (e.g., Charmaz, 2000; Locke, 2001; Strauss, 1987). The second generation of GT scholars (Bowers, Charmaz, Clarke, Corbin, Morse, and Stern) agree that Strauss but not Glaser moved in such directions (Morse et al., 2009). Significantly, such directions are requisite if GT is to continue to be a useful method for feminist research.[9]

The second way in which GT has been always already implicitly feminist is its rootedness in George Herbert Mead's concept of perspective. Much of symbolic interactionism has always been perspectival, fully compatible with producing through research what are today understood as situated knowledges (Haraway, 1991, 1997; McCarthy, 1996). Perspective involves the commitment to representing those we study on their own terms, through their own perspectives. That is, the groundedness of good grounded theorizing lies deeply in the seriousness of the analyst's commitment to representing *all* understandings, all knowledges and actions of those studied—as well as the analyst's own—as perspectival. Feminists have often come to grasp such partialities through considerable pain (Star, 2007).

Thus, the interactionist concept of perspective can be deployed to complicate—to make analyses more radical, democratic, and transgressive. Representing the full multiplicity of perspectives in a given situation (from the heterogeneous "powers that be" to the prisoners of various kinds of panopticons, "minority" views, "marginal" positions, "subjugated knowledges," and/or the "other(s)"/alterity) disrupts the *representational* hegemony that usually privileges some and erases others (Clarke, 2005, pp. 58-60; Denzin, Lincoln, & Smith, 2008). Representing *is* intervening (Hacking, 1983). This, of course, has been at the heart of many feminist projects (e.g., Lather & Smithies, 1997). (It also links to the concept of implicated actors, discussed below.)

Third, I would argue that GT is always already feminist (at least vis-à-vis my grasp of feminisms) because an interactionist constructionism is a *materialist* social constructionism (Law, 1999). That is, many people (mis) interpret social constructionism as concerned only with the ephemeral or ideological or symbolic. But the material world is itself constructed— materially produced, interpreted, and given meanings—by us and by those whom we study. It is *what* we study. The material world, including the nonhuman and our own embodiment, is present and to be accounted for in our interpretations and analyses. This materialism, this importance of things, this sociality of things was also argued by Mead (1934/1962, p. 373), as Blumer (1969, pp. 10–11) and McCarthy (1984) have most elegantly demonstrated.

The fourth way in which GT can be viewed as always already feminist lies in its foregrounding of a deconstructive mode of analysis via open coding. Open coding connotes just that—data are open to multiple simultaneous readings or codes. Many different phenomena and many different properties can be named, tracked, and traced through reams of all different kinds of data. There is no one right reading. All readings are temporary, partial, provisional, and perspectival—themselves situated historically and geographically (e.g., Haraway, 1991; McCarthy, 1996).

When analyzing, we can ourselves attempt to "read" the data from different perspectives and for different purposes. Strauss's concrete practice to produce multiple readings was working in data analysis groups that take up members' project data. Multiple readings are routinely and explicitly sought and produced through such group efforts. Such group work is also the usual pedagogical tradition for teaching and learning GT—to bring multiple perspectives together so that you can more easily produce multiple readings, multiple possible codes. In this way of working, the analyst is constantly banging into and bouncing off the interpretations of others. Of course, this further enhances and legitimates the capacity of the analyst to come up with multiple possible readings on his or her own and to abandon ideas about "right" and "wrong" readings. I would characterize such analytic working groups as "consciousness raising" because they use the same basic social process of laying out multiple experiences and interpretations.[10]

The fifth way in which GT is always already tacitly feminist concerns difference as range of variation. Variation has always been attended to in GT, but the attention has, I argue, been too scant. Strauss (1993) returned to this point in his capstone book and emphasized it as follows:

[Social science activity] is directed at understanding the entire range of human actions, of which there are so many that the dictionary can scarcely refer to them all. That is, an interactionist theory of action should address action generally and be applicable to specific types of action, so that in effect the theory can also help us understand the incredibly variegated panorama of human living. (p. 49)

Through SA (discussed below) I seek to further shift the emphasis in GT from attending primarily to commonalities to attending to this "incredibly variegated panorama of human living," to mapping and analyzing differences of all kinds. Making differences more visible and making silences speak (also often about difference) are two of the explicit goals of SA.

Yet, for all its implicit feminisms, there were and continue to be problems for feminists with traditional forms of GT. These include a lack of reflexivity, tendencies toward oversimplification, the interpretation of data variation as "negative cases" rather than differences worthy of understanding, and, for some, a search for fundamental(ist) "purity" and "Truth" through GT (Clarke, 2005, pp. 11-18). Charmaz's (2006) constructionist GT actively works against these problems.

Making Grounded Theory More Explicitly Feminist

Many scholars have forged GT into explicitly feminist tools for qualitative research over the past 40 or so years (Clarke, 2007; Olesen, 2007). The range of feminist usages of GT is staggeringly broad, and it is truly impossible to review this vast literature here. Instead, I highlight several clusters of contributors who have made GT explicitly feminist in important and enduringly valuable ways: nurse researchers; sociologists; and science, technology, and medicine scholars. Issues of diversity crosscut disciplinarity, and I also discuss both Glaser's and Strauss's positions vis-à-vis gender and race in GT research.

Feminist GT Nursing Research

It comes as no surprise that nurse researchers comprised the first group of scholars to adopt GT. Strauss and Glaser were faculty in the School of Nursing at University of California, San Francisco (UCSF) in the 1960s when they conceived the GT method and published their book, and Strauss remained on the faculty until his death in 1996. Virginia Olesen was also on the faculty and introduced feminist theory and feminist social science perspectives on women's health to sociology and nursing curricula beginning in 1973.[11]

The earliest wave of feminist nursing GT scholarship was undertaken by Holly Wilson, Sally Hutchinson, Phyllis Noerager Stern, Ellen O'Shaughnessy, June Lowenberg, Barbara Bowers, Susan Kools, Ellen Schumacher, and others.[12] It was generally more tacitly rather than explicitly feminist. That is, the research topics often featured concerns particular to girls and women and to caregiving, and they centered on giving voice to ill people and their families, noting gender. Explicitly gendered analyses such as the problematization, production, or performance of gendered identities were rare. Nor did this early work pursue the intersectionalities of gender identities with race and class issues, as feminist research often does (discussed further below).

More recently, many nurse scholars have extended their efforts in more explicitly feminist directions. Among these is Margaret Keamey, whose research on pregnant African American women using crack cocaine was groundbreaking (e.g., Keamey, 2001). An array of studies led to her GT-based *Understanding Women's Recovery From Illness and Trauma* (Kearney, 1999). Suellen Miller (1996) did feminist research on how new mothers developed career reentry strategies. Her and Kearney's (Kearney, Murphy, Irwin, & Rosenbaum, 1995) GT integrative analytic diagrams are among the best in print, superb for teaching theoretical integration. Benoliel (2001) edited a special issue of *Health Care for Women International* on "Expanding Knowledge About Women Through Grounded Theory." Marcellus (2005) offers a review of GT in maternal-infant research and practice (see also Olshansky, 2003). Other feminist work has focused on nursing interventions for domestic violence (Ford-Gilboe, Wuest, & Merritt-Gray, 2005) and foster care (Kools & Kennedy, 2003). Much, if not most, of this work has clear advocacy, intervention, and policy aims, and all would be of interest to feminists across the disciplines focusing on such topics.

Nurse researchers have also written extensively on GT as method. Recent work addresses the shift from traditional to postmodern GT (Kools, 2008; Mills et al., 2007). It also focuses on dimensional analysis as a form of GT (Bowers & Schatzman, 2009; Kools, 2008); taking GT beyond psychological process (Keamey, 2009); GT sampling and reflexivity (Morse, 2007; Neill, 2006); how "people change and methods change" (Corbin, 2009; Corbin & Strauss, 2008); the development of formal theory (Kearney, 2001, 2007); and debates between the Straussian and Glaserian approaches (see note 9). Schumacher (2008) offers an account of her two decades of GT research on family caregiving. She is especially insightful about the conundrums confronted in a sustained research program, such as whether to handle one's own earlier research conclusions and theorizing with the dubiousness generally accorded to "received theory" in GT work. Kearney (2008) compared the GT research trajectories of a nurse and a sociologist both studying depression. The nurse began with more applied concerns and, over the years, moved into theorizing, while the sociologist's trajectory was just the reverse.

Looking to the future of GT in nursing research, Kushner and Morrow (2003) elucidated relations with interactionist, feminist, and critical theories. They found several useful commonalities, including a special focus on vulnerable groups, the explication of researchers' standpoints, respect for participant expertise within the research process, and emancipatory intent. Plummer and Young (2010) argue that GT is especially compatible with feminist inquiry for research on women.

Feminism, Glaser, Strauss, and American Sociology

In terms of the advent of feminism in GT nursing research, Susan Kools (2008) notes that many of the early generation of GT nurse scholars were trained before the postmodern turn by the white men at UC, San Francisco. The same was true for early GT sociologists. Both Glaser and Strauss, as well as Schatzman, had serious problems with the explicit feminist approaches to knowledge production that began circulating in the 1970s. For example, Glaser (2002b), at the request of nurse scholars, wrote on "Grounded Theory and Gender Relevance," reasserting his earlier arguments that gender, like race and other "face sheet data," needs to "earn [its] way into" a GT analysis rather than "forcing" it (p. 789; see also Bryant, 2003; Glaser, 2002a). He ignores how, over the past 40 years, gender and race/ethnicity have become central to the American sociological enterprise. They have been theorized as fundamental social aspects of being and action that are learned, performative, variegated, enculturated, and situated. They are of intrinsic and nonfungible sociological importance, though precisely *how* they may "matter" in any situation remains an empirical question. Moreover, to allow such issues to "earn their way" into GT analysis would require data to be collected that are capable of addressing them, rather than just waiting for them to magically appear. Pursuing such data—and then analyzing it—would both make researchers more accountable and the feminisms and anti-racisms engaged more explicit (see Clarke, 2005, pp. 73-78).

At the request of French feminists editing a volume about how major social theorists engaged or did not engage gender, I wrote an article about

Strauss's unease both with the concept of gender and with addressing gen-
der- or sex-based and race/ethnicity-based inequities in research (Clarke,
2008, 2010a). Through the lifelong commitment of his wife Fran Strauss to
the American Civil Liberties Union and his ongoing engagement with Blumer's (1958) and other interactionists' work on race (e.g., Duster, 1990/2003;
Omi & Winant, 1994), Strauss saw both sets of issues as routinely "on his
table." He engaged them in limited fashion. That is, while sex/gender and
race/ethnicity issues were rarely explicitly theorized in his work, they were
tacitly constitutive elements of some of the situations he studied, methods
and analytic strategies he developed, and theories he generated. For example,
certain ways of doing GT scholarly work, such as the small working groups
and teams, were and remain deeply congruent with feminist precepts. Many
threads of Strauss's work have also been taken up and elaborated in explicitly
feminist and anti-racist ways by his students in ways that echo the reparative
work of feminist Foucauldians (Clarke, 2008; Star, 2007).

My main assertion here is that neither Glaser's nor Strauss's versions of
formal social theory could legitimately include sex/gender or race/ethnicity
perspectives (Clarke, 2008, 2010a). In mid-twentieth-century mainstream
American sociology, such "identity" issues were understood as sources of
bias. They had to be *made* sociological (e.g., DuBois, 1993; Blumer, 1958).[13]
Today, they are viewed as fundamental aspects of social organization and
stratification, not only integral to but *requisite* for adequate theorizing—
nationally *and* transnationally. For nearly 30 years, feminist standpoint theories have further argued that those positioned in the margins actually have
clearer perspectives on certain phenomena (Star, 2007; Hesse-Biber 2007).
Moreover, in the United States today, it is theoretically necessary to *simultaneously* consider issues of race/ethnicity along with sex/gender as these
are historically deeply entwined, along with other identity issues, in ways
that are increasingly understood as intersectional (e.g., Collins, 2004; Dill
& Zambrana, 2009; Schulz & Mullings, 2006; Weber, 2010). Schwalbe and
colleagues (2000) superbly frame generic processes in the reproduction of
inequality. An impressive chapter in the new *Handbook of Grounded Theory*
by Green and colleagues (2007) lays out strategies for enhancing diversity in
GT research, and Charmaz (2005, 2011) strategizes using GT methods for
social justice research. Social theory no longer precludes addressing differences; rather, it demands it.

Feminist Sociological and Other GT Research

Turning to recent feminist GT sociological research, we find a number of projects explicitly pursuing diversity goals. Wingfield (2007) used GT in a fascinating paper on intersectionality titled "The Modern Mammy and the Angry Black Man: African American Professionals' Experiences with Gendered Racism in the Workplace." The professionals she interviewed often had to combat such gendered images from historical racist discourse—or be dealt with stereotypically themselves (see also Settles, Pratt-Hyatt, & Buchanan, 2008). Anthropologist Maternowska and colleagues (2010) analyzed reproductive decision making among recent Mexican migrants in California. They found that migrants' marginalization and isolation along with economic challenges and new access to contraceptives were together changing familial relationships and reproductive decision making.

Taking GT into feminist queer studies, sociologist Laura Mamo (2007) used GT at the intersection of lived experience and technology studies to explore how both cultural discourses and assisted reproduction are used by lesbian-identified women seeking pregnancy through technoscientific means. Mamo argues that lesbians both follow given technological scripts and create their own interpretations of the technologies, thus subverting the expectations of developers, marketers, and service providers. Berkowitz and Marsiglio (2007) studied how gay men who had fathered children outside of heterosexual intercourse negotiated procreative, father, and family identities. Finding change across these gay men's life spans, they note that the men's procreative consciousness was strongly shaped by institutions (such as adoption and fertility agencies) and by ruling relations (such as assumptions about gay men). Negotiation was a major social process in constructing "out" gay and lesbian parent families "beyond the closet"—navigating residual heterosexual dominance in institutions such as schools and in personal interactions—despite greater acceptance at least in some places (Ryan & Berkowitz, 2009). For lesbians frequenting bars, another GT study found trade-offs associated with bar patronage regarding the psychosocial importance of the bar for individual reasons and for a sense of community and the relationship between minority stress and alcohol use (Gruskin, Byrne, & Kools, 2006).

Emotion work (Hochschild, 1969) and intimate care work (Boris & Parrenas, 2010) have long been of interest to feminists. Wolkomir and Powers (2007) used GT in their thoughtful study of the challenges of emotional labor in an abortion clinic. They found that the workers needed to balance helping women and protecting themselves, and they did so by classifying patients in terms of their different needs and personal styles. Clinic workers then generated effective strategies to handle these differences, including boundary setting to buffer what they viewed as inappropriate demands upon them as providers of care. Schrock and Padavic (2007) also use GT to study a challenging workplace—a batterer intervention program. They found that hegemonic masculinity was both produced (in terms of the men's setting boundaries to maintain their "patriarchal dividend") and negotiated (in terms of their taking some responsibility and choosing nonviolence). The distinctive partialities of "success" were fascinating.

Invisible work and the also invisible burdens of doing it have also long been of interest to feminists and others (e.g., Star, 1991, 2007). Landstedt, Asplund, and Gådin (2009) explored teens' perceptions of what is significant for mental health in Sweden, applying a gender analysis. Boys' more positive mental health appeared to be associated with their low degree of responsibility taking and beneficial positions relative to girls. Girls were at greater risk for mental health problems, due in large part to the weight of the invisible work of being more responsible in interactions and performatively. I am unhappily reminded of the classic feminist article "Why I Want a Wife" (Syfers, 1971). *Plus ça change...*

Janet Shim's (2005, 2014) ambitious research combines the lived experiences tradition with feminist science, technology, and medicine studies approaches in GT research. She focuses on two different sets of people concerned with cardiovascular diseases (CVDs) in the United States today: epidemiologists and related researchers who study racial, ethnic, sex/gender, social class, and other distributions of CVDs in populations and people of color diagnosed as having CVDs. Shim's explicitly comparative approach centers on the meanings of race, class, and sex vis-à-vis CVDs—constructed by the epidemiologists on the one hand, and by the people of color diagnosed and living with CVDs on the other (see also Schwalbe et al., 2000). Shim's work demonstrates the fruitfulness of doing feminist GT with a comparative design and then teasing out comparisons both within and between emerging categories (Kathy Charmaz, personal communication, October 2005). Clarke, Mamo, Fosket, Fishman, and Shim's (2010) edited volume *Biomedicalization: Technoscience, Health, and Illness in the U. S.* offers an array of technoscience studies, many of which utilize grounded theory approaches on gender-related topics.

Last, feminist economists have challenged traditional economic theory by developing a gendered reconceptualization of social indicators based on the use of GT with focus-group data (Austen, Jefferson, & Thein, 2003). Such new indicators can be used to reorganize how economic analyses are done in ways that, quite radically even today, include gender.

I must end this section with an apology. While I discuss some works pursued in "far away places," my "lite" review here emphasizes work done by nurses and sociologists who trained at UCSF. I certainly do not mean to imply that these works are in any way "better" than others. Rather, I merely know them better myself. I will discuss the limitations of GT and SA below, before concluding.

What Is Situational Analysis?

In the extension of GT I developed called situational analysis (Clarke, 2003, 2005), *the situation of inquiry itself broadly conceived is the key unit of analysis.*[13] This is radically different from traditional GT, which focuses on the main social processes—human action—in the area of inquiry. In SA, the situation of inquiry is empirically constructed through the making of three kinds of maps and by following through with analytic work and memos of various kinds.

The first maps are *situational maps* that lay out the major human, nonhuman, discursive, historical, symbolic, cultural, political, and other elements in the research situation of concern (Figure 3.1). The goals of this map are first to enhance research design by laying out everything about which at least some data should be gathered. Downstream in the research, situational maps are used to provoke analysis of relations among the different elements. Working *against* the usual simplifications (Star, 1983) in particularly postmodern and feminist ways, these maps capture and provoke discussion of the many and heterogeneous elements and the messy complexities of the situation (see Clarke, 2005, pp. 83-123).

Second, the *social worlds/arenas maps* lay out all of the *collective* actors and the arenas of commitment within which they are engaged in ongoing discourse and negotiations. Such maps offer meso-level interpretations of the situation, taking up its social organizational, institutional, and discursive dimensions. They are distinctively postmodern in their assumptions: we cannot assume directionalities of influence; boundaries are open and porous; negotiations are fluid; discourses are multiple and potentially contradictory. *Negotiations* of many kinds from coercion to bargaining are the "basic social processes" that construct and constantly destabilize the social worlds/arenas

Figure 3.1: Abstract Situational Map: Messy/Working Version (From Clarke [2005] *Situational Analysis: Grounded Theory after the Postmodern Turn.* Copyright 2005 by Sage Publications, Inc. Reprinted with permission of the publisher.)

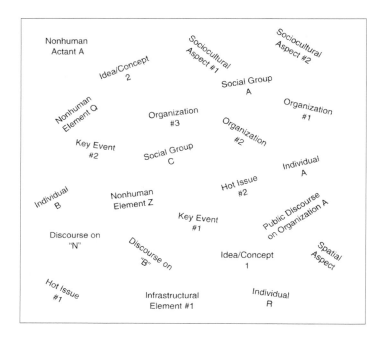

maps (Strauss, 1993). Things could always be otherwise—not only individually but also collectively, organizationally, institutionally, and discursively, and these maps portray such postmodern possibilities (see Clarke, 2005, pp. 109-124).

Third, *positional maps* lay out the major positions taken, and *not* taken, in the data vis-à-vis particular axes of variation and difference, focus, and controversy found in the situation of concern. Perhaps most significantly, positional maps are *not* articulated with persons or groups but rather seek to represent the full range of *discursive* positions on key issues. They allow multiple positions and even contradictions within both individuals and collectivities to be articulated. Complexities are themselves heterogeneous, and we need improved means of representing them (see Clarke, 2005, pp. 125-136). I see this as explicitly feminist as well.

Significantly, SA takes the nonhuman in the situation of inquiry very seriously. The nonhuman can include things, animals, technologies, discourses, and so forth. In doing initial situational maps, the analyst is asked to specify the nonhuman elements in the situation, thus making pertinent materialities and discourses visible from the outset. The flip sides of the second kind of map, the social worlds/arenas maps, are discourse/arenas maps. Social worlds are "universes of discourse" routinely producing discourses about elements of concern in the situation. Such discourses can be mapped and analyzed. Last, positional maps open up the discourses per se by analyzing positions taken on key axes. Discourses can thereby be disarticulated from their sites of production, decentering them and making analytic complexities visible.

Situational Analysis as Always Already Implicitly Feminist

SA is always already feminist both in the ways discussed previously as characteristic of GT (since SA is an extension of GT after the postmodern turn) and also in (at least) the following ways:

1. Acknowledging researchers' embodiment and situatedness
2. Grounding analysis in the lived material and symbolic situation itself
3. Conceptually foregrounding complexities and differences in the data
4. Mapping *all* the actors and discourses in the situation regardless of their power in that situation

First, while traditional GT historically and occasionally today may have a foot in the positivist domain that assumes the possibility of "scientific objectivity" and "truth," constructivist GT and SA do not. That is, neither constructivist GT nor SA assumes that there is a singular transcendent "Truth" in the Enlightenment scientific sense of being True at all times and places. Rather, both assume that different epistemologies—different modes of knowledge production—will produce different "truths" that are congruent with the assumptions and practices involved in producing them and that are historically and geopolitically located (Charmaz, 2006; Clarke, 2005). There are no global verities. Instead, constructivist GT and SA not only assume but explicitly acknowledge the embodiment and situatedness of knowledge producers—both us (the researchers) and them (who and what we are studying)—as we collaborate in the production of new knowledge, which is assumed to be partial (Haraway, 1991, 1997; Lather, 2007, 2008; McCarthy, 1996). Second, SA is always already feminist in its overall analytic focus on the situation itself as the unit of analysis that transforms "objects of study" and their

Figure 3.2 Clarke's Situational Matrix (From Clarke [2005] *Situational Analysis: Grounded Theory after the Postmodern Turn.* Copyright 2005 by Sage Publications, Inc. Reprinted with permission of the publisher.)

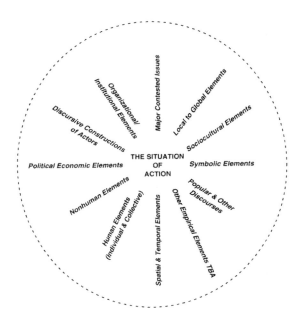

"contexts" into a single ultimately nonfungible unit by refusing the object-context binary. The important so-called contextual elements are not constellated somehow *around* the objects of study but, instead, are actually *inside the situation itself.* They are *constitutive* of it (Figure 3.2).

The concept situation is feminist in part in terms of its *gestalt*—how a situation is always greater than the sum of its parts because it includes their relationality in a particular temporal and spatial moment. A gestalt understanding of situations as generating "a life of their own" offers a very poststructuralist reading, granting a kind of agency to the situation per se similar to the agency discourses have or are in Foucauldian terms. Such agency is most important in understanding SA. Relationalities and situatedness have long been central to feminisms.

A third way that SA is always already feminist concerns the assumptions and representational strategies of focusing on normativity or homogeneity versus focusing on differences, complexities, or heterogeneities. The capacity of GT techniques to fracture data and permit multiple analyses is a key contribution. SA features and enhances this capacity. Foundationally, this involves analyzing *against* the assumptions of the normal curve, the conceptual default drive of Western science, black-boxed inside the hardware of knowledge production and inside the software of social science training. Please visualize a normal curve. The normal curve is a high modern concept embodying Enlightenment thinking and thereby producing knowledge that fits its orderly classificatory preconceptions (e.g., Lampland & Star, 2009). Although the fringes or margins of the normal curve are literally contiguous with the center, we are led to assume they are *not* constitutive of the "normal." In sharp contrast, it is the boundaries/margins that *produce* the center, the peripheries/colonies that *constitute* the core/metropole (Said, 1978). Moreover, in narrowly focusing on what is construed as "the normal," the broader situation in which the phenomenon has been historically and otherwise located recedes to the point of invisibility.

SA replaces such metaphors of normal curves and normativity with relational metaphors of ecology and cartography. Figure 3.3 displays (in two dimensions but please imagine three) a wide variety of differently situated positions: P1, P2 . . . /P19, and so on. This messy positional map conceptually replaces modernist uni-dimensional normal curves with a postmodern multidimensional representation of the variety of positionalities and human and nonhuman activities and discourses within a lived situation. We need to move seriously *toward* complexity and heterogeneity rather than away

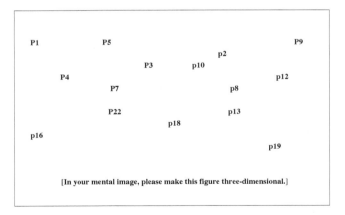

Figure 3.3 Mapping Positionality (From Clarke [2005] *Situational Analysis: Grounded Theory after the Postmodern Turn.* Copyright 2005 by Sage Publications, Inc. Reprinted with permission of the publisher.)

from them, instead of seeking simplification. Otherwise, we merely continue performing recursive classifications that ignore the empirical world (Lampland & Star, 2009). For example, we cannot fathom biodiversity without ambitious sciences of plants and animals and the situated ecologies of their relations. The same holds for humans living on this complex planet.

Such relational modalities of representation do not concern themselves with frequency. Instead, they attend intently to positions and their distribution across situational or topographical maps that do the work of helping us to "see" the full range of positions. In doing SA, one draws maps to help make known, understand, and represent the heterogeneity of positions taken in the situation under study and/or within given (historical and/or visual and/or narrative) discourses in that situation.

The main goal of SA vis-à-vis differences is not only to enhance their *empirical* study but also to describe them more richly. That is, we cannot assume what any kinds of differences mean to those in a given situation, and we need more and better methods to explore the existence, meanings, and consequences of differences within concrete social practices. This may include studying the production and consumption of discourses as practices (e.g., Schwalbe et al., 2000). We need to grasp variation *within* data categories, the range of variation within data, complexities, contradictions, multiplicities, and ambivalences that manifest individually, collectively, and discursively. The situational maps are each and all designed to do precisely this de-essentializing feminist work.

The fourth and last way I would argue that SA is always already feminist is that it requires mapping of *all* the actors and discourses in the situation regardless of their power in that situation. This can be both a feminist and a democratizing move. Many contemporary modes of analysis, including those of Foucault (e.g., 1975) and Latourian actor-network theory (e.g., Law & Hassard, 1999), center on the analysis of (those in/discourses in) power. In sharp contrast, SA goes beyond what could be called "the master discourse" (Hughes, 1971). By *not* analytically recapitulating the power relations of domination, SA analyses that represent the full array of actors and discourses turn up the volume on lesser but still present discourses, lesser but still present participants, the quiet, the silent, and the silenced.

Such analyses can amplify not only differences but also resistances, recalcitrance, and sites of rejection. The concept of *implicated actors* is important here. These are actors explicitly constructed and/or addressed by a social world and for whom the actions of that world may be highly consequential—

but who are either not present or not allowed to be fully agentic in the actual doings of that world. The actions taken "on behalf of" implicated actors are often supposedly "for their own good." Individuals and social groups with less power tend to be implicated rather than fully agentic actors (Clarke, 2005, pp. 46-48; Clarke & Montini, 1993). They often tend to be female or otherwise "othered," possibly including the nonhuman. SA focuses on making the less powerful, silent, and silenced more visible and more analytically central.

In sum, the goal of SA is not prediction but vivid descriptions and strong analytic insights. Theorizing should make thick description and thick interpretation possible. SA studies also seek to specify what has gone and goes unstudied—that which may not be seen or perceived or which may be refused—and is worthy of note regardless (Star, 2007). Thus, making the heretofore invisible visible is a goal congruent with ongoing feminist analytics, and one that takes feminism beyond gender relations when gender relations are not enough (Collins, 2009; Smith, 2007; Weber, 2010).

Making Situational Analysis More Explicitly Feminist

SA has been increasingly taken up since it first appeared in 2005 (Clarke, 2005). Studies using situational mapping along with grounded theory have often done so to better grasp what has usually been understood as the broader social context. For example, Mills, Francis, and Bonner's (2008) "Getting to Know a Stranger: Rural Nurses' Experiences of Mentoring: A Grounded Theory" addressed the problems of recruiting and retraining nurses. In rural areas, they are often the sole health care providers for large geographic regions. The project explored how experienced nurses cultivated novices through recognizing their potential and teaming up in critical situations. In contrast, another study focused on enhancing access to mental health services for potential patients who are culturally diverse. Schnitzer, Loots, Escudero, and Schechter (2009) examined the quite limited help-seeking of ultraorthodox Jewish parents in a Belgian city, which was both highly gendered and framed predominantly in spiritual and religious ways. Mothers largely dealt with daughters' educational and health needs and problems (both mental and physical) and fathers with sons'. They suggest culturally sensitive ways to enhance the accessibility of services which also need, at times, to be gender specific for this population.

The concepts of social worlds and arenas were developed by Strauss and elaborated by me prior to making them part of SA via mapping them

(Clarke, 1991, 1998; Clarke & Montini, 1993; Strauss, 1978, 1993). In brief, social worlds are groups with shared commitments to certain activities, sharing resources of many kinds to achieve their goals and building shared ideologies about how to go about their business. They are interactive units, worlds of discourse, bounded not by geography or formal membership but by the limits of effective communication. Social worlds are fundamental "building blocks" of collective action and the main units of analysis in such studies. In arenas, all the social worlds come together that focus on a given issue and are prepared to act in some way. Clarke and Montini (1993) is an especially accessible exemplar. The article analytically places the technology RU486 in the center and then moves through the specific perspectives taken on it by each of the major social worlds involved in the broader abortion and reproduction arena. By attending to diversities *within* worlds, the paper also demonstrates that social worlds are not monolithic.

Moore's (2007) book, *Sperm Tales: Social, Cultural, and Scientific Representations of Human Semen,* uses GT and SA to analyze representations of sperm from different social worlds/arenas—reproductive sciences, the Internet, children's "facts of life" books, forensic transcripts, sex workers' narratives, and personal expertise. Semen representations, she finds, are distinctively related to the changing social positions of men, masculinities, and constructions of male differences in the different arenas and beyond. Moore (2007) also offers a sophisticated methods appendix with an account of more than a decade of research on these different arenas and of her strategies of triangulation to produce a formal grounded theory (pp. 155-164).

Kohlen (2009) offers an extended SA in *Conflicts of Care: Hospital Ethics Committees in the USA and Germany.* Although such committees were initiated in the United States in the 1980s, only in recent years have German hospitals followed suit. Kohlen compares three different hospitals, finding differences in the committees due to institutional structures, local cultures, and histories. As in the United States, nurses (mostly women) are particularly committed to such work, seeking "real rather than symbolic" engagement toward improving patient care. The nurses framed moral understandings of and standards for patient care that too often were an "elusive quest" in ways similar to accountability in U.S. hospitals (Wiener, 2000). Kohlen (2009) also used SA to identify silences and exclusions in the discourse, finding that nurses did *not* discuss *nursing* problems of care in the ethics committees, not wanting to expose "not only the dying patient in utmost vulnerability, but also the work of nursing including its messy necessities" (pp. 228-229).

Science, technology, and medicine studies continue to draw feminist GT and SA researchers. Clarke and Star (2008) offer an ambitious overview of the social worlds/arenas approach as a theory-methods package, and they review recent work in the field. Although a number of studies have used positional mapping, other than Kohlen's (2009) book, discussed above, to date they have not been feminist projects.

Limitations of Grounded Theory and Situational Analysis

All methodologies feature advantages and pose limitations. Both GT and SA are distinctively *analytic* approaches to taking data apart. GT does this by coding, integrating codes and categories, and generating a substantive theory of action that characterizes the common social processes in the situation. Situational maps do it by abstracting all the elements in the situation and mapping them. Social worlds/arenas maps parse the meso-level organizations and institutions in the situation. Positional maps analyze the contested discourses in the situation, seeking especially to analyze silences.

But the idea of deconstruction is even stronger here. GT and other *analytic* approaches have been criticized for "fracturing" data, for "violating" the integrity of participants' narratives, and for "pulling apart" stories, for example by Riessman (2008, p. 79). I see this not as a weakness or problem but instead as the key to GT's *analytic*, rather than *re-representational*, strength. Analysis and re-representation are two deeply different qualitative research approaches. Re-representation usually centers on the lived experiences of individuals (occasionally on those of collectivities). Analysis centers instead on elucidating *processes* of social phenomena—action. Feminist research needs both—and more (e.g., Riessman, 2008, p. 209n24).

GT can certainly be used to understand and explain individuals' lived experiences per se (e.g., Charmaz, 2010). And, through social worlds analysis, GT and SA help theorize social action at the collective level (e.g., Casper, 1998; Clarke, 1998). But while both attend to the social setting, neither centers on generating rich ethnography, institutional or other. Finally, neither method explicitly targets understanding long-term politico-economic and related change. However, a group of now former students and I theorized the rise of medicine, medicalization, and biomedicalization by generating a historical database (Clarke et al., 2003; Clarke et al., 2010). And I offered methodological strategies for theorizing biomedicalization in its transnational travels, utilizing local and regional historical and visual materials (Clarke, 2010c).

Conclusion

With Lather, I am seeking "a fertile ontological space and ethical practice in asking how research-based knowledge remains possible after so much questioning of the very ground of science . . . gesturing toward the science possible after the critique of science" (Lather, 2007, pp. viii, ix). In feminist hands, both GT and SA can help generate such fertile spaces and ethical practices. Further, "The work of grounded theorists will be enhanced with a return to the recognition, so deeply rooted in the symbolic interactionist bones of GT, that researcher and participant are mutually imbedded in the social context of the research and that data are co-created" (Olesen, 2007, p. 427). And reading and teaching widely in our feminist community of discourse will nurture, sustain, and provoke us both intellectually and politically. This volume is a major resource for such practices.

In terms of future feminist research using GT, my hopes are for more explicitly feminist projects, especially research that questions the very grounds of traditional disciplinary categories and conventions and opens up possible new avenues for enhancing social justice. Here, I am thinking of Austen and colleagues' (2003) exciting deconstruction of "social indicators" in the discipline of economics, which for decades remained impenetrable by feminist perspectives. Another exemplar, especially of epistemic diversity, is Shim's (2005, 2014) nuanced study of the meanings of "race," "class," and "gender" to epidemiologists and people of color with CVDs. While much epidemiology rotely pursues "the usual suspects," the people of color she studied produced their own insightful understandings of how racism, sexism, and class-based discrimination were making their heart conditions worse. Shim hopes that policies in health care, epidemiology, and beyond will be built on such subjugated knowledges toward alleviating health inequalities.

What other kinds of feminist-informed knowledges exist and how might they be channeled by good research into improving social policies and reducing inequalities? Resources toward such goals include Charmaz's (2005, 2011) work on using GT toward social justice ends, Olesen's (2005, 2007) papers on feminist research, and Denzin and colleagues' (2008) book on decolonizing methods. My paper on doing transnational research on biomedicalization, including feminist and gender issues, encourages the use of historical, visual, and other discursive materials (Clarke, 2010c).

I particularly recommend using SA in feminist studies where import is placed on elucidating differences, making silences speak, and revealing contradictions within positions and within social groups. Samik-lbrahim (2000) has argued that GT methodology is especially useful in less-developed countries and settings. The same holds true for SA; hence there is potential utility for both in feminist postcolonial studies. SA would be especially valuable where (nonhuman) infrastructural elements of situations are quite different (availability of roads, water, health care, traditional and changing gender arrangements, and divisions of labor). Researchers need to take such differences into *explicit* account to generate policy recommendations and programmatic interventions (Clarke, 2010c). An example here is local needs assessment research in which the desire is to grasp *both* the specifics of the local situation materially *and* the perspectives of local people on their own needs—remembering that these may well be multivocal, gendered, and contradictory. Thus, SA should be helpful in feminist postcolonial studies and transnational studies wherein the particularities of situatedness are of special import.

I also hope for feminist research using GT and SA in the study of discourses—historical, visual, and narrative—and in multi-site research that combines studies of discursive data with interviews and ethnographic work. I have framed how this can be pursued via integrative mapping (all data sources analyzed together) and comparative mapping (data sources analyzed separately) (Clarke, 2005, pp. 176-177). I would argue also that the time has come for more comparative work, explicitly contrasting the positions articulated in public discourses with those produced by the various sets of actors active in and implicated by those discourses (Lather & Smithies, 1997; Shim, 2005, 2014).

Following in Anselm Strauss's (1987) protofeminist footsteps, I particularly advocate researchers' participation in working groups of various kinds to provoke analysis by having to come to grips with other perspectives, other interpretations of data, commentary on preliminary incarnations of integrated analyses, and so on. Strauss believed so strongly in the working group process that in his 1987 GT book, he actually provides transcripts of the sessions of such groups. Groups explicitly focused on feminist research would further echo consciousness raising and further provoke discussions of feminist theoretical developments and needs (e.g., Lather, 2007). Using

GT and SA in such groups can be done in actual collaborative research (e.g., Lather & Smithies, 1997) or with independent research projects using such groups as analytic worksites (e.g., Lessor, 2000; Wiener, 2007).

Beyond actually using GT and SA in feminist research, my major recommendation for making them—or any other approach—more explicitly feminist is to engage with the work of exciting feminist and other theorists, methodologists, and researchers. Feminist qualitative research is itself, as demonstrated by this volume and its impressive predecessor, a lively community of ongoing discourses. It is a widely distributed and very heterogeneous arena that can be a source of wondrous provocation. It exceeds "conversations" and "collaborations," and it too has a gestalt that is greater than the sum of its parts. For me, reading Patti Lather, whom I see as a theorist of feminist methodologies, always ruptures my taken-for-granted-ness. She vividly portrays dilemmas, conundrums, partialities, contradictions, ethics—the agonies and ecstasies of research. She reminds us that we are merely *trying* to be feminist at this historical moment, "getting lost" along the way, knowing we grasp and acknowledge only a few of the shortfalls of our work. But we go on.

Online Resources

Situational Analysis

http://www.situationalanalysis.com. This is the only website devoted to SA. It offers lists of publications using SA, upcoming conferences and workshops, bibliographies, and more.

Anselm Strauss

http://sbs.ucsf.edu/medsoc/anselmstrauss/index.html. This site focuses on the work of Anselm Strauss, including his grounded theory work. It includes unpublished essays, topical bibliographies, and more.

Relevant Journals

Gender & Society
International Journal of Qualitative Methods
International Review of Qualitative Research
Qualitative Health Research
Qualitative Inquiry

Qualitative Research
Qualitative Sociology
Symbolic Interaction

Notes

1. See especially Glaser (1978, 2002a, 2007), Glaser and Holton (2004), Strauss (1987, 1995), Strauss and Corbin (1990, 1994, 1998), Charmaz (2000, 2006, 2008a, 2009), Bryant and Charmaz (2007), Clarke (2003, 2005, , 2007a,b, 2009), Corbin and Strauss (2008), and Locke (2001).

2. On feminist research, see, e.g., this volume and its first edition (Hesse-Biber, 2007). See also Hekman (2007), Lather (2007, 2008), Naples (2003), Olesen (2005, 2007, 2011), and Smith (2007).

3. The concept of abduction is, appropriately, from pragmatist philosophy where the roots of symbolic interaction and GT also lie (e.g., Locke, 2007; Reichertz, 2007; Richardson & Kramer, 2006; Strübing, 2007; Timmermans & Tavory, in review). I have recently extended the concept in theorizing anticipation as our current modus operandi (Adams, Murphy, & Clarke, 2009).

4. See, on theoretical sampling, Glaser and Strauss (1967, pp. 45–77), Glaser (1978, pp. 36–54), Strauss (1987, pp. 38–39), Strauss and Corbin (1998, pp. 201–215), Clarke (2005, especially pp. 31–35), Charmaz (2006, pp. 96–122), and Morse (2007).

5. At an early National Women's Studies Association conference, held in Bloomington, Indiana, in 1980, there was a panel on "Qualitative Methods and Feminism" (www.nwsaconference. org/archives.html). On that panel, according to Star, were Sandra Harding, Pauline Bart, and herself. Star's presentation was predicated on the dissertation research of Barbara DuBois at Harvard in clinical psychology, which used GT to analyze women's experiences (DuBois, 1983; Star, 2007).

6. In the United States, there has long been what I see as a misuse of the term *pragmatic* largely to equal to *expedience* based in the logics of homo economicus, with some form of capitalism as the only reasonable path. In sharp contrast, pragmatists like Dewey referred to the pragmatic as what would work or be feasible to do, *given the conditions of the situation.* As such, it is more closely akin to Foucault's "conditions of possibility" (Foucault, 1975), elucidating what needs to be taken into account to answer his question, "What is to be done?" (Foucault, 1991, p. 84).

7. See also Atkinson et al. (2003, pp. 148–152) and Denzin (2007). Glaser (1978, 2002a) and Glaser and Holton (2004) argue that GT could also be used with quantitative research.

8. Issues of trust vis-à-vis research have changed. In the mid-twentieth century, neither researchers nor respondents (now called participants) were deemed reliable or trustworthy—generating a vast literature on reliability. Today, we are much more publicly skeptical, exhibiting profound distrust in governments, media, science, corporations, professions—and in research. In feminist literatures, the question of trust is often argued in terms of accountability (e.g., Haraway, 1991, 1997; Hesse-Biber, 2007; Lather, 2007, 2008).

9. The debate between Glaser and Strauss and Corbin, which has implications for feminist research, is extensively taken up in Bryant and Charmaz (2007) and in Morse and colleagues (2009). Morse and colleagues (2009) include a dialogue among the second generation that

ends up asserting that today there are different kinds of GT (pp. 236–247). Denzin (2007) describes Glaserian GT as objectivist, the Strauss and Corbin version as systematic, the Charmaz version as constructivist, and Clarke's as situationist. I think these terms work well. See also Charmaz (2000, 2006, 2008a, 2008b, 2009), Clarke (2005, pp. 12–18; 2007b), Glaser (2002a, 2007), Glaser and Holton (2004), Locke (2001), Morse (2009), and Walker and Myrick (2006).

10. Strauss so much believed in this process that he incorporated transcripts of group analysis sessions into one of his major methods books (Strauss, 1987). See Star (2007) on feminist issues and Wiener (2007) and Lessor (2000) on working groups.

11. See the Anselm Strauss website at http://sbs.ucsf.edu/medsoc/anselmstrauss/index.html. See Glaser's website at www.groundedtheory.com. On Virginia Olesen (2005, 2007, 2011), see http://nursing.ucsf.edu/faculty/virginia-olesen.

12. Stem (2007, 2009), Bowers and Schatzman (2009), Kools (2008), and Schumacher (2008) all provide accounts of this era. Benoliel (1996) analyzed GT nursing research published from 1980 to 1994.

13. After publication of my book, I discovered several other methods also called "situational analysis." What this means in terms of electronic searching for my version of "situational analysis" is that it needs to be done with "AND grounded theory."

References

Adams, V., Murphy, M., & Clarke, A. E. (2009). Anticipation: Technoscience, life, affect, temporality. *Subjectivity*, *28*, 246-265.

Atkinson, P., Coffey, A., & Delamont, S. (2003). *Key themes in qualitative research: Continuities and change.* Walnut Creek, CA: AltaMira Press/Rowman and Littlefield.

Austen, S., Jefferson, T., & Thein, V. (2003). Gendered social indicators and grounded theory. *Feminist Economics*, *9*(1), 1–18.

Becker, H. S. (1963). *Outsiders: Studies in the sociology of deviance.* New York: Free Press.

Becker, H. S. (1970). Whose side are we on? In H. S. Becker, *Sociological work: Method and substance* (pp. 123–134). New Brunswick, NJ: Transaction Books.

Benoliel, J. Q. (1996). Grounded theory and nursing knowledge. *Qualitative Health Research*, *6*(3), 406–428.

Benoliel, J. Q. (2001). Expanding knowledge about women through grounded theory: Introduction. *Health Care for Women International*, *22*(1–2), 7–9.

Berger, P., & Luckmann, T. (1966). *The social construction of reality: A treatise in the sociology of knowledge.* Garden City, NJ: Doubleday.

Berkowitz, D., & Marsiglio, W. (2007). Gay men: Negotiating procreative, father, and family identities. *Journal of Marriage and the Family*, *69*, 366–381.

Blumer, H. (1958). Race/ethnicity prejudice as a sense of group position. *Pacific Sociological Review*, *1*, 3–8.

Blumer, H. (1969). *Symbolic interactionism: Perspective and method.* Englewood Cliffs, NJ: Prentice Hall.

Boris, E., & Parrenas, R. S. (Eds.). (2010). *Intimate labors: Cultures, technologies and the politics of care.* Stanford, CA: Stanford University Press.

Bowers, B., & Schatzman, L. (2009). Dimensional analysis. In J. M. Morse, P. N. Stern, J. M. Corbin, K. C. Charmaz, B. Bowers, & A. E. Clarke, *Developing grounded theory: The second generation* (pp. 86-106). Walnut Creek, CA: Left Coast Press.

Bryant, A. (2003). A constructive/ist response to Glaser. *FQS: Forum for Qualitative Social Research*, 4(1). Available at http://www.qualitative-research.net/index.php/fqs/article/view/757

Bryant, A. (2006). *Thinking informatically: A new understanding of information, communication, and technology*. Lampeter, Ceredigion, UK: Edwin Mellen.

Bryant, A., & Charmaz, K. (Eds.). (2007). *Handbook of grounded theory*. London: Sage.

Casper, M. J. (1998). *The making of the unborn patient: A social anatomy of fetal surgery*. New Brunswick, NJ: Rutgers University Press.

Charmaz, K. (2000). Grounded theory: Objectivist and constructivist methods. In N. Denzin & Y. Lincoln (Eds.), *Handbook of qualitative research* (2nd ed., pp. 509–536). Thousand Oaks, CA: Sage.

Charmaz, K. (2005). Grounded theory in the 21st century: Applications for advancing social justice studies. In N. K. Denzin & Y. S. Lincoln (Eds.), *The SAGE handbook of qualitative research* (3rd ed., pp. 507–536). Thousand Oaks, CA: Sage.

Charmaz, K. (2006, 2014). *Constructing grounded theory: A practical guide through qualitative analysis*. London: Sage, 1st & 2nd eds.

Charmaz, K. (2008a). Grounded theory as an emergent method. In S. N. Hesse-Biber & P. Leavy (Eds.), *The handbook of emergent methods* (pp. 155–170). New York: Guilford.

Charmaz, K. (2008b). The legacy of Anselm Strauss in constructivist grounded theory. *Studies in Symbolic Interaction*, 32, 127–142.

Charmaz, K. (2009). Shifting the grounds: Constructivist grounded theory methods. In J. M. Morse, P. N. Stern, J. M. Corbin, K. C. Charmaz, B. Bowers, & A. E. Clarke, *Developing grounded theory: The second generation* (pp. 127–155). Walnut Creek, CA: Left Coast Press.

Charmaz, K. (2010). Studying the experience of chronic illness through grounded theory. In G. Scambler & S. Scambler (Eds.), *New directions in the sociology of chronic and disabling conditions: Assaults on the lifeworld* (pp. 8–36). London: Palgrave.

Charmaz, K. (2011). Grounded theory methods in social justice research. In N. K. Denzin & Y. S. Lincoln (Eds.), *The SAGE handbook of qualitative research* (4th ed., pp. 359–380). Thousand Oaks, CA: Sage.

Clarke, A. E. (1991). Social worlds/arenas theory as organizational theory. In D. R. Maines (Ed.), *Social organization and social process: Essays in honor of Anselm Strauss* (pp. 119–158). New York: Aldine De Gruyter.

Clarke, A. E. (1998). *Disciplining reproduction: Modernity, American life sciences, and the "problem of sex."* Berkeley: University of California Press.

Clarke, A. E. (2003). Situational analyses: Grounded theory mapping after the postmodern turn. *Symbolic Interaction*, 26(4), 553–576.

Clarke, A. E. (2005). *Situational analysis: Grounded theory after the postmodern turn*. Thousand Oaks, CA: Sage.

Clarke, A. E. (2007a). Feminisms, grounded theory, and situational analysis. In S. Hesse-Biber (Ed.), *Handbook of feminist research: Theory and praxis* (pp. 345–370). Thousand Oaks, CA: Sage.

Clarke, A. E. (2007b). Grounded theory: Conflicts, debates and situational analysis. In W. Outhwaite & S. P. Turner (Eds.), *Handbook of social science methodology* (pp. 838–885). Thousand Oaks, CA: Sage.

Clarke, A. E. (2008). Sex/gender and race/ethnicity in the legacy of Anselm Strauss. *Studies in Symbolic Interaction, 32*, 161–176.

Clarke, A. E. (2009). From grounded theory to situational analysis: What's new? Why? How? In J. M. Morse, P. N. Stern, J. M. Corbin, K. C. Charmaz, B. Bowers, & A. E. Clarke, *Developing grounded theory: The second generation* (pp. 194-233). Walnut Creek, CA: Left Coast Press.

Clarke, A. E. (2010a). Anselm Strauss en heritage: Sexe/genre et race/ethnicite. In D. Chabaud-Rychter, V. Descoutures, A. Devreux, & E. Varikas (Eds.), *Questions de genre aux sciences sociales "normales"* (pp. 245–259). Paris: La Decouverte.

Clarke, A. E. (2010b). In memorium: Susan Leigh Star, 1954–2010. *Science, Technology, and Human Values, 35*(5), 1–20.

Clarke, A. E. (2010c). Thoughts on biomedicalization in its transnational travels. In A. E. Clarke, L. Mamo, J. R. Fosket, J. R. Fishman, & J. K. Shim (Eds.), *Biomedicalization: Technoscience, health, and illness in the U.S.* (pp. 380–405). Durham, NC: Duke University Press.

Clarke, A. E., & Charmaz, K. (Eds.). (2014). *Grounded theory and situational analysis* (Sage Benchmarks in Social Research Series, Vols. 1–4). London: Sage.

Clarke, A. E., & Friese, C. (2007). Situational analysis: Going beyond traditional grounded theory. In A. Bryant & K. Charmaz (Eds.), *Handbook of grounded theory* (pp. 694–743). London: Sage.

Clarke, A. E., Mamo, L., Fosket, J. R., Fishman, J. R., & Shim, J. K. (Eds.). (2010). *Biomedicalization: Technoscience, health, and illness in the U.S.* Durham, NC: Duke University Press.

Clarke, A. E., & Montini, T. (1993). The many faces of RU486: Tales of situated knowledges and technological contestations. *Science, Technology, and Human Values, 18*(1), 42–78.

Clarke, A. E., Shim, J. K., Mamo, L., Fosket, J. R., & Fishman, J. R. (2003). Biomedicalization: Technoscientific transformations of health, illness, and U.S. biomedicine. *American Sociological Review, 68*(2), 161–194.

Clarke, A. E., & Star, S. L. (2008). Social worlds/arenas as a theory-methods package. In E. Hackett, O. Amsterdamska, M. Lynch, & J. Wacjman (Eds.), *Handbook of science and technology studies* (2nd ed., pp. 113–137). Cambridge, MA: MIT Press.

Collins, P. H. (2004). *Black sexual politics: African Americans, gender, and the new racism.* New York: Routledge.

Collins, P. H. (2009). Emerging intersections: Building knowledge and transforming institutions. In B. T. Dill & R. E. Zambrana (Eds.), *Emerging intersections: Race, class, and gender in theory, policy, and practice* (pp. vii–xiii). New Brunswick, NJ: Rutgers University Press.

Corbin, J. (2009). Taking an analytic journey. In J. M. Morse, P. N. Stern, J. M. Corbin, K. C. Charmaz, B. Bowers, & A. E. Clarke, *Developing grounded theory: The second generation* (pp. 35–54). Walnut Creek, CA: Left Coast Press,

Corbin, J., & Strauss, A. (2008). *Basics of qualitative research: Grounded theory procedures and techniques* (3rd ed.). Thousand Oaks, CA: Sage.

Creswell, J. W. (2007). *Qualitative inquiry and research design: Choosing among five traditions* (2nd ed.). London: Sage.

Dahlgren, L., Emmelin, M., & Winkvist, A. (2007). *Qualitative methodology for international public health.* Umea, Sweden: International School of Public Health, Umea University.

Denzin, N. (1989). *The research act: A theoretical introduction to sociological methods.* Chicago: Aldine. (Original work published 1970)

Denzin, N. (2007). Grounded theory and the politics of interpretation. In A. Bryant & K. Charmaz (Eds.), *Handbook of grounded theory* (pp. 454–472). London: Sage.

Denzin, N. K., & Lincoln, Y. S. (Eds.). (2005). *The SAGE handbook of qualitative research* (3rd ed.). Thousand Oaks, CA: Sage.

Denzin, N., Lincoln, Y., & Smith, L. T. (Eds.). (2008). *Handbook of critical and indigenous methodologies.* Thousand Oaks, CA: Sage.

Dill, B. T., & Zambrana, R. E. (2009). *Emerging intersections: Race, class, and gender in theory, policy, and practice.* New Brunswick, NJ: Rutgers University Press.

Dougherty, D. (2005). Grounded theory research methods. In J. A. C. Baum (Ed.), *The Blackwell companion to organizations* (pp. 849-866). Oxford, UK: Blackwell.

DuBois, B. (1983). Passionate scholarship: Notes on values, knowing, and method in feminist social sciences. In G. D. K. Bowles & R. Duelli-Klein (Eds.), *Theories of women's studies* (pp. 105–117). London: Routledge & Kegan Paul.

DuBois, W. E. B. (1993). *W.E.B. DuBois reader.* New York: Scribner.

Duster, T. (2003). *Backdoor to eugenics.* New York: Routledge. (Original work published 1990)

Fassinger, R. E. (2005). Paradigms, praxis, problems, and promise: Grounded theory in counseling psychology research. *Journal of Counseling Psychology.* 52(2), 156–166.

Fonow, M. M., & Cook, J. A. (2005). Feminist methodology: New applications in the academy and public policy. *Signs: Journal of Women in Culture and Society, 30(4),* 211–236.

Ford-Gilboe, M., Wuest, J., & Merritt-Gray, M. (2005). Strengthening capacity to limit intrusion: Theorizing family health promotion in the aftermath of woman abuse. *Qualitative Health Research, 15(4),* 477–501.

Foucault, M. (1975). *The birth of the clinic: An archeology of medical perception.* New York: Vintage/Random House.

Foucault, M. (1991). Questions of methods. In G. Burchell, C. Gordon, & P. Miller (Eds.), *The Foucault effect: Studies in governmentality* (pp. 73–86). Chicago: University of Chicago Press.

Gilgun, J. F. (2013). Grounded theory, deductive qualitative analysis and social work research and practice. In A. E. Fortune, W. Reid, & R. Miller (Eds.), *Qualitative methods in social work* (2nd ed., pp. 107–135). New York: Columbia University Press.

Glaser, B. G. (1978). *Theoretical sensitivity: Advances in the methodology of grounded theory.* Mill Valley, CA: Sociology Press.

Glaser, B. G. (2002a). Constructivist grounded theory? *FQS Forum: Qualitative Social Research,* 3(3). Available at http://www.qualitative-research.net/index.php/fqs/article/view/825

Glaser, B. G. (2002b). Grounded theory and gender relevance. *Health Care for Women International,* 23(8), 786–793.

Glaser, B. G. (2007). Doing formal theory. In A. Bryant & K. Charmaz (Eds.), *Handbook of grounded theory* (pp. 97–113). London: Sage.

Glaser, B. G., & Holton, J. (2004). Remodeling grounded theory. *Forum for Qualitative Social Research,* 5(2). Available at http://www.qualitative-research.net/index.php/fqs/article/view/607

Glaser, B. G., & Strauss, A. L. (1967). *The discovery of grounded theory: Strategies for qualitative research.* Chicago: Aldine.

Green, D. O., Creswell, J. W., Shope, R. J., & Plano Clark, V. L. (2007). Grounded theory and racial/ethnic diversity. In A. Bryant & K. Charmaz (Eds.), *Handbook of grounded theory* (pp. 472–492). London: Sage.

Gruskin, E., Byrne, K., & Kools, S. (2006). Frequenting the lesbian bar. *Women s Health,* 44(2), 103–120.

Hacking, I. (1983). *Representing and intervening: Introductory topics in the philosophy of natural science*. Cambridge, UK: Cambridge University Press.

Haraway, D. (1991). Situated knowledges: The science question in feminism and the privilege of partial perspectives. In D. Haraway, *Simians, cyborgs, and women: The reinvention of nature* (pp. 183-202). New York: Routledge.

Haraway, D. (1997). Modest_Witness@Second_Millenium. In D. Haraway, *Modest_Witness@ Second Millenium. FemaleMan©_Meets_Onco Mouse™: Feminism and technoscience* (pp. 23-48). New York: Routledge.

Hekman, Susan. (2007). Feminist methodology. In W. Outhwaite & S. P. Turner (Eds.), *Handbook of social science methodology* (pp. 534–546). Thousand Oaks, CA: Sage.

Hesse-Biber, S. N. (Ed.). (2007). *Handbook of feminist research: Theory and praxis*. Thousand Oaks, CA: Sage.

Hochschild, A. (1969). Emotion work, feeling rules, and social structure. *American Journal of Sociology, 85*, 551–575.

Hughes, E. C. (1971). *The sociological eye*. Chicago: Aldine Atherton.

Jenks, C. (1995). The centrality of the eye in Western culture: An introduction. In J. A. Walker & S. Chaplin (Eds.), *Visual culture: An introduction* (pp. 1–16). London: Routledge.

Kearney, M. H. (1999). *Understanding women's recovery from illness and trauma*. Thousand Oaks, CA: Sage.

Kearney, M. H. (2001). Enduring love: A grounded formal theory of women's experience of domestic violence. *Research in Nursing & Health, 24*, 270–282.

Kearney, M. H. (2007). From the sublime to the meticulous: The continuing evolution of grounded formal theory. In A. Bryant & K. Charmaz (Eds.), *Handbook of grounded theory* (pp. 127–150). London: Sage.

Kearney, M. H. (2008). Inconstant comparisons: A nurse and a sociologist study depression using grounded theory. *Studies in Symbolic Interaction, 32*, 143-160.

Kearney, M. H. (2009). Taking grounded theory beyond psychological process [Editorial]. *Research in Nursing & Health, 32*, 567–568.

Kearney, M. H., Murphy, S., Irwin, K., & Rosenbaum, M. (1995). Salvaging self: A grounded theory of pregnancy on crack cocaine. *Nursing Research, 44(4)*, 208–213.

Kohlen, H. (2009). *Conflicts of care: Hospital ethics committees in the USA and Germany*. Frankfurt and New York: Campus Verlag.

Kools, S. B. (2008). From heritage to postmodern grounded theorizing. *Studies in Symbolic Interaction, 32*, 73–86.

Kools, S. B., & Kennedy, C. (2003). Foster child health and development: Implications for primary care. *Pediatric Nursing, 29(1)*, 39–46.

Kushner, K. E., & Morrow, R. (2003). Grounded theory, feminist theory, critical theory. *Advances in Nursing Science, 26(1)*, 30–43.

Lampland, M., & Star, S. L. (Eds.). (2009). *Standards and their stories: How quantifying, classifying, and formalizing practices shape everyday life*. Ithaca, NY: Cornell University Press.

Landstedt, E., Asplund, K., & Gådin, K. (2009). Understanding adolescent mental health: The influence of social processes, doing gender and gendered power relations. *Sociology of Health and Illness, 31(7)*, 962–978.

Lather, P. (2007). *Getting lost: Feminist efforts toward a double(d) science*. Albany: State University of New York Press.

Lather, P. (2008). (Post) Feminist methodology. *International Review of Qualitative Research, 1(1)*, 55–64.

Lather, P., & Smithies, C. (1997). *Troubling the angels: Women living with HIV/AIDS.* Boulder, CO: Westview Press.

Law, J. (1999). After ANT: Complexity, naming, and topology. In J. Law & J. Hassard (Eds.), *Actor-network theory and after* (pp. 1–19). Malden, MA: Blackwell. ·

Lempert, L. B. (2007). Asking questions of the data: Memo writing in the grounded theory tradition. In A. Bryant & K. Charmaz (Eds.), *Handbook of grounded theory* (pp. 245–264). London: Sage.

Lessor, R. (2000). Using the team approach of Anselm Strauss in action research: Consulting on a project on global education. *Sociological Perspectives, 43(4),* S133–S147.

Locke, K. (2001). *Grounded theory in management research.* Thousand Oaks, CA: Sage.

Locke, K. (2007). Rational control and irrational free-play: Dual-thinking modes as necessary tension in grounded theorizing. In A. Bryant & K. Charmaz (Eds.), *Handbook of grounded theory* (pp. 565–579). London: Sage.

Mamo, L. (2007). *Queering reproduction: Achieving pregnancy in the age of technoscience.* Durham, NC: Duke University Press.

Marcellus, L. (2005). The grounded theory method and maternal-infant research and practice. *Journal of Obstetrical, Gynecological, and Neonatal Nursing, 34(3),* 349–357.

Maternowska, C., Westrada, F., Campero, L., Herrera, C., Brindis, C. D., & Vostrejs, M. M. (2010). Gender, culture and reproductive decision-making among recent Mexican migrants in California. *Culture, Health and Sexuality, 12(1),* 29–43.

McCarthy, D. (1984). Towards a sociology of the physical world: George Herbert Mead on physical objects. *Studies in Symbolic Interaction, 5,* 105–121.

McCarthy, D. (1996). *Knowledge as culture: The new sociology of knowledge.* New York: Routledge.

Mead, G. H. (1962). *Mind, self, and society* (C. W. Morris, Ed.). Chicago: University of Chicago. (Original work published 1934)

Miller, S. (1996). Questioning, resisting, acquiescing, balancing: New mothers' career reentry strategies. *Health Care for Women International, 17,* 109–131.

Mills, J., Chapman, Y., Bonner, A., & Francis, K. (2007). Grounded theory: A methodological spiral from positivism to postmodernism. *Journal of Advanced Nursing, 58(1),* 72–79.

Mills, J., Francis, K., & Bonner, A. (2008). Getting to know a stranger—rural nurses' experiences of mentoring: A grounded theory. *International Journal of Nursing Studies, 45(4),* 599–607.

Moore, L. J. (2007). *Sperm tales: Social, cultural, and scientific representations of human semen.* New York: Routledge.

Morse, J. M. (2007). Sampling in grounded theory research. In A. Bryant & K. Charmaz (Eds.), *Handbook of grounded theory* (pp. 229–244). London: Sage.

Morse, J. M. (2009). Tussles, tensions, and resolutions. In J. M. Morse, P. N. Stern, J. M. Corbin, K. C. Charmaz, B. Bowers, & A. E. Clarke, *Developing grounded theory: The second generation* (pp. 13–23). Walnut Creek, CA: Left Coast Press.

Morse, J. M., Stern, P. N., Corbin, J. M., Charmaz, K. C., Bowers, B., & Clarke, A. E. (2009). *Developing grounded theory: The second generation.* Walnut Creek, CA: Left Coast Press.

Naples, N. A. (2003). *Feminism and method: Ethnography, discourse analysis, and activist research.* New York: Routledge.

Neill, S. J. (2006). Grounded theory sampling: The contribution of reflexivity [Review]. *Journal of Research in Nursing, 11(3),* 253–260.

Olesen, V. L. (2005). Early millennial feminist qualitative research: Challenges and contours. In N. K. Denzin & Y. S. Lincoln (Eds.), *The SAGE handbook of qualitative research* (3rd ed., pp. 235–278). Thousand Oaks, CA: Sage.

Olesen, V. L. (2007). Feminist qualitative research and grounded theory: Complexities, criticisms, and opportunities. In A. Bryant & K. Charmaz (Eds.), *Handbook of grounded theory* (pp. 417–435). London: Sage.

Olesen, V. L. (2011). Feminist qualitative research in the millennium's first decade: Developments, challenges, prospects. In N. K. Denzin & Y. S. Lincoln (Eds.), *The SAGE handbook of qualitative research* (4th ed., pp. 129–146). Thousand Oaks, CA: Sage.

Olshansky, E. (2003). A theoretical explanation for previously infertile mothers' vulnerability to depression. *Journal of Nursing Scholarship, 35*(3), 263–268.

Omi, M., & Winant, H. (1994). *Racial formation in the United States: From the 1960s to the 1990s.* New York: Routledge.

Padgett, D. K. (2008). *Qualitative methods in social work research.* Thousand Oaks, CA: Sage.

Pascale, C. M. (2008). Talking about race: Shifting the analytical paradigm. *Qualitative Inquiry, 14*(5), 723–741.

Pearse, N., & Kanyangale, M. (2009). Researching organizational culture using the grounded theory method. *The Electronic Journal of Business Research Methods, 7*(1), 67–74.

Plummer, K. (2005). Critical humanism and queer theory: Living with the tensions. In N. Denzin & Y. Lincoln (Eds.), *Handbook of qualitative research* (3rd ed., pp. 357–373). Thousand Oaks, CA: Sage.

Plummer, M., & Young, L. E. (2010). Grounded theory and feminist inquiry. *Western Journal of Nursing Research, 32*(3), 305–321.

Reichertz, J. (2007). Abduction: The logic of discovery of grounded theory. In A. Bryant & K. Charmaz (Eds.), *Handbook of grounded theory* (pp. 214–228). London: Sage.

Richardson, R., & Kramer, E. H. (2006). Abduction as the type of inference that characterizes the development of a grounded theory. *Qualitative Research, 6*(4), 497–513.

Riessman, C. K. (2008). *Narrative methods for the human sciences* (2nd ed.). Thousand Oaks, CA: Sage.

Ryan, M., & Berkowitz, D. (2009). Constructing gay and lesbian families "beyond the closet." *Qualitative Sociology, 32*, 153-172.

Said, E. (1978). *Orientalism.* New York: Random House.

Samik-Ibrahim, R. M. (2000). Grounded theory methodology as the research strategy for a developing country. *Forum: Qualitative Social Research, 1*(1), Art. 19. Retrieved June 15,2011, from http://www.qualitative-research.net/index.php/fqs/article/viewArticle/1129/2511

Schatzman, L., & Strauss, A. (1973). *Field research: Strategies for a natural sociology.* Englewood Cliffs, NJ: Prentice Hall.

Schnitzer, G., Loots, G., Escudero, V., & Schechter, I. (2009). Negotiating the pathways into care in a globalizing world: Help-seeking behaviour of ultra-orthodox Jewish parents. *International Journal of Social Psychiatry, 57*(2), 153–165.

Schreiber, R. S., & Stern, P. N. (Eds.). (2001). *Using grounded theory in nursing.* New York: Springer.

Schrock, D. P., & Padavic, I. (2007). Negotiating hegemonic masculinity in a batterer intervention program. *Gender & Society, 21*, 625–649.

Schulz, A. J., & Mullings, L. (Eds.). (2006). *Gender, race, class, and health: Intersectional approaches.* San Francisco: Jossey-Bass.

Schumacher, K. (2008). Twenty years of grounded theorizing about family caregiving: Accomplishments and conundrums. *Studies in Symbolic Interaction, 32,* 87–102.

Schutze, F. (2008). The legacy in Germany today of Anselm Strauss's vision and practice of sociology. *Studies in Symbolic Interaction, 32,* 103–126.

Schwalbe, M., Goodwin, D. H., Schrock, S., Thompson, S., & Wolkomir, M. (2000). Generic processes in the reproduction of inequality: An interactionist analysis. *Social Forces, 79,* 419–452.

Scott, J. W. (1992). Experience. In J. Butler & J. W. Scott (Eds.), *Feminists theorize the political* (pp. 22–40). New York: Routledge.

Settles, I. H., Pratt-Hyatt, J. S., & Buchanan, N. T. (2008). Through the lens of race: Black and white women's perceptions of womanhood. *Psychology of Women Quarterly, 32,* 454–468.

Shim, J. K. (2005). Constructing "race" across the science-lay divide: Racial projects in the epidemiology and experience of cardiovascular disease. *Social Studies of Science, 35(3),* 405–436.

Shim, J. K. (2014). *Heart-Sick: The Politics of Risk, Inequality, and Heart Disease.* New York: NYU Press.

Smith, D. E. (2007). Institutional ethnography: From a sociology for women to a sociology for people. In S. Hesse-Biber (Ed.), *Handbook of feminist research: Theory and praxis* (pp. 409–418). Thousand Oaks, CA: Sage.

Star, S. L. (1983). Simplification in scientific work: An example from neuroscience research. *Social Studies of Science, 13,* 208–226.

Star, S. L. (1991). The sociology of the invisible: The primacy of work in the writings of Anselm Strauss. In D. R. Maines (Ed.), *Social organization and social process: Essays in honor of Anselm Strauss* (pp. 265-283). Hawthorne, NY: Aldine de Gruyter.

Star, S. L. (2007). Living grounded theory: Cognitive and emotional forms of pragmatism. In A. Bryant & K. Charmaz (Eds.), *Handbook of grounded theory* (pp. 75–94). Thousand Oaks, CA: Sage.

Star, S. L., & Bowker, G. (2007). Enacting Silence: Residual categories as a challenge for ethics, information systems, and communication technology. *Ethics and Information Technology, 9,* 273–280.

Star, S. L., & Strauss, A. L. (1998). Layers of silence, arenas of voice: The ecology of visible and invisible work. *Computer Supported Cooperative Work: The Journal of Collaborative Computing, 8,* 9–30.

Stern, P. N. (2007). On solid ground: Essential properties for growing grounded theory. In A. Bryant ·& K. Charmaz (Eds.), *Handbook of grounded theory* (pp. 114–126). London: Sage.

Stern, P. N. (2009). Glaserian grounded theory. In J. M. Morse, P. N. Stern, J. M. Corbin, K. C. Charmaz, B. Bowers, & A. E. Clarke, *Developing grounded theory: The second generation* (pp. 55–85). Walnut Creek, CA: Left Coast Press.

Strauss, A. L. (1978). A social world perspective. *Studies in Symbolic Interaction, 1,* 119–128.

Strauss, A. L. (1987). *Qualitative analysis for social scientists.* Cambridge, UK: Cambridge University Press.

Strauss, A. L. (1993). *Continual permutation of action.* New York: Aldine de Gruyter.

Strauss, A. L. (1995). Notes on the nature and development of general theories. *Qualitative Inquiry, 1(1),* 7–18.

Strauss, A. L., & Corbin, J. (1990). *Basics of qualitative research: Grounded theory, procedures, and techniques.* Newbury Park, CA: Sage.

Strauss, A. L., & Corbin, J. (1994). Grounded theory methodology: An overview. In N. Denzin & Y. Lincoln (Eds.), *Handbook of qualitative research* (pp. 273–285). Thousand Oaks, CA: Sage.

Strauss, A. L., & Corbin, J. (Eds.). (1997). *Grounded theory in practice.* Thousand Oaks, CA: Sage.

Strauss, A. L., & Corbin, J. (1998). *The basics of qualitative analysis: Grounded theory procedures and techniques* (2nd ed.). Thousand Oaks, CA: Sage.

Strübing, J. (2007). Research as pragmatic problem-solving: The pragmatist roost of empirically grounded theorizing. In A. Bryant & K. Charmaz (Eds.), *Handbook of grounded theory* (pp. 580–602). London: Sage.

Suddaby, Roy. (2006). What grounded theory is not. *Academy of Management Journal,* 49(4), 633–642.

Syfers, J. (1971). Why I want a wife. *Ms Magazine,* 1(1).

Tarozzi, M. (2008). *Che cos'é la grounded theory.* Rome: Carocci.

Timmermans, S. (2006). *Postmortem: How medical examiners explain suspicious deaths.* Chicago: University of Chicago Press.

Timmermans, S., & Tavory, I. (2012). *Theory construction in qualitative research:* From grounded theory to abductive analysis. *Sociological Theory* 30(3), 167–186.

Urquhart, Cathy. (2007). The evolving nature of grounded theory method: The case of the information systems discipline. In A. Bryant & K. Charmaz (Eds.), *Handbook of grounded theory* (pp. 339–362). London: Sage.

Walker, D., & Myrick, F. (2006). Grounded theory: An exploration of process and procedure. *Qualitative Health Research,* 16(4), 547–559.

Weber, L. (2010). *Understanding race, class, gender, and sexuality: A conceptual framework* (2nd ed.). New York: Oxford University Press.

Wiener, C. (2000). *The elusive quest: Accountability in hospitals.* New York: Aldine de Gruyter.

Wiener, C. (2007). Making teams work in conducting grounded theory. In A. Bryant & K. Charmaz (Eds.), *Handbook of grounded theory* (pp. 293–310). London: Sage.

Wingfield, A. H. (2007). The modern mammy and the angry black man: African American professionals' experiences with gendered racism in the workplace. *Race, Gender & Class,* 14(1–2), 196–212.

Wolkomir, M., & Powers, J. (2007). Helping women and protecting the self: The challenge of emotional labor in an abortion clinic. *Qualitative Sociology,* 30, 153–169.

CHAPTER FOUR

BUILDING EMERGENT SITUATED KNOWLEDGES IN PARTICIPATORY ACTION RESEARCH

Bill Genat

Introduction

This article describes an approach to participatory action research that extends the traditional role of the researcher to that of an agent collaboratively and actively engaged in the construction of local knowledge and theory with a particular group of research participants. Initially, the article describes the foundational premises for this approach and a practice framework to guide the researcher. It then describes the social arena of the research act as an interacting system of social worlds of specific stakeholders, each defined by discourse and with particular understandings and investments in a particular framing of phenomena in this social arena and beyond.

Drawing upon Wadsworth's (1997) concept of the critical reference group as 'whom the research is for', the article suggests privileging this stakeholder group within the social arena of the research act and describes how the formulation of a 'participant focus group' drawn from the critical reference group can function as an incubator of new meanings, representation and language and thus the locus for the production of a particular local theory or 'situated knowledge' regarding the phenomena in question. An examination of the epistemological status of such local situated knowledge in comparison with accepted academic theory concludes the article. Theory is understood in this article as the analysis of the relationship of a set of concepts or phenomena, as known or experienced by a particular social group.

Conceptual Framework

Over the years, 'action research' has come to cover a wide range of practices. The common thread linking all action research practice is the requirement

for action to be initiated either by the researcher or the research(er) participants as a component of the research design (Cornwall & Jewkes, 1995; Mills,
2000; Stringer, 2007). While either the researcher or the participants may
undertake the designated action, implicit in an action research project design
is reflection or review of the action component. While the action component
may focus on achieving a direct benefit to the participants, and by some be
seen as an end in itself, it is the learning generated from the action–reflection cycle that provides the critical data of action research (Stringer, 1999).
Clarity about the form of the data, how it will be evoked, recorded, analysed,
interpreted and written up, and by whom, constitutes the crucial process of
the production of knowledge within an action research project.

   This article focuses on one approach to participatory action research
(PAR) and uses three premises to define a PAR project:

   + it investigates the action of research participants in a specific local
     context;
   + it includes cycles of action–reflection that produce experiential learning
     amongst a particular group of research participants in a specific context
     transforming both individuals and their culture within a 'liberationist/
     emancipatory ethos' (Fals Borda, 2001, p. 32);
   + the emergent experiential learning creates a shared conceptual frame-
     work, theory or local knowledge amongst a particular group of research
     participants regarding phenomena in their local context.

   Others use similar premises to define participatory action research (Cornwall & Jewkes, 1995; Fals Borda, 2001; Stringer, 2007). Within this article, I
will draw upon examples from a previously published PAR project with Aboriginal healthworkers (AHW) (Genat et al., 2006) to illustrate the argument.

Practice Framework

Participatory action research, as described above, includes not only applied
action that makes a difference to the situation of a particular group of participants, but also the production of local knowledge regarding how these participants interpret and understand their own situation. When participatory
action research aims to reveal how a group of local people attribute meaning,
interpret and understand their world, the practitioner role embodied by the
researcher is critical to the study. The way the researcher negotiates, engages
and facilitates research with the participant group at the centre of the project

is key to the research outcome. The style of engagement will determine the quality and nature of the relationship, the extent to which participants become co-researchers (hereafter, for the sake of clarity, 'participants' are assumed to be participant co-researchers), the depth of the emergent data and the extent to which the researcher is regarded as an ally trustworthy and capable of sharing and articulating any aspect of these participants' world view.

A practice framework based on the following foundational principles underpins this approach to participatory action research. Ideally, a researcher works to:

+ establish reciprocity and an equal relationship of trust with the key group of research participants;
+ collaboratively develop a research project that is valued and of benefit to the key group of research participants;
+ build solidarity around a research question significant to the key group of research participants;
+ acknowledge, respect, value and privilege local knowledge;
+ facilitate learning and develop local capacity;
+ bring a self-reflexive component to practice by consistently interrogating their own standpoint and use of power along the dimensions of gender, race and class;
+ ensure emergent representations are credible with the key group of research participants.

Such a practitioner framework borrows heavily from the community development literature (Butler, 1991; Jackson et al., 1988; Kelly & Sewell, 1989). The participatory action researcher enacts this practice framework in a particular social arena with a strategic focus on the engagement of the key group of research participants here defined as the participant focus group.

The Participant Focus Group

Whatever the initial interest of the researcher wishing to engage in this version of participatory action research, the research act takes place within a particular social arena (Clarke, 2005). Every inquiry generates a unique social *arena*, an interacting system of social *worlds*, each inhabited by a particular stakeholder group invested in particular discourses. Each of these groups has an interest or 'stake' in how particular phenomena are labelled, known about, represented and understood within and beyond the immediate social arena.

While these groups are not totally homogenous in their views, implicit in the dominant view or 'stake' of each stakeholder group is an investment in, first, their particular understanding and representation of the phenomena in question, and second, the degree of their influence in asserting a particular view of the phenomena as the accepted representation in the social arena both of the research act and beyond.

For instance, within the social arena of a study of how a group of Aboriginal healthworkers working in a urban Aboriginal health service described and interpreted their work activities (Genat et al., 2006), the Aboriginal healthworkers themselves plus groups of nurses, doctors, managers, welfare workers and clients all constituted particular social worlds of discourse with specific views about healthworker practice (see Figure 4.1). Together, these social worlds constituted the social arena of Aboriginal healthworker practice. Prior to the study, most accepted representations of Aboriginal healthworker practice were those of policy-makers, managers, doctors and nurses. As in many health contexts, medical dominance (Willis, 2006) is a key factor in defining the Aboriginal healthworker role.

Policy-makers and program managers are key stakeholders within the social arena of the research act as are potential program recipients. Denzin (1989) suggests that often policy-makers develop interventions and programs on the basis of their own experience rather than the experience of the people whom their policies are meant to benefit. In doing so, they mistake their own

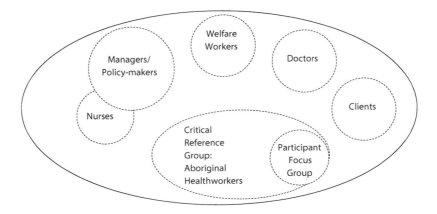

Figure 4.1 The overall social arena and interacting social worlds of aboriginal health worker practice including the participant focus group (PFG).

experience for the experience of others. Within the approach to participatory action research being described here, the experience of the people whom the policies or programs are meant to benefit is of key concern. Often, program recipient perspectives are seen as secondary to the views of experts. 'Lay' views of the phenomena in question may be seen as of lesser import than academic or 'scientific' representations of the 'facts'.

Within social research, where the meanings people bring to the world define the dependent variables, data are inherently unstable. Denzin (1989) asserts that in the social realm there are no 'facts', there is only interpretation. Where representations of the world are highly contested, research becomes a political act. Within the microcosm of the social arena of the research act, Foucault's power/knowledge nexus is at stake regarding how particular phenomena are understood and represented (Foucault, 1972). Each stakeholder group inhabiting a particular social world within the social arena of the research act has a particular perspective describing the phenomena at the focus of the inquiry which is important to reveal. Each stakeholder group is a potential incubator of a broader discourse that works to secure a particular representation of the phenomena in question.

Within the social arena of the research act it is the 'critical reference group' (CRG—Wadsworth, 1997), the particular stakeholder group whose experience and knowledge is unknown or perhaps subjugated, that in this approach to PAR constitute the key or critical group of research participants. It is their experience and interpretation of a particular phenomena that we seek to learn more about in order that both the members of the critical reference group know more about each other and their commonalities of experience and perspective, and in order to enable other stakeholders in the social arena to learn more about how members of the critical reference group experience their world. Within the social arena of the study of Aboriginal healthworker practice, inhabited by doctors, nurses, managers, welfare workers and clients, Aboriginal healthworkers constituted the critical reference group.

Amongst the critical reference group, the aim of the researcher is to recruit a group of participants to whom the research project is highly significant, to the point of being interesting enough to prompt their ongoing engagement as 'participant researchers' or collaborators in the research project over its duration. The researcher seeks their engagement in deciding the framing of the research question, developing an appropriate design and methods of inquiry, analysing the data, and ensuring that the representation of their interpretation of the phenomena in question is authentic and credible. This group of participants (participant researchers) is defined hereafter as the 'participant focus group'.

While it is important to investigate each of the social worlds in the social arena of the research act, it is the participant focus group that the researcher seeks to engage in cycles of action and reflection that produce shared experiential knowledge about their particular situation and context. It is this group in particular with whom the researcher seeks to build an ongoing collaboration and close relationship based on mutual respect and trust over sufficient period of time that key themes can be shared, contested, discussed, refined, recorded and coconstructed as local knowledge. Inasmuch as this framework connects and relates key phenomena shared in common by the participant focus group to explain their local situation, it constitutes their local theory of their situation. Key themes of the shared perspectives among the participant focus group are given credibility through triangulation with data from other members of the CRG. The interaction of the participant focus group is the crucible for the genesis of specific local situated knowledge (local theory).

Within the study of Aboriginal healthworker practice, two participant focus groups emerged initiated by healthworkers, one focused on 'best practice' and the other focused upon increasing the professional status of Aboriginal healthworkers. While my general question as an outside researcher was how do healthworkers describe and interpret their work-related activities, the healthworker's questions were how do we get better at what we do, and, how do healthworkers within the organization gain greater professional status. In this way, the healthworkers' explorations served to inform both their own questions and my general question.

The collection of data from other stakeholders inhabiting particular social worlds is also vital within this approach to participatory action research in order to bring forth multiple perspectives and reveal the multi-vocality and complexity of the social arena of the research. Where time and resources are limited, research with other stakeholder groups can be through more traditional qualitative approaches. Key themes of the participant focus group perspective can subsequently be contrasted with other perspectives circulating in the social arena of the research project revealing disjunctures in the experiences of the critical reference group and discourses operative in the broader social arena or other social worlds amongst (often) more powerful and influential stakeholders.

From a broader sociological theoretical perspective, positioning the participant focus group as the origin point for the construction and production of local situated knowledge locates this approach to participatory action research squarely in the realm of symbolic interactionism (Blumer, 1969). At the heart of the theory of symbolic interactionism is Mead's (1934) understanding that interpretation is central to human interaction in the world thereby shifting the behaviourist learning algorithm from stimulus–response, to stimulus–interpretation–response. Building further on Mead's work, symbolic interactionism understands meaning as always emergent from a being's interaction with their world, both material and social. Establishing a participant focus group from within the CRG with whom to undertake an inquiry into phenomena of particular interest to them, sets up a space of interaction where emergent meaning can be examined, contested, debated, reviewed, recorded and constructed. Applied to the experience of Aboriginal healthworkers, this approach and its principles accords with the decolonizing methodologies outlined by Smith (1999).

The participant focus group sits at the centre of this approach to participatory action research. It is their (often) subjugated knowledge that is privileged in terms of resources devoted to articulating their position and in the construction of the text. Other interpretations, from both other stakeholders in the social arena of the research and from the literature are examined against the foreground of emergent key themes of the local knowledge (theory) of the participant focus group. The researcher devotes particular attention to facilitating the open interaction of this group, building shared understandings, unity and solidarity with these key collaborators in the research project.

In addition to the participant focus group functioning as an incubator of local knowledge and discourse, it also functions as a vehicle for building solidarity and community. While the participant focus group does not represent the CRG, it can function as an activist node in the network of relationships that constitute the CRG. As people within the participant focus group begin to establish some solidarity around the way they view the phenomena at the focus of their research, they will be able to use their links to engage with other nodes of the CRG network to share ideas and develop the discourse around the phenomena under investigation. It is the extent to which the participant focus group is able to maintain and develop productive links with other key groups across the CRG that solidarity within the CRG can be built, at least regarding the phenomena under investigation and how it is represented and understood. These processes facilitate learning and the building of local capacity.

Rationale for the Approach

The above approach to participatory action research is based on the rationale of answering the questions: Who is the research for? Who is the research to benefit? While much is made of undertaking research for the nebulous 'greater good' or to contribute to the overall theoretical 'body of knowledge' in a particular academic discipline, such aspirations are brought into question by contemporary social theory. While we are all beneficiaries of positivism and hypothetico-deductive research, we also know that the production of any knowledge is an outcome of social position, location or situatedness producing a particular way the world is understood, the way questions are formulated, the methods chosen to answer the research question and the interpretation of the results. All research is undertaken by somebody somewhere. There is no 'all-conquering gaze from nowhere' (Haraway, 1991, p. 188).

Now that many of us are over the idea that 'Truth' is somehow waiting to be discovered, we realize that to exist well on the planet we need to live easefully alongside the many truths in play. In this context, the search for abstract theories that add to the 'body of knowledge' seem far less urgent in comparison to generating greater understanding of how people can transform their particular life situation for the better. Within the approach to participatory action research articulated here, the foundational premise is that the research is for the benefit of the critical reference group. These benefits include not only the implicit actions generated within the process, but also the production of local knowledge (local theory) about how the critical reference group experience and interpret the phenomena in question.

If research is to be of benefit to the critical reference group, the research question needs to be owned by some members of the critical reference group. Therefore, a researcher seeking to work with a specific group of people in order to benefit their situation requires a very flexible approach towards developing the research project. Most likely, the researcher will already be aware of some of the issues facing a group of people in a particular context and have his or her own questions. However, to evoke specific questions participants have about their own situation requires the researcher to make strong connections with some of the people and through an engagement with the participant focus group, link to the CRG, the broader group of people sharing a particular situation. Over time, as trust and understanding develop, and as dilemmas are shared, the researcher and researcher participants will be able to frame challenges into potentially researchable questions.

The Social Arena of the Research Act

While it is the research question emerging from the experience of the critical reference group through the participant focus group that will guide the research project, as indicated above, the research question is at the hub of a social arena, a system of social worlds of various stakeholders each who have some interest in the research question. Generally, the system of stakeholders will involve a range of groups linked to the critical reference group in the context of their specific local situation, a system that can be strategically mapped setting out actual stakeholder positions on the basis of the data regarding the phenomena in question (Clarke, 2005). Such mapping is undertaken with the participant focus group. Data collection undertaken with each of the stakeholder groups will reveal their positions about the general situation of the critical reference group and, more specifically, about the research question. The overall research act will provide a means for these disparate perspectives to become better known within this social world and increase the potential for all stakeholders to gain a bigger picture of the issue at hand and possibly, in future, to reconcile disparate views and work collaboratively on the basis of greater shared understanding. The researcher occupying a specific role within this system as lead investigator of phenomena related to the research question will thereby have a basis for a professional relationship with each of the participating stakeholder groups. Potentially, the researcher will be able to take a proactive role in developing a broader perspective among all stakeholders and catalyse future collaborative action based upon the new understandings emergent from the research.

In taking on the role as an interpreter within the social arena of the research act, the researcher requires a clear negotiated understanding of his or her role in the research project with the participant focus group. In relationship to the participant focus group, capacity development is a two-way process. To what extent is the researcher able to represent views of the participant focus group? How might the researcher facilitate the opportunity for members of the participant focus group to represent their own views in forums and meetings with various stakeholder groups? A key element of the practice framework outlined above is for the researcher to 'facilitate learning and develop local capacity'. Strengthening the capacity of the participant focus group to represent themselves in previously inaccessible forums and to articulate their own perspectives in terms that other stakeholders respond to is an important capacity development role of the researcher.

While the researcher at the hub of this social arena links and, potentially, connects the stakeholder groups in the context of a local specific situation, the researcher is also a link to the broader world of research funders and the academy. The researcher has a critical role to play in keeping funders and academics involved, developing their understanding of the research project as it emerges in collaboration with the participant focus group. The degree to which the research can be aligned with the expectation of these bodies will depend significantly on the ability of the researcher to frame the project within the familiar discourse of these groups. Within the broader world, there will be people who hold a strong faith in positivist research and quantifiable measures of the world. The researcher needs a clear understanding of epistemology and how the inquiry process described here can add to every stakeholder's understanding of the phenomena in question. Therefore, the researcher requires a keen insight into the epistemological status of the emergent knowledge from the participatory action research project.

Construction and Production of Emergent Local Knowledge in the Participatory Action Research Process

Initially, in the participatory action research project, the researcher is developing relationships with potential participants from the critical reference group in order to form a participant focus group with whom to construct the research project. While the researcher has her or his own questions regarding phenomena relevant to the critical reference group, the researcher is looking for dilemmas emerging from critical reference group participants that can be expressed as researchable questions; dilemmas that some participants from the critical reference group find so compelling that they are willing to join a participant focus group and take on a commitment to engage with the research project on a regular basis over a sustained period. While for some researchers this approach may seem to be too risky in terms of timelines, funding and reporting requirements, in all likelihood there is a fallback position, a potential alternative approach; if a participant focus group fails to emerge, then, with the consent of the participants, the project could revert to a traditional ethnography or a qualitative research project. Nevertheless, once the participant focus group becomes committed to a research question aligned with the interests of the researcher, negotiations regarding research design, research roles, ethical considerations, data collection, analysis, representation, writing and dissemination can commence and continue to be ongoing through the period of the research project.

While data collection will involve participants from all the stakeholders in the social arena constructed by the research question, it is the data collected from the critical reference group and, in particular, the participant focus group that is central within this participatory action research approach to activating the sociological imagination (Mills, 1959), the exploration of the transformation of personal troubles into public issues. Where the interaction of the participant focus group builds upon one individual's experience and reveals that one person's private troubles are also shared by other participants, in this moment, personal troubles become public issues, creating the 'threefold cord' (Kelly & Sewell, 1988) in which personal information is liberated out of the interior personal world, beyond the tight dyad of the interpersonal, into the 'public' shared domain. Initially the public domain is within the participant focus group. Potentially, through this portal, the information is transmitted beyond into the chaotic outer web of contested, negotiated and celebrated meanings implicated within the myriad shifting relationships of the broader social arena of the research act and public domain.

While the process of sharing these experiences transforms private troubles into public issues, of equal moment is the *voice* of members of the critical reference group. Critical to the role of the researcher is the recognition that the sharing of meanings around similar experiences and the creation of an evolving language through the collective naming of common experiences is the genesis of local situated knowledge, theory and discourse about the phenomena in question. It is in these moments that the role of the researcher as interpreter and recorder of the emergent data is crucial. It is here the accuracy and adequacy of how participant interpretations are named and represented requires a trusting open relationship between the researcher and the participants. The researcher is in a privileged position of power with regard to representation, and the way data is recorded and interpreted. For instance, if the researcher is working with a focus group using a whiteboard to record the way participants describe phenomena, it is important that the participants are able to challenge the way the researcher is rendering their descriptions into language. The researcher needs to provide the opportunity for participants to challenge these renderings by creating a space in the process for review. It is critical the researcher records emic descriptions of phenomena through direct quotations. Regular feedback to participants of primary data in the form of transcripts of participant narratives, and later, as findings in the forms of completed research papers or chapters is critical to credible representation of, ongoing engagement and investment in, and ownership of the research by the participant focus group.

While the interaction of the participant focus group, and other formal and informal interviews with participants from both the participant focus group and the critical reference group will give rise to accounts of their experience regarding the phenomena at the focus of inquiry, of critical import is the question, 'Where in the transcripts of interview and focus group narratives do we find the issues *key* to the common experience of the critical reference group in relation to the phenomena at the focus of the inquiry?' What are the key shared themes within their perspective? While much regarding the mundane will emerge in narratives, data that are nevertheless central to triangulating the minutiae regarding the experience of the participants, how do we crack the code to reveal the critical elements of experience of members of the CRG in relation to the phenomena in question?

In order to achieve this, Denzin (1989) suggests a focus on epiphanies or defining moments of experience, which are:

> Key interactional moments that leave marks on human lives . . . in them, personal character is manifested and made apparent . . . they occur in those problematic interactional situations where the subject confronts and experiences crisis . . . and reveal underlying tensions and problems in a situation. (pp. 15–18)

Stories of these moments may emerge in interview situations, or often in focus group discussions where the sharing of one participant may prompt another to share a singular experience of their own.

Denzin suggests that accounts of these defining moments contain *key experiential elements* of the shared personal crises and problems of the critical reference group that are at the core of broader social issues. While such an epiphanic account coalesces and voices key elements within a participant's experience, a researcher who is either an 'informed reader' (1989, p. 46), or one who maintains on ongoing dialogue with the participant is able to show how these elements make sense when understood in the context of a life or lives. Hence, these key experiential elements provide categories of analysis closer to a participant's experience than many other theoretical approaches.

In this way, accounts of 'key interactional moments' (1989, p. 15) have the potential to articulate critical emic categories of meaning.

In the study with Aboriginal healthworkers (Genat et al., 2006), these analytic methods, of focusing upon accounts of crisis moments emergent within interactions of healthworkers and identifying key elements or themes of experience from within those accounts were used to frame the stories healthworker experience. The following example arose during a meeting of the participant focus group on 'best practice'.

Prior to the meeting, Rita, an Aboriginal healthworker, had spent all day in court waiting to give evidence on behalf of a client facing eviction from her government rental house. In the meeting, Rita expresses not only her frustration at 'wasting' another day in court, but also her feelings of guilt towards other clients who, in her absence, failed to receive their regular home visit and checkup. In her disquiet, she uses the forum to challenge particular facets of healthworker practice:

> I reckon we create dependency . . . I'm not a lawyer, and I've been spend-
> ing all week at court—I'm not a lawyer—I'm a healthworker—and I feel
> like everything that I've learnt, like all the paramedical [clinical] stuff—
> that's not important!—it's all the social stuff—I feel like the social takes
> over—more than the paramedical or anything to do with medical . . . like
> I can see the point of someone going with them [to court]—it's just that
> it seems, it is always the healthworker—and it should be the family, or
> even welfare's job . . . healthworkers—see this is what I mean—it's like
> the jack-of-all-trades . . . when you are doing all these other things . . .
> there's not enough of you . . .

The first theme identified from this text was how the particular holistic approach to practice adopted by these Aboriginal healthworkers exposed them to the myriad results of social disruption faced by many indigenous Australian families. Among others, these included insecure housing tenure, poverty, related social security issues, and family violence. A section in the reported results entitled, 'A holistic approach: The "social" takes over the "paramedical"' further developed this theme and contained other CRG narratives illustrating this issue. For example, a narrative of another AHW:

> This lady is constantly in need—she's got high blood pressure—she can't
> handle her money—I've been taking her to welfare places—getting food

hampers, clothes—I've even been with her shopping to see how she
spends her money to try and help her—she smokes a lot—we need some-
one to work out a budget with her—we've tried it ourselves—we need a
full-on thing with her—she doesn't have enough money for medication—
I've been ringing around for her bills, trying to get extensions—her son's
in prison—we take her there, but now he's been transferred to [a rural
prison] and she wants us to take her there—there's lots of family problems—her de facto is a drunk and is always abusing her—there's people
coming over and drinking—she's got no way of getting round—we've tried
to get her involved in some day outings, but she's not really interested.

Other headings within the reported results derived from Rita's former quote
were:

Vulnerable to Co-option: 'Colleagues don't see our case load as important', which comprised a section about how it is always the Aboriginal
healthworker who ends up as the odd-job person left to complete tasks
other health professionals do not want; and,

Discriminating Dependency: 'She wants my life', a section which elaborated the many demands faced by Aboriginal healthworkers. Indeed,
according to Rita, the scale of the many client demands, a legacy of government welfare dependency enforced historically, was that there was 'not
enough of you'. Thus, this emotional, epiphanic account of Rita shared
in interaction with her colleagues revealed fundamental aspects common
to the Aboriginal healthworker experience. The use of emic categories
of experience captured in the narrative could be used as sub-heading or
themes to structure their particular local knowledge of the phenomena
and their local theory of healthworker practice.

The Epistemological Status of the Research Findings

Implicit within the interpretive analytical standpoint of this approach to
participatory action research, is the assertion that, in social life, there is only
interpretation. According to Denzin, 'Under the interpretive paradigm,
knowledge can be assumed neither to be objective nor to be valid in any
objective sense' (1989, p. 30). Denzin proposes the purpose of an interpretive
approach to research is to enable an 'authentic understanding' (1989, p. 33) of

the problematic, lived experience of ordinary people. Within this approach, the writer uses thick description to evoke verisimilitude; the researcher attempts to draw in the reader and evoke an authentic and empathetic understanding of the key troubling experiences within people's lives.

From this post-structuralist position, and on the basis that credibility or plausibility replaces traditional conceptions of validity (Lincoln & Guba, 1985), Denzin proposes that the politics of the text along with its verisimilitude constitute its legitimacy (1997, p. 10). He quotes Stake: "a text with high verisimilitude provides the opportunity for vicarious experience, the reader, 'comes to know some things told, as if he or she had experienced them'". In this way the evocative text, when read by other stakeholders within the social arena of the research act, touches similar experiences in the life of the reader and enables an empathetic understanding of the experience of the critical reference group.

The epistemological status of the findings of a participatory action research process such as that described here exist as a truth of the participant focus group regarding a particular phenomena at a particular moment in time. While the epistemological status of the findings do not provide the basis for generalizable claims that the experience of the critical reference group in the study represents the experience of similar groups in other places, it is a valid claim that other people in similar situations may recognize similar experiences of their own within the text.

Summary

This article has described an approach to participatory action research that facilitates the construction of local situated knowledges with people whose voices are often subjugated and marginal to the deliberations of mainstream policy and program planners. Key to this approach is the role of the researcher as a facilitator, interlocuter, interpreter, capacity developer, and advocate—as a political actor in the social world of the research act alongside a group of participant researchers constituting the 'participant focus group'. Equally important is the aptitude of the researcher to understand the epistemological status of the findings from such an approach to research, their meaning and status in relation to the existing body of knowledge in the field. This approach to participatory action research builds local theory and knowledge, and positions local participants as advocates for new ways of understanding the world.

References

Blumer, H. (1969). *Symbolic interactionism: Perspective and method.* Berkeley, CA: University of California Press.

Butler, P. (1991). Reflections on good community development. *Community Quarterly, 24,* 5–10.

Clarke, A. (2005). *Situational analysis: Grounded theory after the postmodern turn.* Thousand Oaks, CA: SAGE.

Cornwall, A., & Jewkes, R. (1995). What is participatory research? *Social Science & Medicine, 41*(12), 1667–1676.

Denzin, N. K. (1989). *Interpretive interactionism.* Newbury Park, CA: SAGE.

Denzin, N. K. (1997). *Interpretive ethnography.* Thousand Oaks, CA: SAGE.

Fals Borda, O. (2001). Participatory (action) research in social theory. In P. Reason & H. Bradbury (Eds.), *Handbook of action research* (pp. 27–37). London: SAGE.

Foucault, M. (1972). *The archaeology of knowledge.* New York: Random House.

Genat, B. with Bushby, S., McGuire, M., Taylor, E., Walley, Y., & Weston, T. (2006). *Aboriginal healthworkers: Primary health care at the margins.* Nedlands: University of Western Australia Press.

Haraway, D. (1991). *Symians, cyborgs and women: The reinvention of nature.* New York: Routledge.

Jackson, T., Mitchell, S., & Wright, M. (1988). The community development continuum. In *Community development in health resources collection* (pp. 2–7). Northcote: Preston Northcote District Health Council.

Kelly, A., & Sewell, S. (1989). *With head, heart and hand.* Brisbane: Boolarong.

Lincoln, Y., & Guba, E. (1985). *Naturalistic inquiry.* Newbury Park, CA: SAGE.

Mead, G. (1934). *Mind, self and society.* Chicago, IL: University of Chicago Press.

Mills, C. W. (1959/1993). The sociological imagination. In C. Lemert (Ed.), *Social theory: The multicultural and classic readings* (pp. 379–382). Boulder, CO: Westview.

Mills, G. (2000). *Action research: A guide for the teacher researcher.* Columbus, OH: Merrill Prentice Hall.

Smith, L. (1999). *Decolonising methodologies: Research and indigenous people.* London: Zed Books.

Stringer, E. (2007). *Action research: A handbook for practitioners* (3rd edn). Thousand Oaks, CA: SAGE.

Wadsworth, Y. (1997). *Everyday evaluation on the run.* St Leonards, NSW: Allen and Unwin.

Willis, E. (2006). Introduction: Taking stock of medical dominance. *Health Sociology Review, 15*(5), 421–431.

PART III
EXEMPLARS OF SITUATIONAL ANALYSIS RESEARCH

INTRODUCTION

P ART III OF OUR BOOK is composed of exemplars—outstanding examples—of using situational analysis (SA) in empirical research. It is very gratifying to be able to include such excellent articles, given that the method is relatively new. This is possible because SA builds on the advantages of grounded theory (GT) and helps strengthen and expand it, especially by including discourse analyses. It is also exciting that SA is already appearing in research outside the United States and across varied disciplines and professional venues, in journals of family studies, social work, counseling and psychotherapy, education, public health, health policy, nursing, sociology, science and technology studies, library and information science, and beyond.

In addition to the excellent articles based on SA research, we also include in this volume "reflections" on using the SA method by the authors of the original articles.[1] The idea for reflections was provoked by the first article, "Situating Knowledges," by Jennifer Fosket, a very early, skilled, and candid user of the method. Her article is itself a reflection on SA practices. The other reflections were recruited initially for a session at meetings of the International Congress of Qualitative Inquiry in 2013 and now appear here in revised form.

To orient readers to the SA method, we next briefly discuss how to do each of the three kinds of maps in situational analysis (situational and relational, social worlds/arenas, and positional maps) and the kinds of analytic help they are designed to provide. We then discuss some key mapping issues, including tinkering with map making to produce project maps tailored to one's own research needs. One of the emphases in this volume is on using SA in critical qualitative research, and we discuss how the maps work to assist in critical analyses and introduce those articles included that are exemplars of critical SA. Last, we introduce all five exemplars of SA and discuss their distinctive engagements and contributions to the method.

The Three Kinds of Situational Analysis Maps

SA uses three kinds of maps to explore the different elements that embed our research topics: situational maps, social worlds/arenas maps, and positional maps. Together, these maps lay out the varied elements involved in the area of study including: human and nonhuman actors and actants, institutions and organizations, discourses and symbols, political economies and sociocultural landscapes, and the like. The goal is to bring together multiple perspectives—including multiple types of data commonly used in multi-sited ethnography—without being reductionist and in a way that facilitates exploring relationships among the different elements present in a situation of social action.

The focus on pictorial representation with maps allows researchers to think about their data in new ways. They allow us to represent the messiness of our research, which can be a useful way of initially entering data collection, doing analysis and, later, even overcoming analytic paralysis. They are a good way to think *across* different types of data sources (e.g., field notes, interviews, and documents). They are also a good way to think across levels of research (e.g., micro, meso, and macro levels) to see how relationships and practices actually blur such distinctions (which are today seriously questioned across the social sciences). In the process, the maps allow us to see the multiplicity and contingencies of the varying perspectives we encounter in research. In other words, we can begin to see how our research topic is "situated." We can therefore locate ourselves in the research situation as well, enabling more reflexive social research.

Each of the maps works in somewhat different ways, but all are based on creating pictorial representations of data (in addition to textual representations in memos, a practice rooted in GT). Drawing is important here, so having large pieces of paper, pencils, and erasers helps for a good start. If you prefer to work on screen, this can work well, too—if you are already adept. If not, paper and pencil give much greater freedom and allow you to think about the analysis of the data rather than how to manipulate the technology. Too often people tend to distract themselves with technology as doing analysis may be challenging and anxiety producing.

Situational Maps

Here we briefly focus on how to make messy and ordered situational maps. To make a messy situational map, simply write all the elements present in your situation of inquiry on a big piece of paper. Messy situational maps are meant to be just that, so do not feel you should be confined to making organized lists. These maps are most useful if you think freely and broadly about your research, jotting down any and all elements that come to mind from your data and from your prior knowledge, regardless of how peripheral they may seem. This process is intended to help open up the analytic process, creating room for surprise.

Messy situational maps can then be used as the basis for constructing ordered situational maps and for relational mapping. To do an ordered situational map, you use the model in Figure 2.5 Abstract Situational Map: Ordered/Working Version in Clarke's first paper in Part 1, "From Grounded Theory to Situational Analysis: What's New? How? Why?" In this version, the elements are organized into lists of individual human elements, political economic elements, discursive elements, and so on.

Once an adequate situational map is done, the next step is to start asking questions based on it and memoing your answers. *Relations* among the various elements on the map are the focus here. You might not think to ask about certain relations within the situation, but if you do quick and dirty *relational analyses based on the situational map,* they can be very revealing. To do this, first make a bunch of photocopies of your best version to date of the situational map. Then take each element in turn and think about it in relation to each other element on the map. Literally center on one element and draw lines between it and the others and *specify the nature of the relationship by describing the nature of that line* initially in your mind or aloud. Then, if it is at all interesting, put it in a memo so the idea does not "float away." You should do this systematically, one at a time, from every element on the map to every other. Use as many maps as seems useful to diagram yourself through this analytic exercise. Some people like to use different color markers.

This is the major work one does with the situational map once it is constructed. Doing some of this out loud helps articulate relations more clearly. Using a sound-sensitive tape recorder with this works well. Sometimes outcomes are tedious or silly—but at other times they can trigger breakthrough thinking. This is one of those sites where being highly systematic in considering data can flip over into the exciting and creative moments of intellectual work.

Relational maps can also help the analyst decide which stories—which relations—to pursue. Which relations are the most interesting? The least explored in prior research? How can you get at them better in your interviews and other data collection? Such questions can be especially helpful in the early stages of research when we tend to feel a bit mystified about where to go next, how to "theoretically sample," and what to memo. Theoretical sampling is a research strategy from GT and part of SA as well. It is based on the assumption that as we proceed in our research, we begin to understand a bit more and want to pursue particular topics we either did not know about initially or did not think were that important. One "samples"—seeks more data about something—based on the hunch that it will pay off substantively and theoretically. This is one of the ways in which qualitative research is "iterative"—the project is invented and reinvented over time as the researcher's understanding becomes increasingly sophisticated.

Relational analysis sessions can be very helpful in generating directions for theoretical sampling. A session should produce several relational analyses with the situational maps and several memos. Of course, such careful attention to the messy situational map will likely lead you to change that map and then you will need new photocopies and then ... you are really analyzing.

While situational and relational maps usually analyze a situation at only one particular point in time, these maps can also be used comparatively in historical research (see Clarke 2005:268–276). The articles by Clarke in Part II, and here by Fosket and by Pérez and Cannella all offer situational maps and discuss them in some detail.[2]

Social Worlds/Arenas Maps

The second major mapping strategy in SA is the social world/arenas map. A social world is a group of people who come together through a shared interest on which they are prepared to act and who use similar technologies and discourses in pursuing their mutual concerns. It is a site of commitment of some kind (e.g., a hobby group, a scholarly discipline, a ball team). An arena is an area of sustained interest and concern that brings multiple social worlds together over time. The worlds in an arena can be allies, enemies, odd bedfellows, and so forth, and arenas are commonly sites of dispute and contestation. Social worlds/arenas maps help analysts visualize these two interrelated units of analysis in social research. These maps help researchers think about the kinds of collective, organizational, and institutional elements in their projects, too often ignored in qualitative inquiry. The goal of these maps is to visualize the social relations that either are the subject of our research or that inform and shape the subject of our research.

To make a social worlds/arenas map, start by putting the subject of your research in the middle of the page. Write out the different social worlds that come together around that area of shared concern and draw circles with dotted lines around each. You may note the key discourses and technologies of different social worlds as you go, including these within the circle.

As your map takes shape, start to consider the relationships between different social worlds. Do some social worlds overlap? If so, visualize these relationships between social worlds by having the lines of the circles overlap. The circles of social worlds maps are often drawn with dotted rather than solid lines to show the porosity of organizational life. After all, most of us move in and out of different social worlds many times each day!

Finally, are some groups more or less central to the arena? For social worlds that are more central, make the circle bigger; for social worlds that are more marginal, make the circle smaller. Revising these maps in this way allows you to get a handle on your research. In the process, ask yourself if your research topic is an arena or if it is part of an arena or even multiple arenas. If it is part of an arena, include this in your map using the lines to show how the topic of your research is embedded in and, if relevant, exceeds an arena.

Making a social worlds/arenas map requires a fair amount of knowledge regarding one's research topic. That said, these maps can be started early in the research project and revised throughout as your understanding of your research topic, involved social worlds, and related arenas develops and changes. Just keep in mind that these maps may start as tentative drafts; doing the maps by hand helps embody the provisionality of our understanding in the early phases of research.

Social worlds/arenas maps make it clear that there are more than two sides to a debate by showing the multiple voices involved. In the process, these maps also help us better understand social hierarchies. We see which groups are centrally involved in an arena and which are not. And we can begin to consider why some groups are more central—and perhaps more powerful or influential—than others by looking at the technologies used and the discourses that each different group produces and engages. We can also address how different ideas about an area of sustained concern result from features of the social worlds involved. For example, how do the technologies and discourses used by social world 1 shape how arena X is understood? How does this compare with social world 2? While social worlds/arenas maps usually analyze an arena at only one particular point in time, these maps can also be used comparatively in historical research (see Clarke 2005:276–282).

Adele Clarke and Theresa Montini's (1993) paper "The Many Faces of RU486: Tales of Situated Knowledges and Technological Contestations" was one of the inspirations for Clarke's development of SA method. It demonstrates each of these features of social worlds/arenas mapping (see also Clarke 1991, 2005:39–51, 109–124), as well as developing the concept of *implicated actors* (see also Clarke 2005:46–48). The subject of that research was RU486, an oral abortifacient that eliminates the need for a surgical procedure.

RU486 was itself very differently constructed by each of the different social worlds within the fraught abortion arena in the United States in the early 1990s. Clarke and Montini asked who was active and creating discourses about RU486. They found pertinent social worlds including politicians, political groups, health care providers, pharmaceutical companies, women's health advocates, anti-abortion groups, the FDA, medical professional societies, and others. Researching how each group constructed RU486, they studied the history, techniques, and discourses of these social worlds along the way. Clarke and Montini also asked what social worlds and discourses were missing from the arena. The most striking absence they found were female users of RU486 who were *represented* by other groups but were themselves missing as vocal actors from the arena. Clarke and Montini therefore described female users of RU486 as "implicated actors." Stem cell researchers, too, were implicated actors, choosing not to reveal their involvement.

The article is explicitly structured to show the different perspectives of the many social worlds dwelling in one shared arena on something about which they profoundly disagree. The article begins with an overview of the scientific properties of RU486, then describes each major social world in the RU486 abortion arena at that time *and* their distinctive construction of RU486 per se. This organizational format helped make the very complex situation more accessible to readers because the structure of the argument— and the arena—can be quickly grasped. (The organization is based on the concept of 'boundary object;' see note 3.) It also allowed the authors to detail *different* positions on RU486 held *within* some social worlds, which were not always unified. Such capacity to reveal complexities is a major advantage of the SA method. A full SA analysis of this discourse analysis project is in the text (Clarke 2005:187–204).

The article by Genat in Part II, and here by Fosket and by Pérez and Cannella offer social worlds/arenas maps and discussions.[3]

Positional Maps Focus

The third major cartographic strategy in SA is positional maps. Here the emphasis is on discursive positions taken and not taken in the data on issues of concern, focus, and often but not always contestation. Unlike situational and social worlds/arenas maps, positional maps do not include representations of individual, collective, and/or institutional actors. Rather, these maps focus *exclusively* on *positions in a discourse*. A key assumption of positional maps is that individuals, groups, and institutions can and do often hold multiple and even contradictory positions on a given issue of concern. By focusing on the *full range* of articulated positions, positional maps assist analysts in seeing complexity, variation, and heterogeneity in situations where once only binaries and/or longstanding, oversimplified divisions may have appeared. This often enables analysts to see established lines of controversy and division in fresh ways.

Perhaps the most innovative and analytically useful aspect of positional mapping is the way in which it helps analysts see not only positions that are clearly articulated but also muted and silent positions in situations of inquiry. In doing so, this form of mapping works against reifying dominant voices in our analyses. Identifying these silences can be interesting and important and spark surprising new lines of inquiry.

In constructing positional maps it is critical to be constantly mindful that positional maps are *not* intended to be representations of individuals, groups, or institutions, especially for those not accustomed to analyzing discourses. Instead, as we have described, they are *maps of positions articulated in the discourse* on their own terms. The goal is to represent the full range of positions. Positional maps can be constructed from a range of discursive materials gathered through fieldwork, participant observation, interviewing, texts, and documents of various kinds, including websites, for example.

To make positional maps, however, one needs to have a good grasp of the major issues in the situation of inquiry on which different positions have been articulated. Look to traditional grounded theory coding, memoing, and situational and social/worlds arena maps for guidance. For analysts working on topics of sustained public debate, it might be difficult to identify the central issues on which different positions have been articulated. Instead, what might stand out are simply the positions. This is fine. It is helpful to make note of these and then think about the key issues at stake in the positions you have noted. Pay close attention to *what matters most* in different positions. This can then form the basis for constructing different axes in your positional maps, which tends to be the most challenging aspect of doing this kind of map.

Positional maps typically have two axes along which positions are arrayed. Often the axes can be constructed in terms of "more versus less," but other categories may be used. As we mentioned, one of the more difficult tasks in positional mapping is determining which issues to place on the axes and which two axes to place in the same map. Here it is often easier to start with the biggest, hottest, most controversial issue in the overall discourse and seek the two main criteria argued about. For the RU486 abortion arena, the issues of its safety and morality were both hot and made for an excellent and revelatory map.

You will likely construct many positional maps with different axes before arriving at one or a few maps most helpful to you in seeing the full range of positions taken in the discourse. As you construct your maps, it is important to plot not only articulated positions but also those that remain unarticulated. While many analysts use positional mapping to analyze positions articulated at only one particular point in time, these maps can also be used comparatively in historical research (see Clarke 2005:282–288).

The article by Clarke on feminist SA in Part II, and those here by Fosket, by Pérez and Cannella, and by Washburn all offer positional maps.[4]

Mapping Issues

One of the things we have learned as developers and teachers of SA, and exemplified by the articles here, is that in actual practice, people sometimes use the method a bit differently. Thus, readers will notice that some of the contributors' maps do not precisely follow the strategies for mapping put forth by Clarke (2005). Some have done so in earlier iterations and chose to publish simpler and more readily understandable versions. Others have creatively adapted their mapping to best capture aspects of their own projects. They have tinkered with it to meet the needs and goals of their projects. Clarke (2005:136–140) calls these "project maps" and encourages their use for both presentations and publications. (In fact, the section on project maps in the 2nd edition of the SA text will be longer.)

In terms of following the mapping strategies as laid out in the method versus tinkering on your own, we encourage both. We do believe it is very worthwhile to first follow the SA strategies to see what those maps can and do offer to your project and to develop project maps later on. Each of the

SA maps is designed to do a particular kind of work. Specifically, *situational maps*, which lay out *all* of the elements in the situation being researched, work as excellent "holding devices" so that researchers need not try and remember everything, but have prior maps as useful references. They also work as "reminder devices," nagging for attention. The relational maps can help you see relations between the elements that might otherwise never occur to you or occur too late to be of best use. They can also direct the overall research through specifying the most interesting and least researched relations—a kind of theoretical sampling.

The *social worlds/arenas maps* require the researcher to pay some attention to the organizational and institutional situation—often full of constraints. Foucault (1975) calls this more broadly "the conditions of possibility." Given the givens, what can—and perhaps cannot—be done? These maps also help make some of the institutional history visible in ways often ignored in qualitative inquiry but possibly quite consequential.

Last, the *positional maps* offer two big advantages. First, they push the researcher to look *solely* at the positions in the discourses in the situation—to untie them from individuals and groups and look carefully at the *full range* of positions in the discourse data. Too often, our thinking follows old channels rather than pushing harder analytically to see or seek new understandings. The second major advantage of positional maps is that they allow us to see *positions missing in the data*. That is, as we fill in the grid formed by the two axes with the positions we have found in the data, the *range of possible positions* is laid out. Based on our knowledge of the data gathered to date, we can specify "Position Not Taken" on the map. Some of these will be totally expectable, but others may be surprising and interesting. Are they gaps in our data? Things not to be spoken of? Thus, positional maps are useful in opening up how we analyze.

We also encourage analysts to take off from situational maps and create your own project maps—preferably *after* doing situational maps and garnering the analytic advantages they provide. People have tinkered and created their own maps from all three kinds of situational maps. Many kinds of tinkering with the different maps are possible and we cannot begin to list them. Several articles included in this volume offer tinkered project maps to illustrate. See articles by Genat, Fosket, and Pérez and Cannella.

Researchers may or may not choose to include maps in their publications, and we have two research exemplars that do not include maps (one by Gagnon, Jacob, and Holmes, and the other by French and Miller). All the others do. Both Fosket's and Pérez and Cannella's articles include all three kinds of maps and their own project maps. Washburn's article includes a positional map that is the focus of the whole paper (see also Friese 2010). The SA maps most likely to end up in published articles and book chapters are social worlds/arenas maps and positional maps. Social worlds/arenas maps also tend to provoke great project maps. As you approach final reports and publications, you may want to produce more polished versions of your maps to include—or not. Trying such maps out in a public presentation can be most valuable in determining whether or not to try and publish it and in revising and polishing the map for publication.

An interesting advantage of SA discussed across most of the articles included here is its value in facilitating collaboration. Precisely because mapping is visual rather than narrative, ideas are much more easily sparked and shared. The reflections by the authors also noted that collaborative mapping helped "level the playing field" between faculty and doctoral student researchers. Everyone was pitching in, analyzing together. This evokes Anselm Strauss's collaborative method of teaching GT—working groups that meet regularly, read, and analyze each other's data, read and critique memos, diagrams, research reports, and so on. Let us draw your attention to Strauss's (1987) book *Qualitative Analysis for Social Scientists*, which offers transcripts of some group analysis sessions (including one in which Clarke was a participant). Strauss also pursued a lot of research in teams of three to six researchers, and some of them have written about such efforts (e.g., Lessor 2000; Wiener 2007).

One of the facets of GT that SA wholly adopts is the process of memoing—writing up ideas, thoughts, analysis of a set of data, almost anything valuable to the project. Kathy Charmaz (2014:162–191) devotes an entire chapter to memoing in her book on doing GT. In this collection, Gagnon, Jacob, and Holmes also vehemently argue for memoing as well as talking about the maps during analytic sessions. They felt too much of their discussion regarding data analysis got lost in the excitement of the moment and it would have been well worth it to write more memos.

Using Situational Analysis in Critical Qualitative Research

In the Introduction to this volume, we provided a brief overview of the history of qualitative inquiry largely since WWII. Critical qualitative inquiry has grown dramatically during this period and is especially lively across the social sciences and humanities today. To reiterate, "critical" operates as a very broad umbrella under which are loosely gathered a wide array of approaches including feminist, anti-racist, anti/postcolonial, indigenous, neo-Marxist, Bourdieusian, and many other approaches concerned broadly with social justice and inequalities. The civil rights, feminist, and anti-war movements of the 1960s and 1970s gave such approaches considerable vigor. LGBT, disability rights, and other subsequent movements have both sustained and expanded such critical edges. Inside the academy, the rise of cultural studies, women's studies, ethnic/racial studies, queer studies, and the like did so as well.

Two domains with long and strong critical traditions are health and education—core domains of living deeply affected by political economies. Karl Marx wrote *The Communist Manifesto* with Friedrich Engels (1848). Significantly, Engels (1844) had already researched and written *The Condition of the Working Class in England in 1844* about Manchester—the heartland of the Industrial Revolution. The book laid bare the severe consequences of urbanization and industrialization for workers and their families in terms of worsened conditions of health, sanitation, safety, and longevity. Contrary to the myth, these new industrial workers had lower incomes than rural workers and lived in unhealthier environments. Many thousands of health researchers have followed this critical path, including in qualitative inquiry, over the last century plus (e.g., Birn & Brown 2013; Navarro & Berman 1983; Waitzkin 2011). One of our authors, Dave Holmes, coedited *Critical Interventions in the Ethics of Healthcare* (Murray & Holmes 2009). Thus, it comes as no surprise that we offer several critical articles in health and medical domains, by Gagnon, Jacob, and Holmes on a public health campaign, by French and Miller on creating the entrepreneurial hospital, and by Washburn on biomonitoring.

Education and access to education also became major social issues in the 19th century as the middle classes emerged and formal education could allow upward mobility into it. Public schooling for children gradually became understood as a fundamental right. Higher education dramatically expanded post-WWII transnationally, and colleges and universities exploded with new students thanks to the G.I. Bill in the United States, similar programs in Canada, and expanded access in Britain and Europe.[5]

As political economic patterns globalized over the last half century, the need for education increased, raising fundamental problems in terms of access across social classes transnationally, especially among the impover-ished where basic literacy may be an issue. Perhaps the key critical theorist and practitioner who emerged in this domain was Paolo Friere, whose *Peda-gogy of the Oppressed* (1970) and *Education for Critical Consciousness* (1973) are still fundamental, liberatory, and inspirational readings. It is thus not at all surprising that some of the most critical qualitative research has emerged around educational issues (e.g., Kincheloe & McLaren 1994, 2000; Kinche-loe, McLaren, & Steinberg 2011), and related feminist educational concerns (e.g., Lather 1991, 2007; St. Pierre & Pillow 2000).

Our contributors Gaile Cannella and Michelle Pérez have coedited both the *Critical Qualitative Research Reader* (Steinberg & Cannella 2012) and *Cri-tical Qualitative Inquiry: Foundations and Futures* (Cannella, Pérez, & Pasque 2015), important contributions to new initiatives for using critical qualitative approaches in higher education research and beyond.[6] We draw your atten-tion to a particularly useful paper by Cannella and Lincoln (2012), "Deploy-ing Qualitative Methods for Critical Social Purposes." It begins with an interesting discussion of changes in critical approaches over the past two decades or so, many of which are the result of feminist, anti-racist, and post-colonial critiques of critical theorizing and practice.

The authors then focus on the knotty problem of why critical projects do not necessarily make the kinds of differences in the world that they seek. A particular challenge they detail has been the different expectations of language use and writing for/in the academy compared to for/in the com-munity, popular media, and so on.[7] We want to add our voices to the call for being "public intellectuals," scholars in the academy who *also* step outside and translate their research for broader audiences and pursue non-academic proj-ects as well. Many younger scholars are already finding new and more widely effective spaces and places for critical work in social media and beyond, such as *The Feminist Wire*. Based on years of feminist women's health research, Clarke and her former student Monica Casper contributed to four different editions of *Our Bodies Ourselves* on the Pap smear. Expectations for academ-ics to have "an electronic presence" are growing, and we can go far beyond per-sonal websites in pursuing this. Analyses of current events, movies, YouTube videos, and the like are excellent means of using our critical gaze to open up perception of how various "isms" are taken for granted and naturalized as "just how things are." The pragmatist interactionist mantra that "things could be otherwise" is an excellent reminder.

Exemplars of Critical Situational Analysis

We include in this book several exemplary papers using SA in clearly critical qualitative research projects. First, Michelle Pérez and Gaile Cannella's "Situational Analysis as an Avenue for Critical Qualitative Research" explicitly shows how SA allowed them to pursue critical aspects of their work more successfully. Their research focused on neoliberal public education "reforms" instituted in post-Katrina New Orleans—largely privatization of a formerly public and unionized education system—as instantiations of "disaster capitalism" (Adams 2012; Klein 2007).

Here SA was especially helpful in exploring the often fleeting and shifting discourses and conditions existing within each specific context they examined over time (Cannella & Pérez 2009; Pérez & Cannella 2013). Specifically, SA mapping enabled them to track what was happening as it occurred and preserved their tracings. Pérez and Cannella also found SA valuable in maintaining their focus on emergent design (such as theoretical sampling) and employing multiple critical, feminist theoretical lenses and methodological tools throughout the research process. They found SA allowed a more fluid reading of the situations as they unfolded, as it helped them resist static representations of data.

Another paper that critiques neoliberal developments, French and Miller's "Leveraging the 'Living Laboratory': On the Emergence of the Entrepreneurial Hospital," centers on a new institutional form in Canada in which patients become human capital deployed as hospitals increasingly "sell" themselves as research sites for pharmaceutical and other clinical trials, a large, growing, and increasingly transnational industry (e.g., Cooper & Waldby 2014). Successful hospitals now leverage their "living laboratories"—patient populations—to enhance their marketable reputations as centers of translational research, innovation, and competent care.

French and Miller drew on both interviews and government-sponsored "oncology asset maps"—discursive marketing documents aimed at accelerating the commercialization of public-sector life sciences research. They initially viewed these oncology asset maps as mute discursive evidence because none of their respondents mentioned them. They then decided to actually ask their participants to comment directly on these maps and found a wide range of perspectives on the propriety of deploying patients in such ways that included serious concerns about ethics that were largely not discussed (see also Murray & Holmes 2009).

In their paper, "Governing through (In)Security: A Critical Analysis of a Fear-based Public Health Campaign," Marilou Gagnon, Jean Daniel Jacob, and Dave Holmes's main objective was to expand the use of situational analysis in critical qualitative research projects that specifically analyze discourses and how they operate. They studied a public health campaign to prevent sexually transmitted infections in Québec, Canada, called "Condoms: They Aren't a Luxury." Their data included documents retrieved from this campaign actually developed by commercial advertising organizations to use social marketing strategies.

Gagnon, Jacob, and Holmes identified the major discourses and found fear everywhere. The ads relentlessly constructed young adults as a risky group—the target audience that needs to be brutally shocked into action to abandon risky sexual behaviors and adopt safer sex practices. Drawing on Foucault's (1979; see also Dean 1999) concept of governmentality, they found this created governance through "a state of permanent (in)security" of which they were critical. Validating in the extreme, recent research in Australia, another former "settler colony," by Pedrana and colleagues (2014) found that having "no drama" and using humor instead of fear were keys to success for a similar HIV/STI-prevention mass-media public health campaign—the exact reverse of the negative stereotyping and harping tone of the fear-based Québec campaign.

Introducing the Five Exemplars of Situational Analysis Research

We next describe in greater detail the five excellent articles that appear in the second section of the volume. While Fosket's article "Situating Knowledge" is in itself a reflection on using the method of SA, we include postpublication reflections written for this volume by all the other authors. Here we discuss the contribution of each article vis-à-vis SA method in some depth to underscore their lessons for other users. We suggest that you read about the article here, then read the article and the author(s)' own reflections on using the method.

Jennifer Fosket's "Situating Knowledge"

This is very much a how-to article by one of the earliest adapters of SA (see also Fosket 2004, 2010). Fosket discusses the processes of using SA and doing all three kinds of maps, detailing specific problems she encountered, how she addressed them, and how she kept putting SA back to work in her project. That is, once she figured out a problem, she would go forward, apply the solution, and keep the analysis moving ahead. This kind of iterative use of a method is very common across qualitative research, and learning to "get right back on the horse" after landing on one's nose analytically is key to mastery of a method. In other words, don't stop working in the midst of confronting an analytic problem, but address it and try again. Then stop for the day—with a sigh of accomplishment rather than dismay.

Fosket is particularly eloquent about the agonies and ecstasies of analysis, getting stuck and unstuck, and how to keep track of one's analytic progress when feeling more chaotic than systematic. This is a real-world experiential view of the process of doing research, one of those papers newcomers especially find immensely solacing and reassuring. She also nicely captures the joy and excitement of special moments of discovery in research, memories of which help us get over the difficult humps.[8]

Fosket is a medical sociologist and science and technology studies scholar. The project discussed here was her dissertation research on the then innovative use of chemotherapy drugs, which had previously only been used in oncology medicine for *treatment* of diagnosed breast cancer to also be prescribed for *healthy* women at high risk for breast cancer as a strategy for *prevention*. She studied the very large STAR trial, a clinical trial that compared two different chemotherapy drugs with potential for this innovative use.

This project took Fosket into several social worlds, some of which overlapped, while others did not. However, all were coming together and/or implicated in what Fosket calls the "STAR trial arena." The complexity of her project quickly led Fosket to feel overwhelmed by data she intuitively knew were connected but could not easily see through traditional grounded theory coding and memoing. In turning to situational mapping, Fosket was able to clarify relationships between elements and gain greater insight into the dynamics and contingencies shaping knowledge production in and through the STAR trial. Her very accessible article provides a candid and reflexive account and offers excellent situational, social worlds/arenas and positional maps, and maps tailored to her project—project maps. Her Figure 5.3 beautifully captures all the major social worlds involved in the clinical trial and the stakes each had in it. Fosket offers superb advice for those new to SA, and encourages "thick analysis." This is a terrific article to read—and reread—if you get stuck in your analysis, as she certainly was.

Michelle Pérez and Gaile Cannella's "Using Situational Analysis for Critical Qualitative Research Purposes"

This article originally appeared in Denzin and Giardina's *Qualitative Inquiry and Global Crisis* (Left Coast Press, Inc., 2011), appropriate for their research on neoliberal "educational reform" in New Orleans after the disaster of Hurricane Katrina. They thoughtfully and reflexively provide readers with another excellent "how-to-do-SA" article, also offering all three kinds of SA maps. The authors sought to critically map post-Katrina New Orleans as a site of disaster capitalism, defined as "orchestrated raids on the public sphere in the wake of catastrophic events, combined with the treatment of disasters as exciting market opportunities" (Klein 2007:6; see also Adams 2012). Pérez and Cannella focus on the opportunistic privatization of the previously public education system after the disaster, successfully using SA to create new imaginaries for critical qualitative inquiry. Offering their own strong introduction to critical research, Pérez and Cannella detail the particular traditions on which they drew in this project (see also Sanders 2009).

Of note regarding the SA method, they found that due to the rapidly changing situation in New Orleans vis-à-vis public education post-Katrina, their many iterations of situational maps were particularly useful across the months of their on-site research (e.g., Cannella & Pérez 2009). While there is a chapter in the SA text on using SA in historical research (Clarke 2005:Chap. 7), that is more common across decades. Thus, Pérez and Cannella nicely open up the meaning of historical uses for SA to include situations of rapid change.

Their neat or ordered situational maps drew Pérez and Cannella's attention more directly to organizations they had casually noted on their messy maps, pushing them to gather data on them. They then productively tracked down representatives of those organizations and their media statements. Providing their own adaptations of situational maps and relational maps, as well as social spheres/power arenas and positional maps, Pérez and Canella adapted SA for their own purposes with gusto. They found their power arenas map helped them to both see what and who had been marginalized and hidden and to decide which of the many possible stories they should ultimately choose to tell in their publications. They had sought a method useful for a critical project about global crisis, and SA worked very well. This is most gratifying.

Rachel Washburn's "Rethinking the Disclosure Debates: A Situational Analysis of the Multiple Meanings of Human Biomonitoring Data"

This examines a recent debate in the environmental health sciences over whether research participants should be given the results of chemical exposure tests performed on their bodily fluids when the clinical significance of such tests is still unknown. Washburn shows that while much attention had been given to differing interpretations of bioethical principles among key stakeholders in this testing, important divisions of opinion also existed in other unexamined areas. Through her analysis, she revealed that different understandings about *both* the meanings *and* the usefulness of chemical exposure data were perhaps just as critical as ethical issues in shaping positions on whether and how to share exposure data with participants.

Washburn is a medical sociologist and science and technology studies scholar, and this article is based on her dissertation research (see also Washburn 2013, 2014). Here she used a subset of her multi-site data—interviews with scientists and public health advocates actively involved in decision making about communicating biomonitoring data to those who were monitored. To analyze the debates, Washburn focused on positional maps, struggling mightily to discern the proper axes for the maps, often the most challenging part of doing positional maps. Her mapping revealed three different positions on the *usefulness* of the data to individuals and groups that had previously gone unexplained: (1) that these single measurement data were not useful; (2) that they could be partially useful under certain circumstances; and (3) that all such data are very useful as they clearly document "chemical trespass."

In her reflection, Washburn is explicitly appreciative of how SA helped her organize her data. Handling large amounts of data can be daunting, to say the least (see also Fosket this volume). She had been especially drawn to Strauss's social worlds/arenas theorizing before she found SA and was thrilled to see it built into the method as map making. She also found the explicit inclusion of the nonhuman particularly valuable given that her research is on biomonitoring where specific chemicals and instruments matter significantly.

Like Pérez and Cannella, Washburn valued how the maps worked as holding devices, revealing complexities in the situation over time. Like Clarke and Montini (1993) discussed above, she used social worlds/arenas mapping to grasp the varied meanings ascribed to biomonitoring in different settings and how these meanings also facilitated different kinds of work happening in those settings.[9] Ultimately, Washburn demonstrates how positional mapping can be used to analyze and rethink the terms of an existing public debate. Her article demonstrates that in addition to helping analysts to see silent positions, positional mapping can also work to make muted, but certainly consequential, lines of contestation visible.

Marylou Gagnon, Jean-Daniel Jacob, and Dave Holmes's "Governing through (In)Security: A Critical Analysis of a Fear-based Public Health Campaign"

This article also used SA in a critical inquiry. It was pursued collaboratively, and SA was a new method for all the authors. They reflect retrospectively with appreciation that SA not only encouraged but pushed them to attend to *all* the discourses in their situation rather than immediately focus on a dominant discourse while ignoring the rest. They realized the public health campaigns that concern them always produce multiple consequential discourses, too often not tracked.

In further deconstructing the discourse, Gagnon, Jacob, and Holmes sought to analyze both visible and invisible elements. They identified *both* what was there (i.e., words, images, symbols, logos, messages, etc.) *and* what remained "silent" in the discourse (i.e., marketing agencies, young adults, STI testing clinics and services, sexual education, condom negotiation skills, condom usage and accessibility, etc.). SA, specifically the relational maps, allowed them to track and link the fear-based discourse produced and marketing and advertising agencies, public health agencies, cost-effectiveness goals of prevention campaigns, debates on the use of fear in public health, and constructions of young adults as complacent and risky. They found a particular biopolitical economy at work that was incongruent with the cultural milieu in which it was operating, sadly making such campaigns ineffective.

Gagnon, Jacob, and Holmes's reflection also takes up the important issue of memoing which is part of the practice of both GT and SA. They ardently encourage memoing *at the time of collaborative mapping* based on their retrospective regrets at *not* having done so. For doing so, taping the analytic session might be a great strategy so that the memoing is automatic rather than an interruption. Summing up orally at the end of the analytic session on tape could also help structure the memo. We would also add that memos are not only for tracking analytic and methodological decisions and ideas for further work, but can also provide the foundations for paragraphs and whole sections of articles and chapters. Writing while you are excited about an idea often produces livelier text—sorely needed! Gagnon, Jacob, and Holmes dream, as we do, of a means of digitizing maps that is not too cumbersome and technically fraught. We hope to have some strategies for doing so in the 2nd edition of the SA text (Clarke, Friese, & Washburn forthcoming 2016).

Martin French and Fiona Miller's "Leveraging the 'Living Laboratory': On the Emergence of the Entrepreneurial Hospital"

This article contributes most strongly here to taking the nonhuman—actants rather than actors—seriously as key elements in situations under analysis. They had pursued fieldwork and in-depth interviews on innovation, technology transfer, and commercialization initiatives in a Canadian academic health science system. Among the documentary data were "oncology asset maps," government-sponsored marketing documents aimed at accelerating the commercialization of public-sector life sciences research. Yet the respondents supposedly doing the innovating were not mentioning these items in the interviews. Drawing on SA, they decided to enroll these discursive objects—or better, discursive actants—in the representational process.

Specifically, French and Miller pursued theoretical sampling strategies from GT in which you add or change interview questions based on your research to date to get at something that seems theoretically promising. In their theoretical sampling, French and Miller started explicitly asking participants about the oncology asset maps in the interviews and hit a jackpot. Instead of being inert or neutral organizational documents as they had imagined, these maps were in some ways "hot potatoes" or "elephants in the room." They needed to be asked about to emerge from the shadows and provoked considerable and heterogeneous discussion and debate which their article documents. SA intentionally seeks to "turn up the volume" on "lesser but still present discourses" in a situation (Clarke 2005:175). In this case, the researchers' theoretical sampling intervened by deploying the "mute evidence" to provoke discussion.

Analytically, these discussions also allowed the researchers to link concepts of biopolitics and economics with the participants' own discussions of their work—also no mean feat. They reflected: "Confrontations with the asset map provoked a more head-on, fulsome and thickly descriptive situational analysis of our participants' views of the entrepreneurial mission and vision of their organizations."

The collaboration between Martin French and Fiona Miller was also facilitated by SA. At the time, Miller was both a professor and an experienced GT researcher while French was a doctoral student, and neither knew SA well. They were able to "meet in the middle" over the mapping processes, which were new to both of them. As they analyzed together, the salience of their different approaches and skill levels dissipated. Although it makes total sense that the maps would work well in precisely this way, as teachers and users of SA, we had not anticipated it.

In conclusion, we hope you find the articles and the reflections on using SA by these thoughtful researchers useful in your pursuit of SA projects. Best wishes for good situational analyses.

Notes

1. We thank Norm Denzin for encouraging Adele Clarke to organize a session of reflections on using SA at the 2013 meetings of the IIQI. All the reflections published here except those of Fosket and Washburn were initially presented at that session.

2. Psychologist Tom Strong and colleagues (2012) report on their SA study of how counselors responded to the DSM-IV-TR, a highly contested psychiatrically oriented administrative set of classifications of mental problems. They offer situational, relational, and two different positional maps of their data, which was innovatively generated through an online survey of counselors, invited contributions to a website blog, and in-depth interviews. Strong and colleagues used SA because of its strengths in elucidating differences and helping researchers specify the array of positions taken in a discourse. Indeed, they found many and divergent strategies used to deal with the requirement to use the DSM-IV-TR and a wide array of positions about it, noting particular tensions among counselors who practice from nonpsychiatric approaches to therapy.

3. See Clarke and Star (2008) for an extensive review of works using the social worlds/arenas model, and also Star and Griesemer's (1989) concept of boundary objects, which is part of the social worlds/arenas conceptual tool bag. (See also Star 2010.) Timmermans and colleagues (2015) focus on Star's work, especially boundary objects. Clarke and Friese (2007) focus on social worlds and arenas issues and provide situational and relational maps of Carrie Friese's project on cloning of endangered species and then discuss the challenges of mapping Friese's research project, which did not fit well with the basic social worlds/arenas framework. The clonings were events that happened rarely across established social worlds that were not organized into a cloning arena. This article discusses alternative meso-level frameworks to supplement social worlds/arenas maps in such situations as networks and assemblages. The key argument is the importance of having a strong grasp of the organizational and institutional elements of a situation.

4. Another excellent article using positional mapping is Friese's (2010) substantively complex paper analyzing the debates surrounding the classification of chimeras—offspring of
endangered animals produced through cloning using domestic animals as surrogates. Friese
provides a classic positional map that shows clearly how she generated the different positions
taken in the debate from her interviews and discursive materials. Then she goes beyond classic
SA to incorporate the notion of shared schemas, "knowledge structures that represent objects
or events and provide default assumptions about their characteristics" (DiMaggio 1997:269).
Friese argues that the emphasis on discourse, language, and symbolism in positional maps
can be more fully elaborated using this analytical framework. She then provides an excellent
schematic/positional diagram that organizes the varied positions taken in the debate more
coherently. Friese thus extended the methods of SA, a lovely contribution. See Clarke and
Friese (2007) for Friese's situational and relational maps discussed in note 3. See also Friese
(2009, 2013) and see note 2 for another exemplar.

5. In the United States:

> benefits included low-cost mortgages, low-interest loans to start a business, cash payments
> of tuition and living expenses to attend university, high school or vocational education, as
> well as one year of unemployment compensation. It was available to every veteran who had
> been on active duty during the war years for at least ninety days and had not been dishon-
> ourably discharged; combat was not required. By 1956, roughly 2.2 million veterans had
> used the G.I. Bill education benefits to attend colleges or universities, and an additional 5.6
> million used these benefits for some kind of training program. Canada operated a similar
> program for its World War II veterans, with an economic impact similar to the American
> case. (see http://en.wikipedia.org/wiki/G.I._Bill)

British and French universities gradually expanded as well.

6. A special issue of the *International Review of Qualitative Research* on this topic is planned for
2016 or 2017.

7. We do, however, also deeply value intense scholarly engagements with difficult technical
vocabularies that must be learned with care (see, e.g., Lather 1996). All too often, the work
of social scientists is expected to be accessible and without jargon (theoretical or technical
vocabulary). Natural scientists certainly do not face such absurd expectations. This is another
indication of hierarchies in the sciences. *All* disciplines generate technical vocabularies in their
pursuit and production of knowledge, and *all* scholars need sites where such engagements are
wholly legitimate.

8. For a novel evoking this experience of analytic joy among anthropologists, see King (2014).

9. Washburn is describing what Star and Griesemer (1989) call a "boundary object," an important concept in social worlds/arenas theory and science and technology studies. Boundary
objects are things that exist at junctures where different social worlds meet in an arena of
mutual concern. Boundary objects can be treaties among countries, software programs for
users in different settings, even concepts themselves. Here the basic social process is "translat-
ing the object" to address the multiple specific needs or demands placed on it by the different
worlds involved. Boundary objects are often very important to many/most of those worlds,
hence can be sites of intense controversy and competition for the power to define them. The
study of boundary objects can be an important pathway into complex situations, allowing
the analyst to study the different participants through their distinctive relations with and
discourses about a specific boundary object. Boundary objects can be human or nonhuman.

On the conceptual tool box of social worlds/arenas theory, see Clarke (2005:45–52). On boundary objects, see Star and Griesemer (1989), Clarke and Star (2008), and Timmermans et al. (2015).

References

Adams, V. 2012. *Markets of Sorrow, Labours of Faith: New Orleans in the Wake of Katrina.* Durham, NC: Duke University Press.

Birn, A. E. & T. Brown (Eds.). 2013. *Comrades in Health: U.S. Health Internationalists, Abroad and at Home.* Rutgers, NJ: Rutgers University Press.

Cannella, G. S. & Y. S. Lincoln. 2012. Deploying Qualitative Methods for Critical Social Purposes. In S. R. Steinberg & G. S. Cannella (Eds.), *Critical Qualitative Research Reader* (pp. 104–114). New York: Peter Lang Publishers.

Cannella, G. S. & M. S. Pérez. 2009. Power-shifting at the Speed of Light: Critical Qualitative Research Post-disaster. In N. K. Denzin & M. D. Giardina (Eds.), *Qualitative Inquiry and Social Justice* (pp. 165–186). Walnut Creek, CA: Left Coast Press, Inc.

Cannella, G., S. M. S. Pérez, & P. A. Pasque (Eds.). 2015. *Critical Qualitative Inquiry: Foundations and Futures.* Walnut Creek, CA: Left Coast Press, Inc.

Charmaz, K. 2014. *Constructing Grounded Theory: A Practical Guide through Qualitative Analysis* (2nd ed.). London: Sage.

Clarke, A. E. 1991. Social Worlds Theory as Organizational Theory. In D. Maines (Ed.), *Social Organization and Social Process: Essays in Honor of Anselm Strauss* (pp. 17–42). Hawthorne, NY: Aldine de Gruyter.

Clarke, A. E. 2005. *Situational Analysis: Grounded Theory after the Postmodern Turn.* Thousand Oaks, CA: Sage.

Clarke, A. E. & C. Friese. 2007. Situational Analysis: Going beyond Traditional Grounded Theory. In A. Bryant & K. Charmaz (Eds.), *Handbook of Grounded Theory* (pp. 694–743). London: Sage.

Clarke, A. E. & T. Montini. 1993. The Many Faces of RU486: Tales of Situated Knowledges and Technological Contestations. *Science, Technology & Human Values* 18(1):42–78.

Clarke, A. E. & S. L. Star. 2008. The Social Worlds/Arenas Framework as a Theory–Methods Package. In E. Hackett, O. Amsterdamska, M. Lynch, & J. Wacjman (Eds.), *Handbook of Science and Technology Studies* (pp. 113–137). Cambridge, MA: MIT Press.

Cooper, M. & C. Waldby. 2014. *Clinical Labour: Tissue Donors and Research Subjects in the Global Bioeconomy.* Durham, NC: Duke University Press.

Dean, M. 1999. *Governmentality.* Thousand Oaks, CA: Sage.

DiMaggio, P. 1997. Culture and Cognition. *Annual Review of Sociology* 23:263–287.

Engels, F. 1844. *The Condition of the Working Class in England in 1844.* Leipzig, Germany: O. Wigand.

Fosket, J. R. 2004. Constructing "High Risk" Women: The Development and Standardization of a Breast Cancer Risk Assessment Tool. *Science, Technology & Human Values* 29(3): 291–323.

Fosket, J. R. 2010. Breast Cancer Risk as Disease: Biomedicalizing Risk. In A. E. Clarke, J. Shim, L. Mamo, J. Fosket & J. Fishman (Eds.), *Biomedicalization: Technoscience, Health and Illness in the U.S.* (pp. 331–352). Durham, NC: Duke University Press.

Foucault, M. 1975. *The Birth of the Clinic: An Archeology of Medical Perception*. New York: Vintage/Random House.

Foucault, M. 1979. Governmentality. *Ideology and Consciousness* 6:5–21.

Friere, P. 1970. *Pedagogy of the Oppressed*. New York: Continuum.

Friere, P. 1973. *Education for Critical Consciousness*. New York: Seabury Press.

Friese, C. 2009. Models of Cloning, Models for the Zoo: Rethinking the Sociological Significance of Cloned Animals. *BioSocieties* 4:367–390.

Friese, C. 2010. Classification Conundrums: Classifying Chimeras and Enacting Species Preservation. *Theory and Society* 39(2):145–172.

Friese, C. 2013. *Cloning Wild Life: Zoos, Captivity and the Future of Endangered Animals*. New York: NYU Press.

Kinchelow, J. L. & P. McLaren. 1994. Rethinking Critical Theory and Qualitative Research. In N. K. Denzin & Y. S. Lincoln (Eds.), *Handbook of Qualitative Research* (pp. 138–157). Thousand Oaks, CA: Sage.

Kinchelow, J. L & P. McLaren. 2000. Rethinking Critical Theory and Qualitative Research. In N. K. Denzin & Y. S. Lincoln (Eds.), Handbook of Qualitative Research (2nd ed. pp. 279–314). Thousand Oaks, CA: Sage.

Kincheloe, J. L., P. McLaren, & S. R. Steinberg. 2011. Critical Pedagogy and Qualitative Research: Moving to the Bricolage. In N. K. Denzin & Y. S. Lincoln (Eds.), *Handbook of Qualitative Research* (4th ed., pp. 163–178). Thousand Oaks, CA: Sage.

King, L. 2014. *Euphoria*. New York: Atlantic Monthly Press.

Klein, N. 2007. *The Shock Doctrine: The Rise of Disaster Capitalism*. New York: Metropolitan Books.

Lather, P. 1991. *Getting Smart: Feminist Research and Pedagogy With/In the Postmodern*. New York: Routledge.

Lather, P. 1996. Troubling Clarity: The Politics of Accessible Language. *Harvard Educational Review* 66(3):525–545.

Lather, P. 2007. *Getting Lost: Feminist Efforts toward a Double(d) Science*. Albany: SUNY Press.

Lessor, R. 2000. Using the Team Approach of Anselm Strauss in Action Research: Consulting on a Project on Global Education. *Sociological Perspectives* 43(4):S133–S147.

Marx, K. & F. Engels. 1849. *The Communist Manifesto*. London: The Electric Book Company.

Murray, S. J. & D. Holmes (Eds.). 2009. *Critical Interventions in the Ethics of Healthcare*. Farnham, UK: Ashgate Pubs., Ltd.

Navarro, V. & D. M. Berman. 1983. *Health and Work under Capitalism: An International Perspective*. Baywood, NY: Baywood Pubs., Inc.

Pedrana, A. E., M. E. Hellard, P. Higgs, J. Asselin, C. Batrouney, & M. Stoove. 2014. No Drama: Key Elements to the Success of an HIV/STI-Prevention Mass-media Campaign. *Qualitative Health Research* 24(5):695–705.

Pérez, M. S. & G. S. Cannella. 2013. Situational Analysis as an Avenue for Critical Qualitative Research: Mapping Post-Katrina New Orleans. *Qualitative Inquiry* 19(7):1–13.

Sanders, G. 2009. "Late" Capital: Amusement and Contradiction in the Contemporary Funeral Industry. *Critical Sociology* 35:447–471.

St. Pierre, E. & W. Pillow (Eds.). 2000. *Working the Ruins: Feminist Poststructural Theory and Methods in Education*. New York: Routledge.

Star, S. L. 2010. This is Not a Boundary Object: Reflections on the Origin of a Concept. *Science, Technology & Human Values* 35:601–617.

Star, S. L. & J. Griesemer. 1989. Institutional Ecology, "Translations" and Boundary Objects: Amateurs and Professionals in Berkeley's Museum of Vertebrate Zoology, 1907–1939. *Social Studies of Science* 19:38–420.

Steinberg, S. R. & G. S. Cannella (Eds.). 2012. *Critical Qualitative Research Reader*. New York: Peter Lang Publishers.

Strauss, A. L. 1987. *Qualitative Analysis for Social Scientists*. Cambridge, UK: Cambridge University Press.

Strong, T., J. Gaete, I. N. Sametband, J. French, & J. Eeson. 2012. Counsellors Respond to the DSM-IV-TR. *Canadian Journal of Counselling and Psychotherapy* 46(2):85–106.

Timmermans, S., G. Bowker, A. E. Clarke, & E. Balka (Eds.). 2015. *Boundary Objects and Beyond: Working with Susan Leigh Star*. Cambridge, MA: MIT Press.

Waitzkin, H. 2011. *Medicine and Public Health at the End of Empire*. New York: Paradigm.

Washburn, R. 2013. The Social Significance of Human Biomonitoring. *Sociology Compass* 7(2):162–179.

Washburn, R. 2014. Measuring Personal Chemical Exposures through Biomonitoring: The Experiences of Research Participants. *Qualitative Health Research* 24(3):329–344.

Wiener, C. 2007. Making Teams Work in Conducting Grounded Theory. In A. Bryant & K. Charmaz (Eds.) *Handbook of Grounded Theory* (pp. 293–310). London: Sage.

CHAPTER FIVE

SITUATING KNOWLEDGE

Jennifer Ruth Fosket

n her now classic piece, "Situated Knowledges: The Science Question in Feminism and the Privilege of Partial Perspective," Donna Haraway (1991) reclaims the metaphor of vision to articulate a kind of objectivity which accounts for the historical contingency of all knowledge claims yet simultaneously maintains a commitment to some degree of "truth" to those claims. For Haraway, the seeming contradiction in simultaneously occupying both of these positions can be usefully navigated through this metaphor. Vision, she argues, while often represented otherwise, is necessarily partial as it is embodied within a specifically situated subject.

Haraway (1991, 1999) insists on recognizing the materiality, the embodied-ness of *all* perspectives. There is no longer a view from nowhere, but always a view from somewhere specific, marked, interested and inherently partial. This partial, situated objectivity-vision is politically advantageous because it insists that all positions are located within realms of political maneuvering and social change and reveals how they are so. It also allows particular embodied actors to be held accountable for what it is that they see and do with their vision.

Following on these and other articulations of "situated knowledge," scholars, especially feminist scholars, have conducted "situated" analyses of social phenomena. These have been pursued through foregrounding the perspectives, experiences, and voices of people located at the margins, as well as through de-stabilizations of the assumed "objectivity" of dominant knowledge producers via foregrounding their knowledge as equally cultured,

From Clarke, Adele E. and Kathy Charmaz. 2014. *Grounded Theory and Situational Analysis*, Volume IV, 91–109. © SAGE Publications. Republished in *Situational Analysis in Practice*, by Adele E. Clarke, Carrie Friese, and Rachel Washburn, 195–215. (Taylor & Francis, 2015). All rights reserved.

marked and *situated* as any other. The theoretical implications of situated knowledges and postmodernism more broadly become more problematic, however, in trying to understand the multiplicity of positions, the cultural, economic, historical and social elements that each and all situate a particular knowledge or set of knowledges. This is methodologically problematic simply due to the sheer number of possibilities, the messiness of data collected at multiple and not necessarily congruent sites, and the dearth of traditional methodologies that can help make sense of it.

Recently, Adele Clarke (2003, 2005) theorized an "updated" grounded theory that attends to the problematics and projects of postmodernity thus providing methodological means to make sense of just these kinds of complexities and differences. Clarke articulates new approaches to analysis within a grounded theory framework that she calls situational analyses. Situational analyses utilize various types of maps to provide access points into one's data, to act as tools for drawing linkages between variously conceptualized sites and to propel the researcher into what I have called "thick analysis" (Fosket 2002). In this paper, I discuss the usefulness of Clarke's methodological innovation for empirically studying situated knowledges gleaned through my own experiences of using it to study a large-scale, multi-sited clinical trial.

Framing My Problem: Clinical Trials as Situated Knowledge

I conducted a multi-sited ethnography of a clinical trial in order to explore the emergence of new knowledge and practices aimed at treating *risk* for breast cancer (Fosket 2002, 2004, 2010). Intrigued by the recent emergence of pharmaceuticals aimed at intervening in bodies that were classified as "high risk" for breast cancer in order to reduce that risk, I sought to understand who and what were important to the construction of this new knowledge. To me, this new knowledge seemed to mark a radical shift in how pharmaceuticals are being thought about and used, how high risk for breast cancer is being conceptualized, and how prevention is being understood and enacted. I wanted to explore these shifts in knowledge as they were emerging, to track and make sense of the competing discourses budding around this new phenomenon called *chemoprevention*.

To tackle these questions, I chose to focus on one large-scale chemoprevention clinical trial. Often depicted as the "gold-standard" for biomedical knowledge production, a clinical trial seemed to be an ideal location to explore the construction of knowledge *in action*. I collected data from multiple sites and positions in order to grasp how the trial looked from each. Instead of a few devoted people working full time to conduct the research, the clinical trial I studied actually consisted of numerous people working with varying levels of commitment and time, and included as important play- ers those located in key organizations as well as in other often surprising and sometimes marginal sites and sources. As I began to uncover the layers of experience, action and meaning that constituted the trial, it became increas- ingly evident that, while ultimately producing what appeared to be a coher- ent set of knowledges defined as objective, the knowledges being produced were fragmented, partial, and very much situated.

However, in order to get to a place where I could begin to make sense of what all of this meant, I had to find my methods. I began with a desire to conduct a social worlds analysis that evolved into situated analyses as I delved further into the process. I next describe these methods.

Situated Analyses

A central focus of grounded theory has long been on uncovering the basic social process—the kinds of action—at the heart of the phenomena being studied. In contrast, Clarke (2003, 2005) argues that we need to move beyond a sole focus on action to a more broad and full focus on the entire situation in all of its many complex parts. The theoretical roots of this lie in social worlds/arenas theories first articulated by Anselm Strauss (1978a,b, 1991) and Howard Becker (1982) and elaborated by Adele Clarke (1991, 1998; Clarke & Montini 1993). In his theoretical work which formed the basis for his methodological innovation of grounded theory, Anselm Strauss (1978b) understood social order as negotiated and thus fluctuating, unpredictable, emergent and always contingent. From this emphasis on group action and organizational dynamics, Strauss (1978a) and Becker (1982) proposed social worlds/arenas theory where social worlds constitute the shared realities within which people act, interact, and make meanings of their situations in ways that give rise to shared realities. Within social worlds and the sub- stantive arenas of shared concerns and commitments in which those worlds intersect, knowledge is constructed in an ongoing fashion vis-à-vis the every- day practices of whatever the world is focused around.

Adele Clarke (1991, 1993) asserts that social worlds/arenas theory offers a useful way to understand the historical construction of particular phenom- ena by examining the social worlds that participated in creating it. Within this frame, distinctive constructions of knowledge can be viewed as emerging within particular social worlds which share specific goals and have stakes in constructing knowledge in particular ways. In social worlds/arenas theory, theoretical possibilities open up to view knowledge as collectively constructed in everyday practices. Here, social worlds (rather than individual positions) are understood as resources for knowledge production. As articulated by Clarke, social worlds/arenas theory understands the negotiated nature of knowledge construction as conflictual and shaped by power. This theory provides a dynamic and interactive lens through which to view multiple con-structions of knowledge because it acknowledges the constant contentions going on among *and* within social worlds over how a particular phenomenon will be constructed and the ways in which these interactions are, ultimately, mutually constitutive.

With her conceptualization of situational analyses, Clarke moved these theories further (2003, 2005). Here, social worlds/arenas theory expands to include as consequential elements everything within a given situation. That is, it is not just the social worlds and their human and nonhuman elements that situate and shape knowledge and practices, but histories, discourses, symbols, institutions, material things, and anything else conceived of as present in the situation. Thus, in theorizing the processual and interactional character of knowledge construction, it is important to grasp the interactions and practices engaged in not just by humans, but also by all of the other consequential elements in the situation. What Clarke's theorizing offers is a concrete analysis of knowledge that not only notes how it is situated, but actively deconstructs what constitutes that situation.

Within this framework, an understanding of the work of scientific knowledge production requires an understanding of everything in the situa-tion: the workplaces and their organizations, scientists and other workers, theories, models, research materials, instruments, technologies, skills and techniques, sponsorship and its organization, regulatory groups, audiences, consumers, and so on. Each of the relevant elements is not merely contextual (i.e., background) but conditional. Each element is an integral aspect of the situation itself, constitutive of the practices and contingencies of the research work that constitutes the very construction of knowledge. Even those ele-ments that are not *physically* present in the situation are part of the situation in a very real sense.

In order to analyze these complex and multi-sited situational elements, Clarke (2003, 2005) articulates various types of maps that can be used as methodological strategies in doing situational analyses. Specifically, she describes: situational maps, which plot all of the relevant elements in the situation and enable analyses of their relationships; social worlds/arenas maps, which illuminate the social worlds, collectivities, and arenas of commitment which engage with the situation; and positional maps, which lay out the interests, commitments, and positions explicitly taken (or absent) in various discourses found within the situation.

Clarke describes situational analyses as approaches which, among other things, can help free a researcher from "analytic paralysis." One source of analytic paralysis that emerged for me resulted from questioning how to make sense of the multiple elements emerging as I interrogated various sites of the clinical trial. Following grounded theory, I had been continuously coding and writing memos throughout my data collection process. Indeed, these analytic processes led me to the various sites at which I collected data, helped form the questions I asked interviewees, and probed me deeper into my data. However, at some point, I felt lost amidst mountains of data which I intuitively knew were interrelated, but which I could not initially figure out how to wrap my brain around. In attempting such a potentially disparate and non-unified or universal analysis, I needed tools that could tie elements together, conceptually linking the various situated positions, identifying their interrelationships, and seeing as complexly woven together what might otherwise appear isolated. Situational analyses provided such tools for me. By sitting down in the middle of my living room floor with a huge piece of paper, paralysis broke as I began drawing circles and lines, mapping the various positions and elements that I was grappling with. As I sketched this and subsequent maps, I was clarifying relationships between elements, understanding who and what was important to the situation, and was, for the first time, able to conceptualize the wholeness of what I was studying—rather than fragmented bits of interesting ideas and data.

At the same time as my needs prompted the use of tools, so too did the tools themselves shape my analysis. As I began mapping I clarified and extended my research agenda—realizing how very situated the situation truly was. For me, mapping the various social worlds and other elements in STAR provided great insights into my data. The maps themselves turned out to be valuable artifacts, visually representing the complex array of factors that make up the STAR trial. To illustrate my use of situational analysis, I present and briefly describe here my own use of the first two types of maps, situational and social worlds/arenas, for my research on a clinical trial. (For a greater elaboration of the clinical trial and my conceptualizations and uses of these maps, please see Fosket [2002].) These maps reflect my own partial and situated knowledge and do not exhaust every possibility, but rather represent those elements and actors that emerged as most salient in the fieldwork that I conducted.

Locating the STAR Trial

The clinical trial I studied is called the Study of Tamoxifen and Raloxifene —or the STAR trial. Its purpose was to compare tamoxifen (a breast cancer treatment drug that had recently been FDA-approved for use in healthy women to reduce their risk of breast cancer) with raloxifene (a drug thought to similarly reduce breast cancer risk without as many side-effects). The STAR trial is located within the newly emerging chemoprevention arena. Chemoprevention, the practice of ingesting pharmaceuticals or nutraceuticals to reduce the incidence of disease, is a relatively new phenomenon within the arena of breast cancer. I used the social worlds/arenas map to conceptually locate its emergence at the intersections of groups, organizations, and interests that had, until the trial was begun, maintained separate spheres. Figure 5.1 locates the chemoprevention and STAR trial arenas within larger intersecting arenas. The chemoprevention arena is located at the center of this map. This arena includes the STAR trial and also includes other clinical research and practices currently ongoing around chemoprevention that I do not take up in my research. The chemoprevention arena is itself situated at the intersections of the treatment and prevention spheres of the breast cancer arena. Because chemoprevention involves administering drugs previously used as treatments to prevent breast cancer, it represents an innovative *prevention* endeavor taken up primarily by *treatment* oriented oncologists. Thus, it begins to blur the lines between treatment and prevention in unprecedented ways. I have also included breast cancer genetics as an arena that intersects with treatment, prevention, and chemoprevention arenas as well. Also a newly emerging arena, breast cancer genetics currently represents another example of a site where treatment and prevention lines are becoming increasingly fuzzy, as genetic assessments may trigger more active prevention strategies.

Both the treatment and prevention spheres are part of the larger breast cancer arena which includes myriad other elements, worlds, and arenas that I do not depict here. The breast cancer arena itself is located at the intersections of the women's health and cancer arenas. These two arenas each repre-

Figure 5.1 Locating the STAR trial

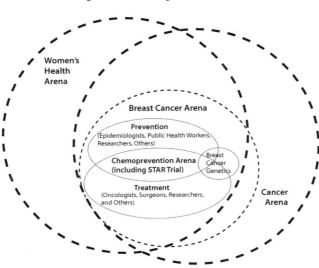

sent much larger arenas in and of themselves. Here they overlap around the breast cancer arena. (They also overlap around arenas of other types of cancer impacting women, not represented here). The women's health and cancer arenas are themselves located in the much larger domain of U.S. health care.

Mapping the Situation: Who/What Matters to STAR

Upon entering the field of STAR, one of the first things I realized was that this "site" itself consisted of multiple sites. It was comprised of many different elements complexly organized and webbed together to form what I ultimately conceived of as the "STAR trial arena." Nonhuman actants (things of various kinds from furniture to technologies to discourses), social actors, body parts, research protocols, organizations and paperwork represent key elements in the constitution of the trial, and critical activists and passionate advocates are central. Additionally, the deeper I delved into the research, the more obvious and important the historical and political situatedness of STAR became. By requiring the researcher to map out all of the "analytically pertinent human and nonhuman, material and symbolic/discursive elements of a particular situation as framed by those in it *and by the analyst*" (Clarke

2005:87), situational maps draw out complexities and reveal which anticipated and unanticipated elements of the situation matter.

Figure 5.2 represents my situational map, highlighting the most salient
elements. The categories used here are not absolute, but reflect what ended
up being most meaningful to me and central to my analysis as I made sense
of my data.[1] An important aspect of situational maps as analytic tools is their
use in uncovering relations between elements.[2] In the remainder of this section, I narrate this situational map, highlighting certain of the key elements
and relationships in-depth.

Multiple cultural discourses, ideologies, and/or rhetorics prevalent in
U.S. society and/or in U.S. biomedicine are key elements to the situation of
STAR because they are consequential in shaping the ways in which breast
cancer is thought about, treated, and its "risks" attended to. The STAR
trial is made possible not just through securing the necessary tools, bodies, resources, researchers and other material needs, but also through the
management of credibility and legitimacy derived through ideological, cultural, and discursive elements (Epstein 1996). Certain cultural ideas about
women's bodies, about the origins of disease and the most appropriate sites
for prevention, about the dangers of risk and the importance of classifying
the normal and pathological distinctly, about what counts as good research
and scientific knowledge, and what the causes, consequences and appropriate responses to cancer are, all create a situation in which STAR appears as
a *credible* solution to a particularly constructed problem of "breast cancer
risk." For instance, I argue that the prominence of a "downstream approach"
to healthcare, an approach that focuses not on prevention of disease but on
its treatment, already well accepted in the U.S., itself contributes to chemoprevention's credibility as a reasonable prevention option. In a framework
already accustomed to treating symptoms of individuals, the idea of treating risk is a logical extension of normative biomedical ideology and practice.
Thus, "downstream medicine" becomes an important discourse in my map.
As another example, "clinical trials" appear as a discourse in my map. By this
I refer to the dominance of clinical trials as the most credible form of biomedical knowledge construction (Marks 2000), and this history and current
stronghold powerfully shape the situation of STAR.

In addition to rhetorics/discourses/ideologies, key social processes are
also important elements in my situational map. Biomedicalization and its
attendant processes of standardization and risk assessments are social processes very much at work in the shaping of the STAR trial. Biomedicalization

is a social process through which increasing aspects of the life world become identified by and imbued with medical and technoscientific meaning and subject to interventions via the vast armamentarium of technoscientific tools, knowledges, and organizations at the disposal of biomedicine (Clarke et al. 2003, 2010; Fosket 2010). In our elaboration of this concept, however, we emphasize that biomedicalization is not just imposed from above, but is part of a cultural system with which individuals also pragmatically and often inescapably engage. In this way, biomedicalization is also an ideology—a way of thinking about and acting toward health and wellness—that is prevalent and consequential in shaping the subsequent knowledges and practices related to health.

The STAR trial is also very much a product of the growing emphasis on risk assessment which is part of biomedicalization. Populations of women previously considered "normal" are transformed into "potentially ill" populations as a result of their classification into "high risk" categories. With

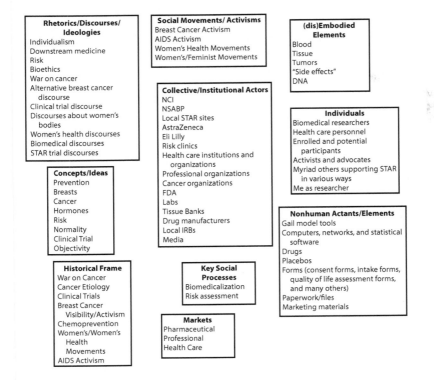

Figure 5.2 STAR trial situational map

biomedicalization comes an increased attention to risk and the transformation of bodies designated at risk through pharmaceutical interventions. These risk assessments are fundamental to the credibility of a trial like STAR in that they create a group of women who are considered at high enough risk to be legitimate users of chemoprevention drugs (Fosket 2004, 2010).

In constructing a situational map, nonhuman elements are important features consisting of materials, tools, and other "things" in the situation. Highly significant nonhuman actants in the STAR arena are the pharmaceuticals themselves, tamoxifen and raloxifene. Computers, computer networks, special software, and the Internet are also all critical nonhuman actants in the situation of STAR. Without computer networks and standardizing specialized software programs, STAR could not function as the multi-sited research project it is.

Blood, tissue, tumors, DNA, and other body parts are taken from women's bodies, and stored, analyzed, transported, isolated, and used in multiple ways as data for STAR. As these elements become preserved, packaged, sent from place to place, banked, etc., they become nonhuman actants in the production of knowledge about chemoprevention and breast cancer risk. However, I also term these "(dis)embodied elements" and highlight them here so as not to efface their human origins. These once embodied elements of research participants' bodies are deeply consequential for STAR as they represent the raw data which shape actions on a daily basis (i.e., if a segment of breast tissue is found to contain cancerous cells, interactions with and participation by the woman to whom that breast tissue belongs will change profoundly). These elements and the knowledge regarding the dangers and/or efficacy of tamoxifen and raloxifene that they reveal, will ultimately guide the representation of the findings of STAR and subsequent actions taken as a result of it.

Many, many different individuals are key players in STAR and appear in the situational map. Each researcher, each woman engaging in the enrollment process, whether or not she ultimately chooses to join, each doctor referring women into the trial, or making the choice not to do so, and every other individual making choices and taking actions that are related to STAR are consequential because it is ultimately the collaborative, interactional, and collective actions of each of these individuals that propel and shape the clinical trial. There are direct relationships between many of these individuals and other elements in the situation: they are linked to organizations listed; they procure and engage with the nonhuman actants and (dis)embodied elements; they are shaped by and act within marketplaces and social processes described; and many of these individuals are also situated within particular collectivities—social worlds whose interests, contributions, and stakes in the trial are elaborated later in my social worlds map (see Figure 5.3).

In addition to those who make a difference in STAR through their everyday actions and interactions around the trial, other individuals represent key players in the situation due to their role in the emergence of chemoprevention, risk assessment, breast cancer, or other arenas that shape the situation of STAR. These include those individuals who posed the theories and instigated, popularized, or paved the way for key research and conceptual shifts that led to chemoprevention and eventually to STAR.

As consequential actors within the organizations, institutions, and social worlds that conduct, monitor, oppose, support, and represent STAR, innumerable individuals could be cited as important to the situation, including the person who monitors the books and signs the paychecks, the person who

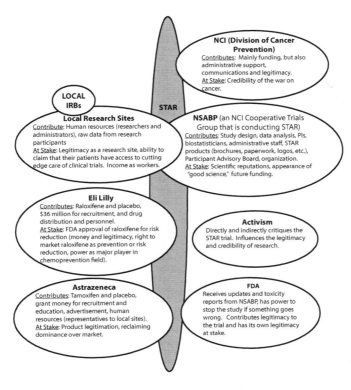

Figure 5.3 STAR trial social worlds map

sustains the lives of those who spend long hours working in the labs that process potential participants' blood samples, and endless others. What is interesting and important about highlighting this is that it demonstrates the sheer numbers of people involved, to varying extents, in the collaborative interactions required to conduct such scientific research. The work of so many visible and invisible individuals plays its part in shaping just how and why STAR emerges in the ways it does. While some individuals are important elements in and of themselves, they are also important in terms of the collective organizations in which they are situated.

There are myriad collectivities and institutions that represent key elements in STAR including the professional organizations to which researchers belong which publish journals and hold conferences where knowledge about STAR is traded; those innumerable collectivities to which individuals important in STAR belong and which shape their ways of being in STAR; and the various institutions and organizations that play key roles in STAR. In addition, other health care organizations and institutions also play key roles in the situation of STAR. They are important to STAR as sources of potential participants, and STAR recruitment efforts target health care providers located in a variety of organizations and institutions. They are also important as groups with whom local sites and NSABP need to cooperate for data collection purposes: pathology reports, mammograms, physical results, etc.

Finally, various media constitute an additional important element in the situation of the STAR trial. Media fundamentally problematize the ways in which knowledge is accessed, disseminated, and constructed. Popular media have been important players in STAR from the outset when national media began to run "news stories" of STAR that double as recruitment opportunities for the NSABP, complete with a 1-800 number to call "for more information" at the end of the news story. In these moves, news items are transformed into marketing strategies, "infomercials" for biomedicine and for the pharmaceutical companies whose drugs are on trial. Since then, coverage has continued and media outlets are considered and used as crucial sites for STAR recruitment. They are also used as tools for activists' critiques. Media are also important as sites of direct-to-consumer advertising of tamoxifen, which shapes the trial in important ways already discussed.

Scientific literature media have also been important sites wherein claims and counter claims about STAR and chemoprevention take place. During the early 1990s, the scientific literature was a source of not insignificant critique of tamoxifan as chemoprevention. The controversies over the early design and conduct of the Breast Cancer Prevention Trial were discussed in letters to the editor of *The Lancet* (e.g., Costa 1993), news articles in *Science* (e.g., Marshal 1995), and other media sources. There was much concern expressed in these articles regarding giving toxic drugs to healthy women to prevent a disease that strikes with relative infrequency, and whether the evaluation of the "risk" of drugs should be different for prevention than for actual cancer therapy (e.g., Love, 1995; Pitot, 1995; Bush & Helzlsouer, 1993).

Another important way to think about collectivities is in terms of social movements. The collective organizing of social movements in health and illness must be considered key elements within any biomedical situation as these movements have brought about profound changes in the ways that biomedicine, including biomedical research, is thought about and practiced. Several social movements are pivotal to the situation of STAR, most importantly breast cancer movements, women's health movements and AIDS activism. These movements are important for the changes they have provoked in policy, institutions, treatments, and in discursive constructions of health, wellness, disease, research, and the meanings and rights of patients. STAR has most certainly been shaped by the historical gains of these movements as well as by current activism.

Discourses, social processes, markets, nonhuman actants, individuals, collectivities and social movements all represent central elements constituting the situation of STAR. While many of these elements also and simultaneously come together around various other issues, this particular conglomeration of actors, actants, social forces and processes are those which I conceive as mattering to STAR. As this analysis highlights, clinical trials like STAR do not take place in a vacuum as biomedicine and biomedical research are not separate from, but are intimately part of, larger cultural and social contexts. Next, I focus in even more closely to elaborate the key social worlds that constitute STAR.

Mapping the STAR Trial Arena

While the situational elements described in the previous section are constitutive of the situation of STAR, this is only true in so far as there are committed groups, individuals, and organizations that engage in the work of making STAR an actual arena of action. Social worlds are the sites of action around STAR within which the elements already described come to matter. Social worlds mapping involves identifying the collective commitments and actions organized into social worlds that come together to constitute the social arena of interest (Clarke, 2005). Within social worlds analyses (e.g., Clarke & Montini, 1993), one begins by empirically specifying the key players (individuals and groups) who are active around the phenomena of interest, as well as those important in the historical construction of the phenomenon.

STAR is an arena consisting of intersecting social worlds concerned about the issue of breast cancer chemoprevention. Figure 5.3 represents a simplified version of my social worlds map of STAR, including who they are, their stakes and contributions. There are a couple of important things to notice in viewing this map. First, the filled in oblong running down the middle of the map represents the STAR trial. The circles that overlap with this oblong represent social worlds "officially" linked to STAR—that is, those who have an organizational role in STAR, are considered a part of the trial by those who designed it and/or have a legal and/or fiscal role in the trial. Those social worlds *not* shown as overlapping represent social worlds that I conceptualize as crucial to the STAR arena, but that are not "official" participants. Additionally, some of the circles overlap with each other and others do not. The overlapping circles represent social worlds that are interconnected in some official capacity—fiscally, organizationally, and/or in terms of personnel.

Discussion

The elements, social worlds and arenas represented by these maps and described in the previous sections illuminate my efforts at situating the knowledge constructed in clinical trial research regarding women's bodies, risks, and the appropriateness of biomedical intervention. The maps enabled me to organize and make sense of the data I had collected and the preliminary thoughts I was having about a vast number of things that, unrelated in many ways, all shared common linkages to the production of knowledge at the site of the STAR trial. Once visually available to me in the form of a map, I could begin to systematically flesh out each element, understand its relationship to STAR and to other elements, know what needed to be elucidated about them, and decide on next steps in my research process. In these very concrete ways, the methodological maps aided my process of undertaking a situational analysis of a clinical trial. In this discussion section, I further explore ways in which situational maps can help materialize some of the sometimes elusive goals of feminist and postmodern theory in the concrete practices of empirical research.

Difference and Complexity

One of the striking benefits of situational mapping is the ability to make sense of and analytically compare and contrast non-congruent data sources. Conducting a multi-sited ethnography that was revealed to be increasingly complex as I undertook its mapping meant that my data derived from heterogeneous sources through heterogeneous methods. I conducted archival research in medical journals on the emergence of chemoprevention drugs; textual analyses of FDA proceedings as well as popular media articles; in-depth qualitative interviews with various types of participants; participant observation at meetings; and analyses of images. Whereas another project might hone in on one of those data sources as primary and use the others for framing or contextual background information, for me, each source was considered of comparable importance to my understanding of the situation of STAR. The maps allowed for this heterogeneity as each element can be added in the map and considered as part of the analysis.

This is increasingly valuable to sociology and social studies of science in particular as more and more cross-disciplinary collaborating and intellectual borrowing means that research studies are often composed of a hybrid of methods—sociologists including serious historical analyses, utilizing anthropological ethnographic methods, and/or analyzing texts or cultural representations. Situational analyses provide an important tool for engaging with such transdisciplinarity in ways that at the same time produce richly sociological analyses.

Simultaneously to providing tools for analyzing such postmodern projects, situational analyses are also valuable in helping to initiate such projects and create useful complexity and depth to what might otherwise be thin. In my mapping of the STAR trial, multiple elements arose that I had not previously considered important and propelled me in new directions, delving me deeper into the complexity of the situation of STAR.

Relationships and Blurring the Macro/Meso/Micro

One of the central uses of situational analyses is to discover, through mapping, relationships between elements. Clarke (2005:142) writes of situational mapping, "All mapping strategies are at base relational. This is a radical aspect of the approaches offered here compared to 'normal' social science and positivist approaches that are at base atomistic, based on supposedly isolable 'variables' and intentionally decontextualizing (for lack of a better term)."

Additionally, because these elements can be heterogeneous, these relationships are often relationships amongst elements located at distinct conceptual levels. In this way, situational maps help to blur distinctions between micro/macro/meso levels. They help to understand dynamic interrelationships between elements at all of these levels and how many may exist at multiple levels simultaneously.

For instance, through doing relational analyses using my situational map, I was able to see linkages between discourses and social processes of consumerism, practicalities of clinical trial research practice and the nonhuman elements of the study pills. Women participants in STAR are required to take two pills a day, one each of the drug they have been randomized to and a placebo made to look like the drug they were not randomized to. This is an interesting necessity brought on by the marketing of pharmaceuticals, such that tamoxifen, sold under the brand name Nolvadex® by AstraZeneca and raloxifene, sold under the brand name Evista® by Eli Lilly, are each purposefully created to look distinctive and thus inspire brand recognition. Yet such distinction works at cross-purposes to a double-blind randomized controlled clinical trial, where *not* recognizing what brand is being taken is paramount. Instead of providing anonymized drugs, the pharmaceutical companies provide their own drug *and* a placebo that looks just like it. This "solution" exemplifies the dominance of consumerism, where logos proliferate, and the right to market one's brand is not to be hindered even during clinical trials.

Relativism, Positionality, and Reflexivity

While situational analyses maintain a commitment to researching a particular phenomenon of interest from multiple perspectives, one of the benefits of situational analyses is that such projects do not assume or imply a theory of relativism. Haraway argues, "Relativism is a way of being nowhere while claiming to be everywhere equally. The 'equality' of positioning is a denial of responsibility and critical enquiry" (Haraway, 1991:191). Within Clarke's articulation of situational analyses, positional maps in particular provide this kind of attendance to the differences in power and responsibilities that shape the various positions investigated.

Within positional maps, the analyst explicitly marks the actants and knowledges in the situation as *interested*. It is not possible within this type of analysis to claim a "view from nowhere" because the researcher is literally specifying the positions taken by those that constitute the situation. Through each of the types of maps, the research is constantly situating the people and things of import to the situation within real worlds of interests, politics, passions, histories, and more. In this way, it is not just *other* positions that become glaringly obvious, but one's own as well.

Inevitably, in conducting this kind of situational analysis, the researcher must consider themselves as elements in the situation. In this way, reflexivity becomes an intimate part of the research agenda. Clarke (2003, 2005) asserts in her description of situational mapping that researchers' own experiences of researching should be considered data in mapping. In uncovering the situatedness of the STAR trial, I needed to see the ways in which I am part of that situation. This was evident in thinking through how my presence and particular situatedness in the world of breast cancer shaped the research in fundamental ways—it shaped who I had access to and what kinds of things those that I interviewed were ready to share. My entrance into the world of breast cancer politics began in 1993 when I attended my first Breast Cancer Action (BCA) meeting with my teacher and friend, Christine LaFia, who had recently been diagnosed with breast cancer. We soon became active participants in the organization, drawn to its radical and feminist politics and unflinching telling of difficult truths about breast cancer. In 1996 Christine died of breast cancer and my experiences with her illness, dying and death drew me even more passionately into the world of breast cancer scholarship and activism. In the almost ten years since, I have continued to be a part of Breast Cancer Action, always as a member and sometimes as an activist volunteering at various venues. Indeed, some of my fieldwork experiences at national conferences were paid for by BCA where I was both a fieldworker and an activist, collecting data for my research and writing excerpts for BCA's website. I have made many friends through my work with BCA, and received invaluable support and expertise for this research. Mostly I have found this connection and my clearly messy involvement with my object of study of benefit to my research. I am constantly learning from the activists I engage with and know much more about the arena of breast cancer than I could ever possibly know if I were not so involved.

However, I am also aware that my positioning poses some dilemmas. I am clearly not a neutral observer. My very first foray into the world of chemoprevention was to write a letter to the editor criticizing the emergence of chemoprevention for breast cancer as an extreme example of individualizing prevention and shifting prevention policy away from locating fundamental causes of breast cancer. I have not strayed too far from this position since. Though my mind has been changed and certainly expanded in numerous areas, I began this research an interested participant in the field and these interests are surely evident throughout my research.

In addition to this larger dilemma, my positioning within my field of study also posed practical dilemmas. Many people who I interviewed formally or informally at conferences and meetings knew of my connection with Breast Cancer Action. While this connection opened many doors (indeed, a couple of people explicitly stated they were only agreeing to be interviewed by me *because* of my connection to BCA), it also closed others or made for suspicion and skepticism. I had people refuse to participate in my research because my connection with breast cancer activism was seen to situate me as irremediably biased on the issues I was studying.

Howard Becker (1967) describes circumstances in which as social scientists we find ourselves critiqued for aligning with the interests of some of those who we study and thus producing biased knowledge claims about particular social phenomena. I find this analysis most useful for understanding my own position within my field of inquiry. He argues that the circumstances in which such accusations of partiality emerge, and those situations in which they do not emerge, are revealing for what they tell us about credibility. The social scientist is apt to find her or his knowledge claims de-legitimated when the knowledge produced represents, or appears to represent, the perspectives of marginalized groups or individuals, the less powerful elements in the situation. In contrast, representing the perspective of dominant groups rarely incites such critique of partiality or interestedness. "We can use the notion of a *hierarchy of credibility* to understand this phenomenon. In any system of ranked groups, participants take it as a given that members of the highest group have the right to define the way things really are" (Becker, 1967: 241). There is an assumption that those at the top have privileged access to information and thus any knowledge derived from such superordinates will automatically be more credible than those produced by subordinates. Moreover, Becker argues that these assumptions are imbued with morality such that we feel beholden to respectfully accept the definitions of reality imposed by those in dominant positions. Thus, within this framework, by refusing to reproduce this hierarchy of credibility and by asserting heterogeneous definitions of reality including some from the perspectives of non-dominant groups and individuals, my own productions of knowledge are vulnerable to dismissal on the grounds that they are "biased."

In addition to my experience in the field detailed above, situational analyses provoke me to explore how the preconceptions, ideas, passions, and interests shape the very conceptualizations of the problem to begin with. In mapping the trial, I have most definitely emphasized not just those elements that seemed most important to me, but also those that are most interesting to me. What is interesting about a situational map is that you can include even elements that you did not end up researching. In this way, the maps can make more evident one's own biases as a researcher. Seeing an element there that I know I chose not to pursue forces me to ask myself why not. In this way, constant reflexivity is integral to situational analyses and any notion of relativism is replaced by bold awareness of positionality.

Conclusion

Utilizing situational analysis, my research highlights concrete ways in which the situation shapes the production of knowledge—or, in other words, illuminates situated knowledge in action. The knowledge that can be, and is being, produced by STAR is contingent upon the everyday work practices of those producing that knowledge. And those everyday practices are con-strained and enabled by the various situational elements shaping the work —shaping various interpretations of what is politically and ethically feasible, what is economically practical, scientifically do-able (Fujimura 1987) and so on. Utilizing situated analyses, my project makes vivid the "situated" part of situated knowledge, highlighting various ways in which situatedness shapes knowledge production in the everyday practices of conducting STAR.

Notes

1. Also, this situational map does not exhaustively list all of the elements in the situation, but rather lists those that ended up most central to my analysis. Previous versions of the map contained elements that ultimately did not remain pertinent.

2. Part of the work involved in this technique is to draw lines between each element and the other elements and identify what the relationships are—the nature of the line. I undertook this process to fruitful ends, but the resultant mass of lines and words defies visual reproduc-tion here. It also provoked memos about the relationships.

References

Becker, Howard S. [1967] 1970. Whose Side Are We On? Reprinted as pp. 123-134 in Howard S. Becker. *Sociological Work: Method and Substance*. New Brunswick, NJ: Transaction Books.

Becker, Howard S. 1982. *Art Worlds*. Berkeley: University of California Press.

Bush, Trudy & Kathy Helzlsouer. 1993. Tamoxifen for the Primary Prevention of Breast Cancer: A Review and Critique of the Concept and Trial. *Epidemiologic Reviews* 15:233-243

Clarke, Adele E. 1991. Social Worlds/ Arenas Theory as Organizational Theory. Pp. 128-135 in David R. Maines (Ed.) *Social Organization and Social Process: Essays in Honor of Anselm Strauss*. Hawthorne, NY: Aldine de Gruyter.

Clarke, Adele E. 1998. *Disciplining Reproduction: Modernity, American Life Sciences, and 'the Problems of Sex.'* Berkeley: University of California Press.

Clarke, Adele E. 2003. Situational Analyses: Grounded Theory Mapping After the Postmodern Turn. *Symbolic Interaction* 26(4):553–576.

Clarke, Adele E. 2005. *Situational Analysis: Grounded Theory After the Postmodern Turn*. Thousand Oaks, CA: Sage.

Clarke, Adele E., Jennifer Fishman, Jennifer Fosket, Laura Mamo & Janet Shim. 2003. Biomedicalization: Technoscientific Transformations of Health, Illness, and U.S. Biomedicine. *American Sociological Review* 68 (April): 161–194.

Clarke, Adele E. & Theresa Montini. 1993. The Many Faces of RU486: Tales of Situated Knowledges and Technological Contestations. *Science, Technology and Human Values* 18(1):42–78.

Clarke, Adele E., Janet Shim, Laura Mamo, Jennifer Fosket & Jennifer Fishman (Eds.) 2010. *Biomedicalization: Technoscience and Transformations of Health and Illness in the U.S.* Durham, NC: Duke University Press.

Costa, Alberto. 1993. Tamoxifen Trial in Healthy Women at Risk of Breast Cancer. *Lancet* 342:444.

Fosket, Jennifer Ruth. 2002. *Breast Cancer Risk and the Politics of Prevention: Analysis of a Clinical Trial*. Ph.D. dissertation in Sociology, Department of Social and Behavioral Sciences, University of California, San Francisco.

Fosket, Jennifer Ruth. 2004. Constructing High-Risk Women: The Development and Standardization of a Breast Cancer Risk Assessment Tool. *Science, Technology & Human Values* 29(3):291–213.

Fosket, Jennifer Ruth. 2010. Breast Cancer Risk as Disease: Biomedicalizing Risk. Pp. 331–352 in Adele E. Clarke, Laura Mamo, Jennifer Fosket, Jennifer Fishman & Janet Shim (Eds.) 2010. *Biomedicalization: Technoscience and Transformations of Health and Illness in the U.S.* Durham, NC: Duke University Press.

Fujimura, Joan H. 1987. Constructing Doable Problems in Cancer Research: Articulating Alignment. *Social Studies of Science* 17:257–93.

Haraway, Donna. 1991. Situated Knowledges: The Science Question in Feminism and the-Privilege of Partial Perspective. Pp. 183–202 in her *Simians, Cyborgs, and Women: The Reinvention of Nature*. New York: Routledge.

Haraway, Donna J. 1999. The Virtual Speculum in The New World Order. Pp. 49–96 in *Revisioning Women, Health, and Healing: Feminist, Cultural, and Technoscience Perspectives*, Ed. Adele E. Clarke and Virginia L. Olesen. New York: Routledge.

Love, R. R. 1995. Tamoxifen Chemoprevention: Public Health Goals, Toxicities for All and Benefits to a Few. *Annals of Oncology* 6: 127–128.

Marks, Harry M. 2000. *The Progress of Experiment: Science and Therapeutic Reform in the United States, 1900-1990.* Cambridge, MA: Cambridge University Press.

Marshall, Eliot. 1993. Search for a Killer: Focus Shifts from Fat to Hormones. *Science* 259: 618–621.

Pitot, Henry C. 1995. The Tamoxifen Controversy: Clinical Chemoprevention Agent and Experimental Carcinogen. *Proceedings of the Society for Experimental Biology and Medicine* 208:139–140.

Strauss, Anselm L. 1978a. A Social Worlds Perspective. *Studies in Symbolic Interaction* 1:119–228.

Strauss, Anselm L. 1978b. *Negotiations: Varieties, Contexts, Processes and Social* Order. San Francisco: Jossey Bass.

Strauss, Anselm L. 1991. *Creating Sociological Awareness: Collective Images and Symbolic Representation.* New Brunswick, NJ: Transaction Pubs.

CHAPTER SIX

USING SITUATIONAL ANALYSIS FOR
CRITICAL QUALITATIVE RESEARCH PURPOSES

Michelle Salazar Pérez & Gaile S. Canella

In our contemporary condition of global neoliberal hypercapitalism in which new forms of imperialism are constituted in the name of democracy, education, and even social justice, conceptualizations and practices of critical qualitative social science are a necessity. Research perspectives and methodologies are required that challenge universals, normality, and truths while avoiding oversimplifications and generalizations. Power is complex, intersecting, and always/already everywhere. We have come to realize that we may need to eliminate beliefs about research that have labeled individuals and groups and resulted in power/control/intervention by one group over others. Our research will most likely require partnering with traditionally marginalized and silenced communities as well as recognizing systemic, institutionalized power structures that dominate society(ies). To construct a critical social science that would reconceptualize what we can know and how we take actions in solidarity with/for those who have been traditionally marginalized, research methodologies are needed that do not require restricted boundaries. Rather methods are called for that are emergent, reflexive, and malleable in order to mirror the complexity of the issue, structure and/or system being studied. Situational Analysis (SA), developed by Adele Clarke (2005), offers great potential as such a method.

Introduction to Situational Analysis

Emerging from the field of medicine, SA is a feminist, postmodern research method rooted in conceptualizations of grounded theory. Social phenomena are studied employing qualitative methodologies like inductive coding and cat-

From Denzin, Norman K. and Michael D. Giardina. 2011. *Qualitative Inquiry and Global Crises*, 97–117. © Taylor & Francis. Republished in *Situational Analysis in Practice*, by Adele E. Clarke, Carrie Friese, and Rachel Washburn, 216–240. (Taylor & Francis, 2015). All rights reserved.

egorizing techniques (Clarke, 2005). Although phenomenological research typically attempts to produce data from interviews and/or ethnographic practice to study human action, SA makes possible a more complete construction of the full situation, including the discourses that both legitimate and are created by the situation. Without being bounded by a particular set of rules, SA offers a way in which to organize and frame a study focusing on discourse (or what Clarke describes as already produced data) with the flexibility necessary to address the unanticipated issues that may surface. The assumptions and processes involved in SA include: (1) valuing and legitimating multiple knowledges; (2) reflexivity (e.g., the researcher as instrument, as subjective, and producer of knowledge); (3) the use of the narrative, visual, and historical as revealing social life; (4) the use of cartography or mapmaking as an *analytical tool* throughout an emergent research process; and (5) the provision of a thick analysis to address complexity, differences, contradictions, and heterogeneity rather than attempting to develop formal theory.

SA allows for qualitative inquiry to focus on the way in which discourses: (1) are negotiated in social relationships and interactions; (2) manufacture "identities and subjectivities" (Clarke, 2005, p. 155); and (3) construct "power/ knowledge, ideologies, and control" (Clarke, 2005, p. 155). Maps are used as tools to examine these three ways of understanding discourse by inductively analyzing the content found in the data while using supplementary qualitative research approaches to facilitate a hybridity of methods. The content used to construct maps is found in the discourses that directly address the situation, those related to the situation, and the positions explicitly expressed or absent (Clarke, 2005).

Because the construction of situational maps is a postmodern analytical method, the process requires reflexivity and multiple readings of discourses from various sources to continually develop and revise research focus and design. Clarke instructed three types of maps in the initial construction of SA: situational, social spheres/power arenas, and positional. Situational maps allow the researcher to articulate the elements associated with a particular issue. Social spheres/power arenas maps illustrate analyses of how people organize relationships within structured conditions.[1] Positional maps represent the range of locations found in discourse practices, including exclusions and erasures of individuals, groups, concepts, knowledges, and perspectives. The method does not require that all types of maps be used, and the maps chosen or analytical processes may be modified. Further, a researcher engaged with/in a particular investigation may create new maps as needed.

The purpose of this chapter is to explain the use of SA for both initial research questions/design and as a data construction and analysis process tool. We describe the process as it was used to construct and implement a research study of early childhood public education in post-Katrina New Orleans.

Situational Analysis and Initial Research Design

To begin any form of qualitative research that can be considered trustworthy and credible (Lincoln & Cuba, 1985), the researcher must immerse her- or himself within the context. Exposure to the discourse practices that are constructing and being constructed by the circumstances facilitate decisions regarding both research questions and the types of data that should be used to address those questions. Media awareness, personal community engagement, and informational meetings are examples of the forms of engagement that contribute to the construction of a plan for research.

Using Situational Maps to Determine
Initial Research Questions

Situational maps allow the researcher to broadly articulate the elements (both human and nonhuman) emerging from the context that are associated with a particular issue (Clarke, 2005). The initial focus of our New Orleans study was developed by creating three types of situational maps: a topic map, a messy map, and an ordered map. Although there are two types of situational maps described by Clarke (the messy map and the ordered map), as we began to explore initial research questions, a more basic foundation for analysis seemed to be needed. Therefore, we first developed what we called a *"topic* situational map." We used this type of map to focus our attentions toward the extremely broad environmental context. A *messy* map then identified the broader discourses related to the situation and the key individuals, groups, organizations, and/or institutions that participate in, are a part of, make invisible, or produce constructions of the issues that emerge (Clarke, 2005). A messy situational map includes "all the analytically pertinent human and nonhuman, material, and symbolic/discursive elements of a particular situation *as framed by those in it and by the analyst"* (Clarke, 2005, p. 87; emphasis in the original). Once the initial messy map had been created, an ordered situational map was used to organize the ideas in a more systematic fashion and provide additional, more specific examples of individuals, groups, and issues to present a better picture of the discourses related to the situation.

Map 1: Topic Map

Topics for this map (Figure 6.1) were selected based on brainstorming from broad personal experiences with issues impacting education for young children related to disaster in New Orleans as we lived there after Hurricane Katrina. Volunteering, attending public community meetings, having conversations with families and former teachers, and conducting general readings of discourses found in the media are examples of these experiences.

An example of the way in which key issues were chosen to be part of the initial topic map can be illustrated with one of our volunteer experiences that occurred in a fourth-grade classroom in a New Orleans public school. One morning, an administrator required that the teacher give a survey to her students, which the teacher then asked us to administer to the class as a whole. The content of the survey was extremely personal and intrusive as it inquired about the children's experiences during and after Hurricane Katrina. Once

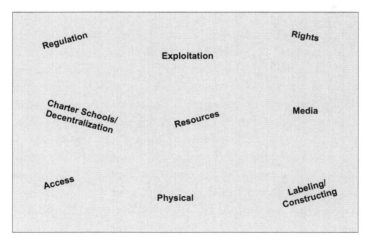

Figure 6.1 Initial topic map: Public discourses and lived experiences, specifically relating public education, disaster, and young children. Adapted from "Messy Situational Map: Nurses' Work under Managed Care," by A. E. Clarke, 2005, *Situational Analysis: Grounded Theory after the Postmodern Turn*, p. 95.

it was complete, the children were asked to resume with a Louisiana Educational Assessment Program test preparation activity. In reflecting on
this experience, it seems that requiring students to fill out a survey for an
undisclosed research purpose with little privacy given and no anonymity can
be viewed as exploitative. Therefore, this situation provides a rationale for
choosing "exploitation" as one of the overall issues impacting young children
in New Orleans, and, as a result, was chosen to be part of the initial topic
map. Additional issues on the map were chosen on a similar basis. A reflexive
reading/analysis of the issues chosen to be placed on the initial topic map led
to the development of the specific purpose for the study: How are discourses
created that influence access to an equitable public education for all young
children following disaster? This specific purpose is the focus of the second
messy situational map.

Map 2: Messy Situational Map

Our second situational map (Figure 6.2), labeled a "messy situational map" by
Clarke, includes specific situations related to the purpose of the study. The
content of this map was determined from a reflexive rereading/analysis of
the initial topic map and the discourses associated with additional volunteer
experiences, attending public community meetings, and further rereadings of
the discourses found in the media. Although every topic listed on this messy
situational map was not addressed in detail during the course of the study
(which would be the case in most studies), each topic was chosen because it
represented part of the overall situation impacting young children and public
education in New Orleans during the time period being considered.

For one year, we attempted to immerse ourselves in the everyday culture
of New Orleans by attending community meetings and events. This was
especially true for the first author related to community organizations. One
organization was a group called Concern, Community, and Compassion (C3),
a grassroots group that meets regularly and advocates for the right to fair
public housing in New Orleans. C3 also mobilizes resistance for other causes
relating to social justice such as protecting homeless civil rights and fighting
against civic repression (an issue that has intensified since Hurricane Katrina
with a heightened police presence, especially in low-income neighborhoods
and communities of color). Accounts witnessed during this involvement with
C3 influenced the decision to consider housing as an issue directly related to
equity for young children and is therefore included in the messy map. Other

Figure 6.2 Messy situational map: Discourses created that influence access to an equitable public education for all young children following disaster. Adapted from "Messy Situational Map: Nurses' Work under Managed Care," by A. E. Clarke, 2005, *Situational Analysis: Grounded Theory after the Postmodern Turn*, p. 95.

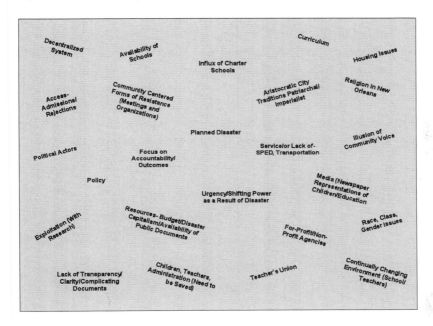

issues selected to be part of this map were determined by similar experiences or with general readings of discourses found in public documents.

Map 3: Ordered Situational Map

The ordered situational map frames and organizes the issues addressed in the messy map. The organization process for developing the ordered map is in itself a form of analysis. A series of headings is suggested in order to group the issues from the messy map. These include: individual human elements/ actors, collective human elements/actors, discursive constructions of individual and/or collective human actors, political/economic elements, temporal elements, major issues/debates, other kinds of elements, nonhuman elements/actants, implicated/salient actors/actants, discursive construction of nonhuman actants, sociocultural/symbolic elements, spatial elements, and related discourses (Clarke, 2005). However, the phrasing/meaning of the headings may be modified (and are not all required) so that the map can appropriately fit the context of a study. As the issues from the messy map are revisited to create the ordered map, some may become more specific in description (as depicted in Figure 6.3A and Figure 6.3B in the highlighted elements). Additionally, developing and revising the ordered map: (1) Frames issues/actors/actants impacting young children and public education in New Orleans as related to disaster; (2) assists in examining the social relationships and interactions found in the discourses; and (3) begins the process of identifying possible constructs of "power/knowledge, ideologies, and control" (Clarke, 2005, p. 15).

Examining the content of the ordered map created during the initial design of the study then assisted us in developing the specific research questions:

Individual Human Elements/Actors- *Key individuals and significant (unorganized) people in the situation*		
Governor Kathleen Babineaux Blanco*	Teachers	Members of school boards*
Administrators Political actors	Parents*	Students
Collective Human Elements/Actors- *Particular groups; specific organizations*		
Cowen Education Institute*	Teacher's Union	
Conservative Think Tanks (Thomas B. Fordham Foundation/Heritage Foundation)*		
Charter Schools/School choice groups*	Business Leaders*	
Community centered forms of resistance (meeting s and organizations)		
Discursive Constructions of Individual and/or collective human actors-*As found in the situation*		
Social world constructions of young children and communities of color (needing to be saved)*		
Illusion of community voice		
Political/Economic Elements- *The state; particular industry/ies; local/regional/global orders;*		
political parties; politicized issues		
Resources- Budget/disaster capitalism	Decentralized System	For profit/non-profit agencies
General Policy*	Lack of transparency/clarity/ complicating documents	
Specific Policy Agenda (e.g. federal funding for charter schools)		
Temporal Elements: US National Historical Frame- *Historical, seasonal, crisis, and/or trajectory aspects*		
Planned Disaster	Capitalism*	Neoliberalism*
School Choice/Charter School movement in the US*		
Major Issues/Debates (Usually Contested) -*As found in the situation; and see positional map*		
Influx of charter schools (privatization of public schools)	Services (or lack of- SPED/transportation)	
Access- admissions/rejections	Focus on Accountability/Outcomes	

Figure 6.3A Part one of ordered situational map: Discourses that influence access to an equitable public education for all young children following disaster. Adapted from "Ordered Situational Map: Nurses' Work under Managed Care," by A. E. Clarke, 2005, *Situational Analysis: Grounded Theory after the Postmodern Turn*, p. 97.

Figure 6.3B Part two of ordered situational map: Discourses that influence access to an equitable public education for all young children following disaster. Adapted from "Ordered Situational Map: Nurses' Work under Managed Care," by A. E. Clarke, 2005, *Situational Analysis: Grounded Theory after the Postmodern Turn*, p. 97.

Other Kinds of Elements- *As found in the situation*

Housing Issues   Exploitation of (with research)   Physical experiences*   Policing*

Nonhuman Elements/Actants- *Technologies; material infrastructures; specialized information and/or knowledges; material "things"*

Charter schools (as a concept/structurally)*   Curriculum   Disaster*

Availability of public documents

Implicated/Salient Actors/Actants- *As found in the situation*

Young Children*

Discursive Construction of Nonhuman Actants- *As found in the situation*

Urgency/Shifting power as a result of disaster   Charter schools (privatization) as an answer to public
                                                                 school rebuilding/reform*

Construction of curriculum as centered on testing*   Illusion that public documents are easily accessed (or
                                                                 even exist)*

Sociocultural/Symbolic Elements- *Religion; race; sexuality; gender; ethnicity; nationality; logos; icons; other visual and/ or aural symbols*

Race, class, gender issues and public school   Religion in New Orleans

Aristocratic city traditions (patriarchal/imperialist)

Spatial Elements- *Spaces in the situation, geographical aspects, local, regional, national, global spatial issues*

Continually changing environment (schools/teachers)   Availability of schools

Related Discourses (Historical, Narrative, and/or Visual) - *Normal expectations of actors, actants, and/or other specified elements; moral/ethical elements; mass media and other popular cultural discourses; situation-specific discourses*

Representation of young children in the media (Newspapers)   "Great Experiment" discourses*

Illusion of choice*   Discourse of elevated violence since Katrina; Killer City*

+ How are young children being discussed/represented in the charter school discourse surrounding public education in post-Katrina New Orleans?

A. What and who is included?
B. What and who is excluded (being left out)?

+ What are specific lived experiences that illustrate social justice/injustice and/or increased/decreased opportunities related to this discourse for young children and disaster?
+ How are these situations related to the way in which young children are constructed publicly?

The ordered map also helped determine the major and supplementary sources that would be used to collect, construct, and analyze data specifically to answer the research questions. One would expect that additional public gatherings, media, and state documents would provide a depth of information as well as interviews related to personal experience. However, because of our concern with the imperialist practices embedded within the notion of ethnographic interviews that claims to "know" the "other," we chose to use documents and public conversations as data sources rather than constructing new information by gathering from individual persons. The sources included: major data sources like the *Times Picayune* (the local newspaper) articles since August 29, 2005 (the day the hurricane made landfall as a Category 3 storm), the Louisiana Department of Education website and documents, New Orleans Public School and New Orleans Recovery District websites and policy documents; supplemental data sources (as illustrations of issues generated from the major sources) like New Orleans Charter School websites, New Orleans Parent Guide, and a range of additional public meetings. Our decision not to interview individuals is/was independent of the use of situational mapping. Although SA does require a variety of data sources to capture the complexity of the context, decisions regarding these sources are fluid within the method.

Data Collection, Construction, and Constant Analysis

SA requires that all data sources, both major and supplementary, be utilized simultaneously to address each specific question developed for the study as all are related and impact the overall understanding of the situation. As new maps are fashioned and data emerge, research design and procedures are/can be revised. As data are collected, situational, social spheres/power arenas, and positional maps are created resulting in new constructions of data (as the body of maps) and continued analysis and revision. Further, the method is fluid, allowing for new versions of map components and even conceptualizations of new types of maps.

Situational Maps
Messy Maps

Since SA allows for and facilitates the continual revisiting and revisioning of maps throughout the research project, data collection and analysis can begin with maps created during initial design of the research questions, like the situational maps that we constructed to provide focus to our research questions for the New Orleans early childhood study. The development of additional situational maps, as well as the revision of initial maps, is then shaped by the data retrieved from major and supplementary sources and the researcher's engagement with that data.

We also suggest that the researcher determine an organizational method to facilitate rereading, tracking, and location of bits of data (in our study, e.g., example personal stories, circumstances in a particular school, quotes from public officials). SA involves a large amount of information that cannot be specifically shown on maps that tend to represent the whole of a particular circumstance. Therefore, we chose to use "constant comparison" (Lincoln & Guba, 1985, p. 335) to facilitate map construction. First, we describe the detailed process (including constant comparison as a method for organizing data) used to create situational maps throughout the study. The two additional types of maps suggested by Clarke, social spheres/power arenas and positional, were also used during constant analysis. However, as the process for constructing these two types of maps is often dependent on analysis of situational maps, these types of maps are described in more general terms.

The following is a description of how a messy map was constructed and information from the map coded for analysis using one component of the New Orleans study: articles from the *Times Picayune* determined using "charter school" as the search term.

- The researcher first immersed herself in the content of the articles retrieved, beginning with articles immediately following Hurricane Katrina.
- Emerging discourse themes were placed in an informal fashion on the messy map. The map was given a label, Messy Map 1-A. The 1 symbolizes the first group of maps (in various studies, there could be additional groupings as the discourses are analyzed) and the A represents the first map in the series of a group.
- Note cards were then created for each item listed on the messy map. An example of the way in which an individual card was coded is Map 1-A (e.g., the corresponding map), TP (the source, *Times Picayune)*, CS (the search term, *Charter School)*, and all dates of the articles that correspond to the item on the map. When there were multiple articles from the same newspaper with the same date, the articles were coded

Figure 6.4 Example note card for a messy map. Illustrates the way in which an index card that corresponds to a messy map might be fashioned.

Messy Map 1-A, TP, CS,
10-12-05a, 12-08-06c

Element/Discourse from Messy Map: Equity

Equity is talked about in terms of distribution of funding and access to safe and functional facilities.

as 10-12-05a, 10-12-05b, and so on. Also, if a particular theme emerged in multiple articles, the multiple dates were recorded on the card. Therefore, a particular card representing a discourse theme listed on a messy map may have the code Map1-A, TP, CS, 10-12-05a, 12-08-06c. See Figure 6.4 for an example of a note card that corresponds to a particular messy map.

♦ After making note cards for each element listed on the initial messy map, a memo, or narrative, is provided on each card to explain the rationale for choosing the particular discourse for the map along with any other information pertinent to that term/issue (e.g., multiple representations of the term in the discourse, links to a specific group).

♦ After rereading a particular set of data used to create an initial messy map and a revisiting of the information on the corresponding note cards, the data were analyzed by revising the messy map to show possible shifts in the focus of the discourses relating to the text.

Analysis has been "saturated" (Clark, 2005, p. 108) when all possibilities for composure of the situational messy map and multiple readings of major and supplementary sources have taken place.

Relational Analysis with Messy Maps

Clarke (2005) also describes relational analysis as a tool for analyzing relationships among discourses listed on a messy map. Although this type of analysis may be used for some portions of a study, the method may not be employed for every messy map developed. To conduct relational analysis, one must first have a general understanding of all the discourses associated with an initial/revised messy map. Then, each term on the messy map will be used as a focal point to determine the relationships that exist (or may not exist) among the issues. Lines can be drawn from the chosen focal point to the related elements on the map. Using the content of the topic map originally created as part of initial design in the New Orleans study, Figure 6.5 is an example of a relational analysis messy map; the focal point of "access" is related to "charter schools/decentralization," "resources," and "rights."

Three note cards were created in this example to describe the relationship that exists between the focal point access and each of the related terms chosen. The note cards denote the corresponding relational map with similar memo and coding as described previously (see Figure 6.6).

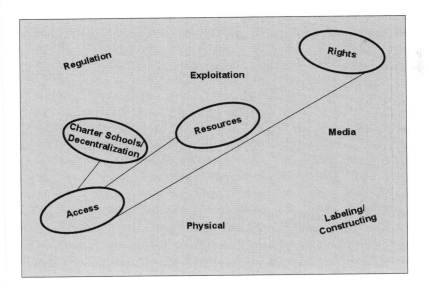

Figure 6.5 Relational analysis map. Illustrates the relationship between access, charter schools/decentralization and rights. Adapted from "Relational Analysis Using Situational Map: Focus on Nurses' Emotion Work," by A. E. Clarke, 2005, *Situational Analysis: Grounded Theory after the Postmodern Turn*, p. 105.

Figure 6.6 Example note card for relational analysis map. Illustrates the way in which an index card that corresponds to a relational map might be fashioned.

Relational Analysis with Messy Map 1-A
Focal Word "Access"
Relationship: Access and Charter Schools/
Decentralization

A general reading of the discourses has shown that some charter schools deny access to children through admission requirements.

Specific examples of this relationship is found in

TP, CS, 10-05-06a
TP, CS, 04-12-07c

Once all elements on the map have been placed at the center of analysis and note cards have been made, additional messy and relational maps are fashioned to uncover further issues and relationships among them. Eventually, this process will facilitate decisions concerning which "stories" (Clarke, 2005, p. 102) to pursue based on connections (or lack of connections) made between elements listed on each map.

Ordered Situational Map

The ordered map serves as a tool to organize, structure, and provide further detail of the content from the messy maps. (Again, see Figure 6.1 and Figure 6.2 for ordered maps created for the initial design of our New Orleans study.) Although categories have been developed by Clarke (2005) to assist in creating the ordered map (e.g., sociocultural/symbolic elements and political/economic elements), these can be used as suggested or modified to fit a particular set of data and/or messy map focus. As the elements from messy maps are revisited to generate the ordered map, some descriptions of the issues may become more specific (for instance by including names of organizations or political figures that are part of the overall understanding of a situation but that have not been included in the messy maps). The process of developing and revising the ordered map in itself is a form of analysis as it assists in: (1) framing the issues/actors/actants impacting the situation;

(2) examining the social relationships and interactions found in the discourses; and (3) beginning the process of identifying possible constructs of "power/knowledge, ideologies, and control" (Clarke, 2005, p. 155). The number of ordered maps constructed for constant SA varies with the study and cannot be preplanned.

Social Spheres/Power Arenas Maps

Social spheres/power arenas maps (See Figure 6.7) are "cartographies of collective commitments, relations, and sites of action" (Clarke, 2005, p. 86). These types of maps illuminate power and the way in which people organize (whether voluntarily or involuntarily) in relation to larger structural situations by acting [out], producing, and responding to discourses (Clarke, 2005, p. 109). Clarke explains:

> Discourses per se are not explicitly represented on social worlds/arenas maps. This is not because they are not present in worlds and arenas but

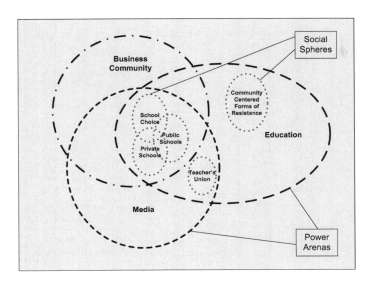

Figure 6.7 Example social spheres/power arenas map. Illustrates the way in which power arenas like education, the business community, and the media interact with social spheres like school choice, private schools, public schools, the teacher's union, and community-centered forms of resistance. Adapted from "Social Worlds/Arenas Map: RU486 Discourse Project," by A. E. Clarke, 2005, *Situational Analysis: Grounded Theory after the Postmodern Turn*, p. 195.

because social worlds *are* universes of discourse (Strauss, 1978) in arenas constituted and maintained *through* discourses. Instead, the focus of
social worlds/arenas maps is on *collective social action.* (p. 114)

This type of map depicts social spheres and power arenas that interact
with each other, overlap, and include the individuals/groups seemingly absent
from discourses to give a broader picture of the situation. Again, we chose to
combine map construction with unitized constant comparison creating
memos on note cards to describe the discourses that make up each major
social sphere/power arena. Multiple revisions were made as discourses were
analyzed through map construction, ultimately changing the focus and
appearance of the social spheres/power arenas map and helping to determine
which "stories to tell" (Clarke 2005 p. 111) or to give focus.

Positional Maps

Positional maps (see Figures 6.8 and 6.9) are used to represent the range of
positions found in discourses (including issues, absence where one might
expect presence and contradictions). Clarke (2005) emphasizes that these
maps are *not* symbolic of (or meant to analyze) a specific person, group, or

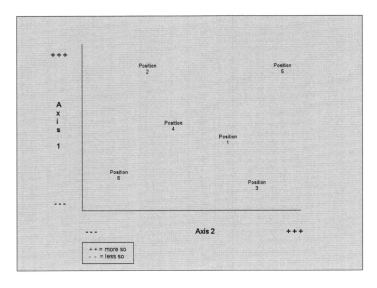

Figure 6.8 Example template of a positional map. From "Abstract Positional Map," by
A. E. Clarke, 2005, *Situational Analysis: Grounded Theory after the Postmodern Turn,* p. 129.

Figure 6.9 Fabricated example of a positional map. Illustrates the differing positions on education defined as test scores and broad definitions of education. Dominant and marginalized positions are also represented in abstract form. Adapted from "Positional Map: Clinical Efficiency and Emotion Work in Nursing Care," by A. E. Clarke, 2005, *Situational Analysis: Grounded Theory after the Postmodern Turn*, p. 130.

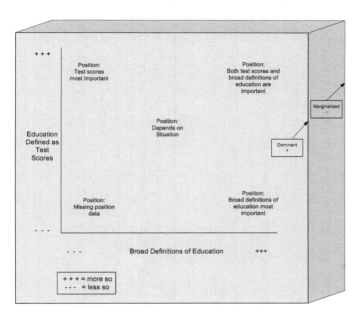

institution's position but rather "represent the heterogeneity of positions" (p. 126) found within discourses. The elements placed on the axes of the map and the positions (or lack of positions) charted are determined based on the examination of discourses already illuminated by situational maps and/or social spheres/power arenas maps. Figure 6.8 provides a template for a positional map, and Figure 6.9 is a fabricated example of a positional map that illustrates the differing positions on the "definition of education" (as testing or as understood more broadly). Additionally, Figure 6.9 takes on a three-dimensional shape to highlight dominant and marginalized understandings of education (e.g., silenced knowledges, erased people, disqualified skills).

Attending to Research Questions

Once all data sources and maps are fully analyzed both individually and comprehensively (through the process of constructing maps, creating note cards/

memos, and reflexive revisions), the discourses found to be related to each specific question, along with additional situations/issues that may emerge, can be part of the overall findings, contingencies, and discussion of the study. Additionally, specific kinds of data may emerge as addressing particular questions more thoroughly; serving as the research instrument, we suggest that the investigator purposely and reflexively focus on the research questions through both journaling and directed rereadings. To illustrate, in our example study in New Orleans, the 151 articles from the "charter school" search resulted in three initial messy situational maps constructed from a focus on the discourses found in: (1) the title of the articles; (2) the major points of each article that include/exclude young children; and (3) the issues that seem to be left out of the content of each article. The initial messy maps developed for each of these three categories specifically address the first question related to the ways that "young children are represented," "included," and/or "excluded." Further mapping was conducted to assist in allowing for a more in-depth understanding of the discourses and to assist in determining illustrative experiences that would be chosen from supplementary resources. Research questions can be addressed specifically, as in situational interaction with each other, and reflexively throughout the study.

Critical Qualitative Research and Using SA in Times of Global Crisis

SA is a reflexive, fluid, and open research methodology that offers avenues for critical qualitative research that can unveil the complexities of societal systems and inequities, whether related to public policy, institutional structures, or other societal constructs that constitute hegemonic conditions. Although micro situations can undoubtedly be explored using this form of phenomenological analysis, the contemporary global circumstances that have resulted in complex networks of power, disaster capitalism, and neoliberal intrusions into every aspect of life require a range of research methodologies that can be used to reveal the complexities of power. SA can certainly provide one such lens.

Note

1. As critical scholars, we chose to insert the "power" construct. Clarke's initial work uses social spheres/arenas without the necessary concern for power).

References

Clarke, A. E. (2005). *Situational analysis: Grounded theory after the postmodern turn.* Thousand Oaks, CA: Sage.

Lincoln, Y. S., & Guba, E. G. (1985). *Naturalistic Inquiry.* Newbury Park, CA: Sage.

Additional References Using Situational Analysis

Clarke, A. (2003). Situational analysis: Grounded theory mapping after the postmodern turn. *Symbolic Interaction, 26,* 4, 553-576.

Clarke, A. (2006). Feminisms, grounded theory, and situational analysis. In S. Hesse-Biber (Ed.), *The handbook of feminist research: Theory and praxis* (pp. 345-370). Thousand Oaks, CA: Sage.

Clarke, A. (2007). Grounded theory: Conflicts, debates and situational analysis. In W. Outhwaite & S. P. Turner (Eds.), *Handbook of social science and technology studies* (pp. 838-885). Cambridge, MA: MIT Press.

Clarke, A. & Friese, C. (2007). Situational analysis: Going beyond traditional grounded theory. In K. Charmaz & A. Bryant (Eds.), *Handbook of grounded theory.* London: Sage.

Clarke, A., & Star, S. L. (2007). The social worlds/arenas/discourse framework as a theory-methods package. In E. Hackett, O. Amsterdamska, M. Lynch, & J. Wacjman (Eds.), *Handbook of science and technology studies* (pp. 113-137). London: Sage.

Gagnon, M., Jacob, J. D., & Holmes, D. (2010). Governing through (in)security: A critical analysis of a fear-based public health campaign. *Critical Public Health, 20,* 2, 245-256.

Mills, J., Chapman, Y., Bonner, A., Francis, K. (2007). Grounded theory: A methodological spiral from positivism to postmodernism, *Journal of Advanced Nursing, 58,* 1, 72-79.

Mills, J., Francis, K., & Bonner, A. (2008). Getting to know a stranger—rural nurses' experiences of mentoring: A grounded theory. *International Journal of Nursing Studies, 45,* 4, 599-607.

Reflection: On Using Situational Analysis for Critical Qualitative Research Purposes

Michelle Salazar Pérez & Gaile S. Cannella

Acknowledging Critical Research Purposes

For at least thirty years, scholars from a range of fields, perspectives, and locations have generated research that would unveil/challenge/transform inequities and injustices created within the diverse and complex relations of power. This work has been/can be labeled feminist, poststructural, queer, postcolonial/indigenous, and critical (theory and pedagogy). While some scholars disagree with the very suggestion that such perspectives are related, even they find it difficult to challenge the notion that all are concerned with relations, complexities, and impositions of power in ways that privilege or harm, normalize or disqualify, even destroy and erase.

Historically, a large body of scholarship and research has emerged that is foundational to this project that is often broadly labeled "critical." This ranges from the postcolonial/indigenous work of Said (1979), Gandhi (1998), Spivak (1999), and Smith (2001) to the poststructural work of Foucault and other Continentalists, to the intersectional work of feminists of color such as Collins (2008), just to name a core few. Often these diverse epistemological perspectives are used to philosophically ground research questions, designs, and analysis as lenses that would challenge traditionally white, male, Western constructions of research and theorizing. Additionally, as the field of qualitative research has expanded in all directions and locations, those who have been concerned with ever-present relations of power—as political, personal, economic, and even environmental—have most often used the broad-based field of qualitative inquiry as their site of academic practice (Cannella & Lincoln 2012).

A large body of work can be found that critiques dominant research conceptualizations and practices and calls for a critical social science (e.g., Popkewitz 1990) that would rethink research. However, even from within this broad history, the complexity and contingent nature of relations of power as produced and producing results is a form of science that is difficult both conceptually and in practice. Further, critical qualitative researchers struggle to determine approaches to use in constructing or collecting, organizing, and interpreting the complex and often large bodies of data necessary for the exploration and potential transformation of particular power relations. We found that situational analysis (SA) (Clarke 2005) facilitated this work for us.

The approach is grounded in a deconstructive purpose that seeks to make differences visible and silences speak, while robustly allowing for instability, rupture, and negotiation within the research process. In our research examining the charter school movement in post-Katrina New Orleans (Pérez & Cannella 2010), SA served as a visual method that helped us unveil power relations masked within texts and public activities within a context in which large amounts of data were shifting (being constructed, disappearing, performed) at the speed of light (Cannella & Pérez 2009). Further, diverse maps and the flexibility of the process (and possibilities for visual construction) literally made possible the visual connections of traditionally marginalized knowledges/lenses with research data (Pérez & Cannella 2013). In this case, we used black feminist thought (e.g., Collins 2008).

Research Context and the Use of Situational Analysis

Our arrival in post-Katrina New Orleans in the summer of 2007 brought both great excitement (to be a part of a community with important past social justice and civil rights activist roots) and apprehension (concern about how we would conceptualize a critical qualitative research project that would become Michelle's dissertation). We sought to expose the public education circumstances of what had become a deeply socially oppressed and ecologically devastated region. The charter school movement as a performance of disaster capitalism (Adams 2012; Klein 2007) and its role in further limiting children's access to an equitable public education ultimately became the focus of the research. While the public education system was not held in high regard by the communities it served prior to the failure of the levees, in 2005, the charter school movement then pushed stakeholders' and children's voices even further to the margins than before Katrina. Using disaster as the excuse for firing vast numbers of education personnel and dismantling the union, school system "reform" became the mechanism used to privatize every facet of public education.

Situational analysis was the method we used to document these activities. The flexible, changeable mapping method facilitated direct application of black feminist perspectives (Collins 2008), combining constructs like the matrix of domination with various texts from New Orleans newspaper articles/visual media outlets, state education documents, field notes from local public meetings, and journal reflections. In the disaster context in which information changed rapidly, SA provided a vehicle through which change, debates, and complex issues could be represented (and permanently maintained) across a range of temporal circumstances and periods. The maps even became documents themselves for comparison from one time period to another, for discussion within collaboration in our regular meetings, and as reminders/stimulators for journal reflection.

Most Useful Maps

The research design, data construction, and analysis for the study focused on the use of messy and ordered situational maps, social worlds/arenas (repurposed as social spheres/power arenas) maps, and positional maps. The use of each device was purposeful based on either what we felt was the most appropriate for analyzing a particular focal point or to assist us when we needed to engage in a broader vision of the circumstances.

Messy Maps

These maps were especially useful for delving into all aspects of the situation. The current bigger picture could be made visible, while at the same time future possibilities could be generated. Further, messy maps allowed for consideration of all discourses found within the situation, both human and nonhuman, even if all were not ultimately used as focal points of the study (e.g., how public housing residents were disenfranchised by school decentralizing). Although messy maps mainly served the function of foundational analysis, as the research unfolded and at times changed direction, new messy maps were continually conceptualized and revised alongside more complex maps.

Ordered Maps

A more thorough examination of discursive constructions within/by/used to legitimate the charter school movement was made possible using ordered maps. We were prompted by the discourses emerging from our messy maps to determine who the main actors/actants were within the situation, how they were discursively produced, and what agendas they served. For instance, since our messy maps included elements like the appointment of state and local district leaders with non-education backgrounds, the generation of ordered maps facilitated the search for and listing of specific names of those in leadership positions and the organizations they represented. Additionally, ordered maps furthered our intersectional analysis (Collins 2008) as we considered how intertwining power matrices surrounding race, class, gender, and sexuality, among other identity markers, were being constructed or made invisible within the discourses. Generation of ordered maps, then, assisted in providing depth and direction for data collection and continued analysis.

Social Spheres/Power Arenas Maps

In addition to gaining both broad and specific knowledge of the situation from the creation of messy and ordered maps, other qualitative research methods such as participant observation, unitizing and constant comparison of media discourses, and reflexive journaling facilitated the development of a social spheres/power arenas map. This map was useful in that it provided analysis of the social spheres that emerged from the data (rhetoric of community input, firing of local teachers, etc.) and how power arenas like urgency, lab/experiment, and opportunity discourses worked in relation to/with these social spheres to (re)produce intersectional matrices of domination. This type of SA map also accounted for the marginalization of young children and teacher's voices. The social spheres/power arena map in particular served as an analytic tool in determining which stories to tell based on the themes that emerged from combining SA with other critical qualitative research methods and to unveil the power structures produced by/functioning within the discourses.

Positional Maps

Similar to our conceptualization of a social spheres/power arenas map for the study, combining SA with other qualitative methods such as constant comparison and participant observation resulted in the utilization of a positional map. It was generated based on the perspectives of those who were critical of, or supported, the circumstances produced by the charter school movement (such as greater emphasis on standardized testing, system decentralization, and children's lack of access to equitable educational experiences). The positional map was useful as it allowed illustration of oppositional viewpoints and even, when redesigned to become three-dimensional, the representation of traditionally hidden/masked viewpoints.

Notes on Experiences with Situational Analysis

Our experiences with mapping and (re)conceptualizing through situational analysis led to unexpected uses and researcher actions including the following.

SA as a Research Design Tool

From the outset of the project, we utilized messy and ordered situational maps to help us conceptualize the initial purpose and research design. Living in the community made it possible for us to immerse ourselves in daily conversations and activities that facilitated awareness of the dominant forms of language and actions being used to legitimate reform. Situational messy mapping was then used to create visualizations of these experiences that led to the construction of research topics (later made more specific with research questions). Further, maps were created for potential data sources and methods of data construction. Messy maps are uniquely suited to recording broad-based local contexts and experiences so that an overall view can be created clarifying purpose of local research as well as the necessary design components.

Situational Analysis as Generating Possibilities for Collaboration

We found that working together collaboratively on map design/analysis was extremely beneficial. As maps were constructed and we each brought our unique experiences to the discussions, a deeper, more complete, yet multifaceted picture of the charter school movement was possible. Additionally, collaborative map production enabled yet another layer of reflective practice as we challenged each other to think further about the research process.

Making the Research One's Own

As we felt it was intended by Clarke (2005), using SA in a way that fit the specific context of the study was key. As such, we considered the postmodern rethinking of grounded theory and map-making exemplars as reference points, not as a strict, fixed methodological process to be rigidly followed.

As an example, once we began to generate a positional map with the various standpoints related to the implementation of state standardized testing, Gaile proposed the reconceptualization of the map to result in a three-dimensional format. For this particular study, this third dimension facilitated the inclusion of the marginalized and often invisible perspectives of young children and other public education stakeholders within the standardized testing debate. While created within the practice of situational analysis for particular purposes, the range of maps and the varying degree to which text, visualizations, and positionings are possible results in greater flexibility and new research possibilities.

Critical Qualitative Research Using Situational Analysis

Cartography throughout the research was iterative as we viewed SA map making as an open-ended, ever-evolving process. Messy maps especially were made in abundance as the research expanded, taking into consideration larger amounts of data that emerged from experiences in the community and the analysis of sources. Maps were rethought and reconceptualized numerous times as we reflected on new information that came to light, making our analyses at times disordered, untidy, and muddled. However, these are exactly the states and conditions that we would expect for critical qualitative research, inquiry that is messy because power relations are complex, laden with data, and always contingent. SA is not easy, requiring depth of philosophical understanding as well as extensive time for data collection, construction, exploration, and analysis—exactly what we would also expect for critical qualitative research that would ultimately be transformative. SA is certainly one valuable tool for scholars who hope to practice critical qualitative inquiry.

References

Adams, V. 2012. *Markets of Sorrow, Labors of Faith: New Orleans in the Wake of Katrina.* Durham, NC: Duke University Press.

Cannella, G. S. & Y. S. Lincoln. 2012. Deploying Qualitative Methods for Critical Social Purposes. In S. R. Steinberg & G. S. Cannella (Eds.), *Critical Qualitative Research Reader* (pp. 104–115). New York: Peter Lang.

Cannella, G. S. & M. S. Pérez. 2009. Power Shifting at the Speed of Light: Critical Qualitative Research Post-disaster. In N. K. Denzin & M. D. Giardina (Eds.), *Qualitative Inquiry and Social Justice: Toward a Politics of Hope* (pp. 165–186). Walnut Creek, CA: Left Coast Press, Inc.

Clarke, A. E. 2005. *Situational Analysis: Grounded Theory after the Postmodern Turn*. Thousand Oaks, CA: Sage.

Collins, P. H. 2008. *Black Feminist Thought: Knowledge, Consciousness, and the Politics of Empowerment* (3rd ed.). New York: Routledge.

Gandhi, L. 1998. *Postcolonial Theory: A Critical Introduction*. New York: Columbia University Press.

Klein, N. 2007. *The Shock Doctrine: The Rise of Disaster Capitalism*. New York: Metropolitan Books.

Pérez, M. S. & G. S. Cannella. 2010. Disaster Capitalism as Neoliberal Instrument for the Construction of Early Childhood Education/Care Policy: Charter Schools in Post-Katrina New Orleans. In G. S. Cannella & L. D. Soto (Eds.), *Childhoods: A Handbook, Critical Histories and Contemporary Issues, Rethinking Childhood Series* (pp. 145–156). New York: Peter Lang.

Pérez, M. S. & G. S. Cannella. 2013. Situational Analysis as an Avenue for Critical Qualitative Research: Mapping Post-Katrina New Orleans. *Qualitative Inquiry* 19(7):1–13.

Popkewitz, T. S. 1990. Whose Future? Whose Past? Notes on Critical Theory and Methodology. In E. G. Guba (Ed.), *The Paradigm Dialog* (pp. 46–66). Newbury Park, CA: Sage.

Said, E. 1979. *Orientalism*. New York: Vintage Books.

Smith, L. T. 2001. *Decolonizing Methodologies: Research and Indigenous Peoples*. New York: Zed Books.

Spivak, G. C. 1999. *A Critique of Postcolonial Reason: Toward a History of the Vanishing Present*. Cambridge, MA: Harvard University Press.

CHAPTER 7

RETHINKING THE DISCLOSURE DEBATES: A SITUATIONAL ANALYSIS OF THE MULTIPLE MEANINGS OF HUMAN BIOMONITORING DATA

Rachel Washburn

Introduction

I t is now possible to measure trace levels of environmental chemicals (e.g. pesticides, metals, plasticizers, and flame retardants), their metabolites, and/or related byproducts in human fluids and tissues through a process called human biomonitoring (Albertini et al. 2006; Gallagher, Hubal, and Edwards 2010; Needham 2008). Though originally developed to monitor the chemical exposures of factory workers in the early 1900s, over the past several decades, the tools and techniques used in biomonitoring have been substantially refined. What were once considered onerous procedures that produced unreliable results have become more automated with the introduction of high-throughput computer-assisted instruments. As a result, scientists can now measure more chemicals at lower concentrations with better accuracy than has previously been possible (Sexton, Needham, and Pirkle 2004, 45). However, these developments have not been met with a commensurate body of knowledge on the human health implications of chemical exposures and, as a consequence, scientists can now produce far more biomonitoring data than they know how to interpret (National Research Council 2006).

This predicament is certainly not novel in the era of genomics and data mining. However, in the case of biomonitoring, it has led to robust debates among scientists, regulators, and environmental health activists regarding if and how to communicate individual-level data to research participants. Some scientists argue that individual-level data should not be shared with research participants on the grounds that these data do not yet have clear implications for individual health and thus may cause unwarranted concern and anxiety. They also contend that the provision of individual-level results to research participants inappropriately gives what is fundamentally

From Washburn, Rachel. *Critical Public Health*, Volume 23, No. 4, December 2012, 452–465. © Taylor & Francis. *Republished in Situational Analysis in Practice*, by Adele E. Clarke, Carrie Friese, and Rachel Washburn, 241–269. (Taylor & Francis, 2015). All rights reserved.

intended for public health surveillance and research purposes the guise of a clinical tool (Williams et al. 2008). Others, however, argue that if research participants give their bodily fluids for analyses, they have the 'right-to-know' about their exposures, regardless of the current interpretive uncertainties. Guidance from Institutional Review Boards (IRBs) in the USA is equally mixed. Some IRBs suggest providing individual-level data to study participants, while most require only the provision of group-level data or nothing at all. This means that currently in the USA, there is wide variation in the type of information research participants in biomonitoring studies may receive (Brown et al. 2010).

What explains these contradictory opinions and uneven practices? The most commonly held explanation, and the one that has been forwarded in a small but influential body of work, posits that the unevenness is attributable to conflicting interpretations of bioethical principles and contrasting politics regarding the role of research participants in the scientific enterprise. For example, environmental scientist and advocate Julia Brody and her collaborators (2007) argue that the four bioethical principles of autonomy, nonmaleficence, beneficence, and justice can all be interpreted to support the communication of individual-level biomonitoring data as the most appropriate and morally defensible course of action (see also Brown 2007; Brown et al. 2010; Buck et al. 2010; Wilson et al. 2010; Wu et al 2009). Furthermore, these authors suggest that the practice of withholding this information from research participants relies on 'ethical standards' that are, simply put, 'outdated' (2007, 1552). Others see things differently. Bioethicist Myron Harrison (2007, 6) asserts that while 'the principle of autonomy supports the "right-to-know"' . . . the principles of beneficence, nonmaleficence, and veracity seem to support nondisclosure.' He goes on to add that 'it is highly unlikely that an individual gains any benefit in knowing his personal test results as opposed to the readily available group mean given to the community (certainly, valuable knowledge)' (see also Deck and Kosatsky 1999; Foster and Agzarian 2007; Williams et al. 2008).

Environmental health scientist Rachel Morello-Frosch and her collaborators (2009, 2011) shed additional light on this debate by suggesting that decisions regarding the communication of biomonitoring data to research participants also stem from investigators' orientation to the research enterprise and the types of relationships they cultivate with the communities they study. These authors point out that in community-based participatory research, where research is viewed as a joint venture between scientists and communities, findings are typically shared and interpreted with study participants. However, they argue that in a 'clinical ethics' model where scientific experts control the research process, personal biomonitoring data are only shared with participants if deemed clinically significant.

In this article, I aim to contribute to this body of scholarship by demonstrating that although the disclosure debates have been framed in terms of differing ethical perspectives, a more profound source of disagreement derives from fundamentally different ways of evaluating the meaning and significance of biomonitoring data. Of particular importance is the question of whether measurements performed on individual biological samples (blood, urine, etc.) collected at a single point in time constitute *useful information*. I focus here on 'single measurement' data because many biomonitoring surveillance and research programs use cross-sectional study design in which only one sample is available.

Based on an analysis of qualitative interviews with scientists, health officials, and environmental health advocates, as well as observational fieldnotes and textual materials, I find that there are at least three different positions on the extent to which single measurement data constitute useful information. The first position, most often articulated by analytical chemists, toxicologists, and epidemiologists, holds that single measurement data, at the individual level, often do not provide useful information for the purposes of assessing health risk and accurately classifying exposure, and therefore, are of questionable value for both scientists and research participants. The second position, which was articulated by epidemiologists, toxicologists, and environmental health advocates, views single measurement data as having limitations, but still useful in particular contexts for particular purposes. Specifically, this position sees utility in single measurement data for the purposes of encouraging individuals to take action to reduce their exposures and within the context of trying to promote trusting relationships between researchers and research communities. The third, and final, position holds that *all* biomonitoring data are useful for the purposes of documenting what has been termed 'chemical trespass,' or the unwanted presence of environmental chemicals in human bodies: here the mere detection of exposure constitutes useful information. Epidemiologists and environmental health advocates articulated this position.

In what follows, I describe each of these positions in greater detail. In doing so, I hope to encourage analysts of the disclosure debates and concerned stakeholders to see different positions on the communication of individual-level biomonitoring data to research participants as stemming not simply from differing interpretations of bioethical principles, but also fundamentally different ways of evaluating and assigning meaning to biomonitoring data. I find that while ethical principles and perspectives may serve as criteria in the evaluation of these data, they are certainly not the sole criteria used by all stakeholders. Rather, as the findings described below demonstrate, a variety of criteria and definitions of usefulness are brought to bear on the evaluation of biomonitoring data, which reflect different epistemological orientations, political agendas, and priorities. Acknowledging these important points of difference may offer a path towards greater consensus on if and how to communicate individual-level biomonitoring data to research participants.

Methods

This article is based on an ongoing qualitative sociological study of the history and contemporary politics of human biomonitoring in the USA. Data were collected from June 2005 to July 2012 through semi-structured interviews, participant observation, and the collection of textual materials. I have interviewed scientists (working in academia and government agencies), environmental health advocates, a journalist, a technician at a commercial laboratory, and individuals who have participated in biomonitoring studies. The findings presented in this article are based on an analysis of a subset of data from this larger study. Specifically, it relies on interviews with scientists and environmental health advocates, as well as participant observation at planning meetings for the California Biomonitoring Program, and textual data (described in greater detail below). I limited the data-set for analysis based on the goal of understanding how discourses produced by those involved in making decisions about the communication of biomonitoring data evaluate and assign meaning to these data.

Data Collection
Interviews

This paper draws on qualitative interviews conducted with 27 individuals from the following categories: epidemiologists ($n = 12$), analytical chemists ($n = 7$), environmental health advocates ($n = 7$), and a toxicologist. Participants for this study were selected based on their involvement in the production or use of biomonitoring data, and were identified through a review of scientific publications (books and journal articles), government reports and websites, and environmental health advocacy organization websites. Following ethics approval, individuals were recruited by email or by phone, and interviewed in person and in some cases over the phone. The interviews lasted between 45 and 90 minutes and covered a range of topics related to participants' professional background and thoughts on the meaning and most appropriate uses of biomonitoring data, as well as the communication of biomonitoring data to research participants.

The interviews were recorded and transcribed verbatim by a professional transcriptionist with the permission of participants.

Participant Observation

Participant observation was carried out at professional conferences, scientific meetings, advocacy-sponsored events, a clinic in Northern California where biomonitoring was offered to patients, and a graduate-level environmental health course. I also attended five all-day planning meetings of the California Environmental Contaminant Biomonitoring Program (also referred to as the California Biomonitoring Program). This program was initiated in 2006 following the passage of California Senate Bill 1379, and is intended to provide data on the chemical exposures of a representative sample of California residents. Part of the legislation also requires that individual-level biomonitoring data be provided to participants of the program, should they request this information. I have downloaded and analyzed all available transcripts from the 18 meetings that have occurred to date (July, 2012). These meetings provide a rich site for examining how the meaning and usefulness of biomonitoring data are framed in discourses.

Texts

Several types of textual data have also been collected for this project. These include government reports, scientific journal articles, books and book chapters, popular press reports, position papers, environmental health advocacy reports, and meeting transcripts. I also analyzed the content of websites written by industry groups and environmental health advocacy organizations.

Data Analysis

The analysis presented in this article is based largely on situational analysis, a recent supplement to grounded theory (Clarke 2003, 2005, 2009). Among the analytical techniques used situational analysis are situational, relational, and positional maps. Data analysis began with a modified version of traditional grounded theory coding (Strauss 1987; Strauss and Corbin 1998). Transcripts, fieldnotes, and collected texts were coded to identify substantive themes. This resulted in an initial set of over 100 codes. These codes were then grouped into categories, which were explored in analytic memos. Based on the analytic memos, a second round of more focused coding was conducted. I paid particular attention to descriptions of how biomonitoring works, the contexts and conditions under which biomonitoring data are more or less valid, and problems that affect the quality of the data.

Based on the second round of coding, I created several positional maps. These maps are intended to help the analyst 'lay out the major positions taken, and *not* taken, in the data vis-à-vis particular axes of variation and difference, concern, and controversy found in the situation of concern' (Clarke 2003, 560 emphasis in original). It was through this process that the *usefulness* of single biomonitoring measurements emerged as a particularly salient and analytically helpful axis along which to distinguish the three major discursive positions described in this paper.

As with all qualitative research studies, the analyst is understood as an instrument in the study, and as such, the findings presented here reflect the author's analysis and interpretation of the data.

Positions on the Usefulness of Single Measurement Biomonitoring Data

Figure 7.1 is a map of the major positions taken in the data organized along two axes: (1) the extent to which single biomonitoring measurements constitute 'useful information,' and (2) the value of communicating individual-level biomonitoring data to research participants. The positions on this map represent positions taken in discourses, not those held by specific individuals, groups, or institutions. Within my data-set, several individuals and groups articulate different and even contradictory positions regarding both the extent to which single measurement data constitute useful information and the value of communicating these data to research participants.

Position A: Single Measurement Data Generally Not Useful

Position A holds that single biomonitoring measurements generally do not provide useful information at the individual level. For this position, usefulness is evaluated based on two criteria that both reflect the norms and practices of knowledge production within analytical chemistry, toxicology, and epidemiology. They are: (1) the extent to which measured chemical concentrations in bodily fluids and tissues can be used to accurately characterize and classify typical exposures and (2) the existence of health-based guidelines through which measured concentrations may be interpreted. With respect to the first criterion, position A emphasizes the distinction between a measured concentration of a chemical in bodily fluids and/or tissues, on the one hand and exposure, on the other. This position views measured concentrations as signals of exposure, not equivalent to the measurement of exposure. One analytical chemist put it this way: 'people sometimes forget that with biomonitoring, we do not measure exposures. We measure concentrations. And here is one of the major challenges in biomonitoring' (Statement made at California Biomonitoring Program meeting, 10 November 2011 transcript, 53).

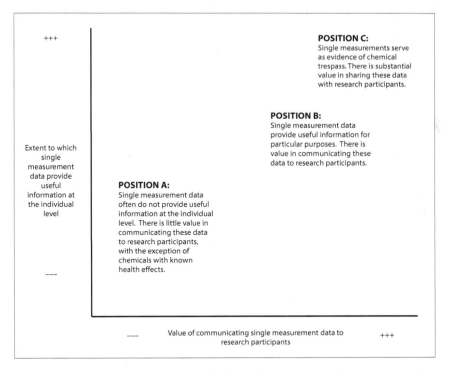

Figure 7.1 Positions on the extent to which single measurement biomonitoring data provide useful information at the individual level and the value of communicating these data to research participants.

Given the episodic nature of human contact with many environmental chemicals, position A points out that on any given day, at any given time, the measureable concentration of a chemical in human fluids and tissues may not reflect an exposure that occurred the previous day, week, month, or year. Single measurement data provide a 'snapshot in time,' and for transient chemicals (i.e. those that are metabolized and excreted quickly), 'could very well not represent reality' (Statement made by epidemiologist at California Biomonitoring Program meeting, 29 July 2009, transcript, 123). The potential failure to capture the 'realities' of exposures is precisely what drives position A to view these data as having questionable utility within the context of exposure assessment. The only conditions through which individual-level data constitute useful information are repeated sampling, which helps to capture daily, weekly, and monthly exposure variation and/or aggregation across hundreds or even thousands of individuals. This position was also expressed in the following ways:

> The level measured in an individual will be influenced by a large number of factors, and typically only one measurement is available. This is especially the case for chemicals with short half-lives in the body, where daily (or even hourly) fluctuations in biomarker levels in an individual will not be captured by the one measurement and may misrepresent the typical level in the individual. (LaKind et al. 2008, S19)

> There are a lot of sources of variability in biomonitoring measurements, particularly with respect to short half-life compounds in the body. . . . So, how well does a given sample actually classify exposure? . . . We [found that we] can correctly classify that exposure about 46 percent of the time. So, we're basically running at 50 percent or not much better than chance, with a single measurement. (Fieldnotes, statement made by epidemiologist at California Biomonitoring Program meeting, 26 July 2012)

Here we see the articulation of what could be termed analytical usefulness, or the extent to which biomonitoring data can be used to accurately assess and classify an individual's typical exposures. Based on the variability described above, particularly for transient, or nonpersistent compounds, position A holds that single measurement data often do not provide analytically useful information at the individual level. This in turn also leads position A to see single measurement data as having little use for research participants. This position was expressed in the following way:

> Having a list of chemicals, to me, doesn't really mean much, especially for these nonpersistent chemicals. You collect a urine sample in the morning and you collect it in the evening and you may have huge variability. So what are you going to make out of that number? ... Having a laundry list of values, *it wouldn't be useful.* (Interview, analytical chemist)

The second criterion position A uses to evaluate the usefulness of biomonitoring data is the existence of established health effects associated with chemical exposures, which could be termed *diagnostic usefulness.* Here, usefulness is based on the extent to which scientists and/or clinicians may use biomonitoring data to assess the individual health implications of chemical exposures: the more that is known about the health effects of chemical exposures, the more useful the data. Given the lack of established clinical guidelines for many of the chemicals currently monitored through biomonitoring, position A holds that single measurement data are numbers often without discernable clinical meaning, and as a consequence, these data do not constitute useful information, particularly for research participants. For example, one toxicologist stated:

> ... Knowing is a funny word, and knowing a number in the absence of someone being able to tell you anything really meaningful about it is not really knowing very much of anything. (Interview)

This statement crystallizes the paradoxical nature of single measurement data at the individual level for position A. These data certainly signal exposure(s), but what do they tell us beyond that? As one epidemiologist stated: 'Does a low mean low? Does as high mean high?' (Fieldnotes, California Biomonitoring Program meeting, 29 July 2012). The key question as posed here is: What do these measurements actually help us to know about exposures? For the positions described below, the answer to this question is that these data are evidence that environmental chemicals (or other markers) can be found in human fluids and tissues. While position A would not disagree, the mere detection of environmental chemicals and/or their metabolites in human fluids and tissues is not necessarily viewed as analytically or diagnostically useful information. For position A, if data are not useful in these ways, they are not considered useful for other purposes. Rather, the data are simply numbers without a discernable meaning.

Position B: Single Measurement Data Useful for Some Purposes

Position B shares many of the concerns described above, but takes a very different approach to evaluating the usefulness of single measurement data. This position holds that while these data may have questionable analytic or diagnostic usefulness, they may still be useful for other purposes. Position B identifies two specific purposes in which single measurement data provide useful information and aid in achieving broader goals this position holds to be important. The first is the promotion of individual empowerment, specifically related to health, and the second is the promotion of trusting relationships between researchers and research participants. With respect to the first goal, single measurement data are considered useful information based on the reasoning that these data may inspire a sense of empowerment among individual recipients and, perhaps more importantly, will encourage these individuals to take action to reduce their exposures, either through individual or collective means. Here we see the articulation of two types of usefulness: *personal usefulness* and *precautionary usefulness*. I use the label *personal usefulness* to refer to the extent to which the receipt of personal biomonitoring data may enhance individuals' self-knowledge and provide a sense of choice and control. I use the term *precautionary usefulness* to refer to the extent to which biomonitoring data may be used as the basis for taking precautionary steps to reduce chemical exposures, either through individual or collective actions. This position was expressed in the following ways:

> It's so hard to take individual measurements and tell anybody anything about what they mean. But I think that overall the *biomonitoring informa-tion is really useful* for exactly what you're talking about [taking action]. Information is power. (Fieldnotes, statement made by toxicologist at California Biomonitoring Program meeting, 17 March 2011, emphasis added)

> [Receiving individual results] allows people to act in a way that's consis-tent with their own values . . . if you have the information, you have the power. And if you don't have it, you don't have that—the opportunities to

do that. (Fieldnotes, statement made by environmental health scientist at California Biomonitoring Program meeting, 17 March 2011)

In these statements, we see position B (particularly in the first statement) making the case that while single measurement data may not have analytic or diagnostic usefulness, in the context of research participants' lives, these data have personal usefulness. Here the uncertainties and variability associated with single measurement data so important to position A are minimized in light of the potential that these data may empower research participants.

Additionally, position B also considers single measurement data useful information for the purposes of creating and maintaining trusting relationships with research participants, which could be termed *relational usefulness*. Biomonitoring data represent something tangible researchers can give back to research participants, and in the contemporary US health culture, where value is placed on 'knowing one's numbers' even when they may not indicate a clear course of action, research participants often express the desire to receive personal biomonitoring data (Altman et al. 2008; Haines et al. 2011). Providing this information to research participants, position B contends, is an important way to show care and respect for participants, and has relational usefulness. This was expressed in the following ways:

> The process [of reporting individual results] really increased the trust in the researchers, between the study community and the researchers. (Fieldnotes, statement made by environmental scientist and advocate, California Biomonitoring Program meeting, 17 March 2011)

> I think what's important . . . is to make sure you don't take from the participants. And I think this new philosophy of reporting results back, you know, sending letters to participants, not just parachuting in, taking a sample, and leaving. This new philosophy . . . *has really moved forward the whole process of interaction with participants.* (Fieldnotes, statement made by epidemiologist, California Biomonitoring Program meeting, 17 March 2011, emphasis added)

In the second statement, we also see the way in which ethical perspectives and principles shape the evaluation of single measurement data for position B. Here the data are useful because they enable researchers to perform an ethical obligation to give back to research communities. This also has relational use-fulness because it helps to foster better interactions between researchers, research participants, and the communities from which participants are drawn.

Position C: Single Measurement Data Highly Useful

For position C, *all* biomonitoring data are viewed as providing useful information because these data are viewed as concrete evidence of chemical exposures. These data confirm that environmental chemicals can cross bodily membranes and make their way into human tissues and fluids, which has historically been difficult to prove through other exposure assessment methodologies. For this position, biomonitoring data tell a story about the vulnerability of human bodies to the wide array of chemicals now used in industrial processes and consumer products, as well as the failure of government agencies to adequately regulate and test these chemicals before they enter the marketplace. For position C, the analytic flaws associated with single measurement data cited by position A do not garner much attention or concern, and are certainly not considered a legitimate basis for questioning the usefulness of these data. Here biomonitoring data are interpreted as signals of exposure and, perhaps just as importantly, what are perceived to be deep flaws in how we regulate chemicals in the USA. In this way, position C evaluates single measurement data as having what could be termed *political usefulness,* or the extent to which these data can be used to accomplish specific political goals (see also Morello-Frosch et al. 2009, 2011). This position was expressed in the following ways:

> I mean biomonitoring is—you know you can't use the word 'proof' in science very easily but here's one place where you can. This is proof that we're exposed. (Interview, environmental health advocate)

> Toxic chemicals and the fact that we all carry these chemicals in our body is evidence of a kind of failure of many of our prevention policies. (Field-notes, statement by environmental health advocate, California Biomonitoring Program meeting, 17 March 2011).

For position C, chemical exposures are understood as a type of bodily contamination and trespass, 'an injustice to be righted.' As such, biomonitoring data, and the exposures they evidence, signal the need for action, not simply at the individual level, but also on behalf of government agencies charged with testing and regulating environmental chemicals. One environmental health advocate articulated this position in an interview in the following way:

> We certainly come down on the side that we do feel it's [exposures] a trespass against us, an injustice to be righted . . . one thing that we're hoping to see down the line is at the least we're going to require a lot more testing of chemicals before they're introduced into commerce so that we can have some reasonable assurance—we won't have proof but we can have some reasonable assurance that we think they're going to be safe before we start to introduce them into the environment and into our bodies.

Stemming largely from the view that chemical exposures constitute a form of bodily contamination, position C strongly supports the communication of biomonitoring data to research participants. Indeed, discourse from position C treats access to biomonitoring data as the right of all individuals who give bodily fluids or tissues for testing. This position was expressed in the following way:

> We really want people to get the information back. We see it, you know, as something that's a useful tool for scientists but that it's also a right-to-know issue and that if you are providing a sample of blood, hair, urine, breast milk, or whatever, you have a right to know what your results were and to have those results explained to you. (Interview, environmental health advocate)

In this statement, position C also suggests that biomonitoring data are personally useful for research participants because these data offer information about one's body.

In sum, for position C, single measurement data are useful both politically and personally. By conclusively demonstrating human exposures to environmental chemicals, biomonitoring data have political usefulness because they support the argument that the US chemical regulatory system has failed to adequately protect citizens from potentially hazardous substances. These data also have personal usefulness for the reasons stated above.

Discussion

This article sheds new light on the recent disclosure debates by showing that perhaps the most salient issue shaping decisions about the communication of individual-level biomonitoring data to research participants is the extent to which these data are deemed *useful*. However, despite its centrality in these decisions, my analysis also shows that there is little consensus on how to define and evaluate usefulness. This is largely because usefulness itself is a rather slippery concept that can reflect a wide array of epistemological orientations, research goals, ethical perspectives, and political priorities. Indeed, among the three positions described above, we see the articulation and use of at least six different kinds of usefulness which I have provisionally labeled *analytic, diagnostic, personal, precautionary, relational*, and *political*. In evaluating single measurement data, each position draws on different kinds of usefulness. Position A relies primarily on analytic and diagnostic usefulness, which leads this position to the conclusion that single measurement data at the individual level are generally not useful. Position B, however, emphasizes personal, precautionary, and social/relational usefulness and, as such, holds that these same data are useful for the purposes of empowering research participants and fostering more trusting relationships with research communities. Lastly, position C draws on personal, precautionary, and political usefulness in its evaluation, which leads this position to the conclusion that single measurement data are of substantial use.

These findings both support and differ from those described by Brody et al. (2007) and Morello-Frosch et al. (2009, 2011) who have similarly mapped the range of perspectives and practices with respect to the communication of biomonitoring data to research participants. These scholars describe three major frameworks that currently shape communication practices in the USA, each of which reflect different ethical perspectives and approaches to the research enterprise. These include: (1) clinical ethics, an approach where decisions about disclosure rest with scientific experts and where these decisions are based on what is known about the relationships between exposure and adverse health effects; (2) community-based participatory research, where decisions about disclosure are made jointly by scientists, participants, and the study community; and (3) and citizen-science 'data judo,' an approach used by environmental health advocacy groups in which decisions about disclosure of biomarker data are shaped mainly by the goal of building support for chemical policy reform (Morello-Frosch et al. 2009). The positions described in this article clearly reflect some aspects of these three frameworks: position A reflects aspects of the clinical ethics framework; position B reflects aspects of community-based participatory research; and position C reflects aspects of citizen-science data judo.

Despite some similar findings, the approach taken by Brody et al. (2007) and Morello-Frosch et al. (2009, 2011) differs from the one taken in this study in subtle but analytically consequential ways. These scholars set out to map current communication practices and the moral principles and political perspectives that underpin them and, as such, their frameworks are organized largely according to these criteria. At the heart of their analysis is their proposition that decisions to share individual-level biomonitoring data with research participants are motivated largely by researchers' perspectives and politics regarding the research enterprise. The more researchers view research as a democratic exercise, the more likely they are to involve research participants in research design as well as the interpretation and dissemination of findings. While I do not dispute this analysis, I find that it leaves the heterogeneous meanings of biomonitoring data, which also shape decisions to communicate these data to research participants, relatively unexamined. The findings described in this article indeed suggest that the meaning of numbers and measurement varies across 'context[s] and communities of interpretation' (Espeland and Stevens 2008: 404). What may be characterized as a relatively useless number for one position is highly meaningful and useful for another. Moreover, we see the articulation of several kinds of usefulness. The positions described in this article are distinguished based on how they each evaluate the usefulness of single measurement biomonitoring data, including the kinds of usefulness brought to bear in their evaluation. Whereas in Brody et al. (2007) and Morello-Frosch et al.'s (2009, 2011) analyses, the three frameworks are distinguished largely in terms of how they each view the value of reporting of biomonitoting data to research participants.

The findings presented here also support research conducted by Caux et al. (2007), which examined different occupational health stakeholders' perspectives on the use and meaning of biomarkers of exposure, effects, and susceptibility in Quebec. These scholars found that there were at least two 'narratives of science,' which shaped how different stakeholders understood the meaning of biomarkers. Stakeholders who articulated the 'first narrative' assumed that biomarkers have intrinsic scientific meaning that is not subject to interpretation. Here 'biomarkers are "scientific" . . . they are perfect and powerful' (Caux et al. 2007, 348). However, for those who expressed the 'second narrative' of science, which emphasized the constructed nature of science, the meaning of biomarkers was understood as subject to interpretation and consensus among the scientific community. In both Caux et al.'s study and the one described in this article, individuals who are not directly involved in the production of biomonitoring data are more likely to express the view that the data have clear and intrinsic meaning. Conversely, those most intimately involved in this process often express the most uncertainty about the meaning of the data.

Taken together, the findings of Brody et al. (2007), Caux et al. (2007), Morello-Frosch et al. (2009, 2011), and those described in this article highlight the importance of context in evaluating and assigning meaning to biomonitoring data. After all, biomonitoring data are merely numbers, which are rendered more or less useful in different contexts and for different purposes. Given the array of settings and purposes biomonitoring data are currently being used in and for, it is not surprising that debates around the interpretation and communication of these data have emerged. In the USA, biomonitoring is used within the contexts of population surveillance, health research, occupational health and safety, environmental health advocacy, and grassroots community efforts. Within each of these contexts, biomonitoring data are utilized in different ways and serve different purposes. This matters because the purposes for which the data are used often shape notions about what constitutes useful information and the most appropriate criteria on which to make such determinations.

Given this heterogeneity, it is critical that debates about the communication of biomonitoring data not be reduced simply to disagreements over bioethical principles. Doing so can have the unintended consequences of not only confining deliberations to a narrow set of questions, but also polarizing positions as either 'ethical' or 'unethical.' Instead, increased attention ought to be paid to the different ways in which biomonitoring data are currently evaluated within different contexts and the assumptions that underpin these assessments. This will undoubtedly contribute to an increased appreciation for different stakeholder perspectives, but may also lead to greater consensus on whether and how to communicate biomonitoring data to research participants.

Finally, the findings described in this article have particular relevance for public health practice, given the central role epidemiologists play in coordinating biomonitoring surveillance and research programs. Because of their close contact with research participants, epidemiologists are often confronted with the challenges and consequences associated with either providing or not providing research participants with individual-level bio-monitoring data in ways that many others involved in biomonitoring are not. Scholarship on genetic testing may offer some potentially fruitful models for epidemiologists faced with making these decisions. Researchers working in this area report findings similar to those described in this article: there is little agreement about the utility of many genetic tests, and utility itself has many meanings and is evaluated in diverse ways (Grosse and Khoury 2006; Foster, Mulvihill, and Sharp 2009; Hedgecoe 2008; Smart 2006). Bredenoord et al. (2011) and Ravitsky and Wilfond (2006) propose two models for making decisions about the communication of data to research participants based on both ethical principles and the evaluation of the utility of the data in question. Both models treat the disclosure of data that lack clinical utility but may have personal meaning to research participants as an area of ethical ambiguity. Both models support the disclose of such data, but make clear that such decisions ought to be based on specific study contexts, including resources and relationships between researchers and research participants.

Conclusion

This article contributes to the existing literature on the recent debates about the communication of individual-level biomonitoring data to research participants. It describes findings from a qualitative, sociological study of the different positions that have been articulated to date on the usefulness of single measurement biomonitoring data and the advisability of providing these data to research participants. These findings suggest that the usefulness of biomonitoring data is currently evaluated in multiple ways, reflecting the application of different standards, norms and principles (some of which may be ethical in nature). I show that different positions on the usefulness of single measurement data in turn also shape positions on the value of communicating these data to research participants: the more useful the data are deemed to be, the more likely the position sees value in the disclosure of these data. These findings both support and differ from those previously reported by other scholars. They also suggest that resolving debates about the disclosure of individual-level biomonitoring data to research participants will likely require greater consensus on the meaning and utility of the data.

Acknowledgements

This research was supported by funding from the University of California Toxic Substance Research and Teaching Program, the University of California, San Francisco Graduate Division, and the Bellarmine College of Liberal Arts at Loyola Marymount University. I thank all of the respondents who contributed to this study their time and perspectives on biomonitoring. I also thank Peter Davidson, Carrie Friese, Katie Hasson, Martine Lappe, Theresa MacPhail, and Jade Sasser for their helpful comments on earlier drafts of this paper. Thanks are also due to the two anonymous reviewers who offered fruitful comments and suggestions. Earlier drafts of this paper were presented at the 2011 annual meeting of the Society for Social Studies of Science (Cleveland, OH) and the 2012 annual meeting of the American Sociological Association (Denver, CO).

References

Albertini, R., M. Bird, N. Doerrer, L. Needham, S. Robison, L. Sheldon, and H. Zenick. 2006. "The Use of Biomonitoring Data in Exposure and Human Health Risk Assessments." *Environmental Health Perspectives* 114 (11): 1755–1762.

Altman, R. G., R. Morello-Frosch, J. G. Brody, R. A. Rudel, P. Brown, and M. Averick. 2008. "Pollution Comes Home and Gets Personal: Women's Experience of Household Chemical Exposure." *Health and Social Behavior* 49: 41 7–435.

Bredenoord, A. L., N. C. Onland-Moret, and J. J. M. Van Delden. 2011. "Feedback of Individual Genetic Results to Research Participants: In Favor of a Qualified Disclosure Policy." *Human Mutation* 32 (8): 861–867.

Brody, J. G., R. Morello-Frosch, P. Brown, R. A. Rudel, R. G. Altman, M. Frye, C. Osimo, C. Perez, and L. Seryak. 2007. "'Is It Safe': New Ethics for Reporting Personal Exposures to Environmental Chemicals." *American Journal of Public Health* 97 (9): 1547–1554.

Brown, P. 2007. *Toxic Exposures: Contested Illness and the Environmental Health Movement.* New York: Columbia University Press.

Brown, P., R. Morello-Frosch, J. G. Brody, R. J. Altman, R. Rudel, L. Senier, C. Perez, and R. Simpson. 2010. "Institutional Review Board Challenges Related to Community-based Participatory Research on Human Exposure to Environmental Toxins: A Case Study." *Environmental Health* 9 (39).

Buck, A. J., J. E. Vena, B. M. McGuinness, M. A. Cooney, and G. Louis. 2010. "Communicating Serum Chemical Concentrations to Study Participants: Follow Up Survey." *Environmental Health* 9 (20).

Caux, C., D. J. Roy, L. Guilbert, and C. Viau. 2007. "Anticipating the Ethical Aspects of the Use of Biomarkers in the Workplace." *Social Science and Medicine* 65 (2): 344–354.

Clarke, A. 2005. *Situational Analysis: Grounded Theory After the Postmodern Turn.* Thousand Oaks, CA: Sage.

Clarke, A. E. 2003. "Situational Analysis: Grounded Theory Mapping After the Postmodern Turn." *Symbolic Interaction* 26 (4): 553–576.

Clarke, A. E. 2009. "From Grounded Theory to Situational Analysis: What's New? Why? How?" In *Developing Grounded Theory: The Second Generation*, edited by J. M. Morse, P. N. Stern, J. Corbin, B. Bowers, A. Clarke, and K. Charmaz, 194-221. Walnut Creek, CA: Left Coast Press.

Deck, W., and T. Kosatsky. 1999. "Communicating Their Individual Results to Participants in an Environmental Exposure Study: Insight from Clinical Ethics." *Environmental Research* 80 (2): S223–S229.

Espeland, W. N., and M. L. Stevens. 2008. "A Sociology of Quantification." *European Journal of Sociology/Archives Europeennes de Sociologie* 49 (3): 401–436.

Foster, M. W., J. J. Mulvihill, and R. R. Sharp. 2009. "Evaluating the Utility of Personal Genomic Information." *Genetics in Medicine* 11 (8) 570–574.

Foster, W. G., and J. Agzarian. 2007. "Reporting Results of Biomonitoring Studies." *Analytical and Bioanalytical Chemistry* 387 (1): 137–140.

Gallagher, J. E., E. A. C. Hubal, and S. W. Edwards. 2010. "Biomarkers for Environmental Exposure." In *Biomarkers: In Medicine, Drug Discovery, and Environmental Health*, edited by V. S. Vaidya and J. V. Bonventre, 517–547. Hoboken, NJ: Wiley.

Grosse, S. D., and M. J. Khoury. 2006. "What Is The Clinical Utility of Genetic Testing?" *Genetics in Medicine* 8 (7): 448–450.

Haines, D. A., T. T. Arbuckle, E. Lye, M. Legrand, M. Fisher, R. Langlois, and W. Fraser. 2011. "Reporting Results of Human Biomonitoring of Environmental Chemicals to Study Participants: A Comparison of Approaches Followed by Two Canadian Studies." *Journal of Epidemiology and Community Health* 65: 191–198.

Harrison, M. 2007. "Applying Bioethical Principles to Human Biomonitoring." *Environmental Health* 7 (Supplement 1 S8).

Hedgecoe, A. 2008. "From Resistance to Usefulness: Sociology and the Clinical Use of Genetic Tests." *BioSocieties* 3 (2): 183-194.

LaKind, J. S., L. L. Aylward, C. Brunk, S. Dizio, M. Dourson, D. A. Goldstein, M. E. Kilpatrick, et al. 2008. "Guidelines for the Communication of Biomonitoring Equivalents: Report from the Biomonitoring Equivalents Experts Workshop." *Regulatory Toxicology and Pharmacology* 51 (3): S16–S26.

Morello-Frosch, R., P. Brown, J. G. Brody, R. G. Altman, R. A. Rudel, A. Zota, and C. Perez. 2011. "Experts, Ethics, and Environmental Justice: Communicating and Contesting Results from Personal Exposure Science." In *Technoscience and Environmental Justice: Expert Culture in a Grassroots Movement*, edited by G. Ottinger and B. R. Cohen, 93–118. Cambridge, MA: MIT Press.

Morello-Frosch, R., J. G. Brody, P. Brown, R. G. Altman, R. A. Rudel, and C. Perez. 2009. "Toxic Ignorance and Right-to-Know in Biomonitoring Results Communication: A Survey of Scientists and Study Participants." *Environmental Health* 8 (6).

National Research Council. 2006. *Human Biomonitoring for Environmental Chemicals*. Washington, DC: National Academy of Sciences.

Needham, L. L. 2008. "Introduction to Biomonitoring." *Journal of Chemical Health and Safety* 15 (6): 5–7.

Ravitsky, V., and B. S. Wilfond. 2006. "Disclosing Individual Genetic Results to Research Participants." *The American Journal of Bioethics* 6 (6): 8–17.

Sexton, K., L. Needham, and J. Pirkle. 2004. "Human Biomonitoring of Environmental Chemicals." *American Scientist* 92: 38–45.

Smart, A. 2006. "A Multi-dimensional Model of Clinical Utility." *International Journal for Quality in Health Care* 18 (5): 377–382.

Strauss, A. L. 1987. *Qualitative Analysis for Social Scientists*. Cambridge: Cambridge University Press.

Strauss, A. L., and J. Corbin. 1998. *Basics of Qualitative Research: Techniques and Procedures for Developing Grounded Theory*. Thousand Oaks, CA: Sage.

Williams, B. L., D. B. Barr, J. M. Wright, B. Buckley, and M. S. Magsumbol. 2008. "Interpretation of Biomonitoring Data in Clinical Medicine and the Exposure Sciences." *Toxicology and Applied Pharmacology* 233: 76–80.

Wilson, S. E., E. R. Baker, A. C. Leonard, M. H. Eckman, and B. P. Lanphear. 2010. "Understanding Preferences for Disclosing of Individual Biomarker Results among Participants in a Longitudinal Birth Cohort." *Journal of Medical Ethics* 36: 736–740.

Wu, N., M.D. McClean, P. Brown, A. Aschengrau, and T.F. Webster. 2009. "Participant Experiences in a Breastmilk Biomonitoring Study: A Qualitative Assessment." *Environmental Health* 8 (4).

Reflection: On Mapping Human Biomonitoring

Rachel Washburn

In this reflection, I describe how I have used situational analysis (SA) in my ongoing sociological research on human biomonitoring, a technique used to measure trace levels of environmental chemicals and their breakdown products in human fluids and tissues. Over the past few decades, biomonitoring has become a progressively popular tool in the environmental health sciences. It is especially appealing to environmental health scientists and activists who see it as reducing the uncertainties associated with quantifying exposures based on measurements of chemicals in the outside air, water, soil, food, and so on.

As a medical sociologist with a particular interest in how science and technology shape and are shaped by how we think about the body, health, and disease, I have found biomonitoring a fascinating topic of inquiry. Its use has given rise to new understandings about the mobility of a wide range of environmental chemicals and the permeability of human bodies to these chemicals. This has stirred new debates on several fronts, including the causes of exposures and the adequacy of chemical regulations. There is also profound disagreement about the precise meaning and significance of biomonitoring data, particularly for individual-level health. All of this has worked to complicate questions regarding what and how to communicate results to individuals who participate in biomonitoring studies. Should participants receive personal biomonitoring results in spite of uncertainties? If so, how should this information be framed? What are the consequences of providing personalized exposure results when we know that most exposures are largely the result of broad economic and political processes?

When I began research on biomonitoring in 2005, I wanted to understand how it was being used in different settings, what biomonitoring data meant to those involved, and its consequences for scientific practices, policy, and understandings of the body, health, and disease. Addressing these questions meant taking a multi-sited ethnographic approach, through which I quickly gathered a large volume of data. Like Fosket (this volume), I, too, found the three main mapping strategies offered in SA incredibly helpful in organizing and analyzing my data. It gave me a systematic approach for identifying the major elements in my situation of inquiry and seeing the complex relationships among these elements. Positional mapping proved especially helpful in allowing me to see muted lines of contestation, particularly around the meaning and significance of biomonitoring data. In what follows, I provide a brief description of the field I entered in the early 2000s. I then describe how I used the three types of maps to open and deepen my analysis of the politics of biomonitoring in the United States.

Studying Human Biomonitoring in the Early 2000s

In March 2001, the Centers for Disease Control and Prevention (CDC) published a landmark biomonitoring report, describing Americans' exposures to more than two dozen environmental chemicals, including heavy metals, pesticides, and phthalates (commonly used plasticizers) (Centers for Disease Control and Prevention 2001). Though the report garnered only modest press coverage, it struck a chord with environmental health scientists and advocates across the United States. For the first time, it was clear that Americans were exposed not just to chemicals used in industrial and agricultural processes, but also to those present in a wide array of common consumer products. Further, these exposures were ubiquitous across the population.

In the decade following the release of this report, the CDC continued to study Americans' exposures to an increasing number of chemicals and published its findings in three additional major reports (Centers for Disease Control and Prevention 2003, 2005, 2009).[1] The last was published in 2009 and included measurement data for more than 200 chemicals. Advocacy organizations in the United States and elsewhere also joined the effort to document human chemical exposures by conducting their own small-scale exposure studies with the assistance of private laboratories. In the United States, between 2001 and 2010, over a dozen such studies were conducted with participants from mostly upper-middle-class backgrounds, including politicians and actors, who had no obvious occupational or residential chemical exposures. These studies, and a few conducted by news organizations, confirmed the CDC's results and provided an intimate look at the lives of the exposed. Published material accessible on organization websites featured participants' photos, short biographies, exposure data, and reactions to personalized results (see Alliance for a Clean and Healthy Maine 2007;

Houlihan 2006; Houlihan et al. 2003, 2005; Oregon Environmental Council 2007; Schreder 2006).

The *Oakland Tribune* featured an especially striking portrayal of the exposed in a three-part series published in mid-2005 titled "What's In You" (Fischer 2005). The series told the story of the Holland Hammonds, a white, middle-class family of four from Berkeley, California, who agreed to have their bodily fluids analyzed for a suite of environmental chemicals. Analyses showed that in addition to having detectable levels of heavy metals, PCBs, and phthalates in their bodily fluids, the family had surprising levels of flame retardants in their blood. Especially high was Rowan, the twenty-month-old son. The story included the family's reaction to their results as well as the journalist's investigation of the sources of such exposures and the science on their consequences for human health. Included in the series was a half-page intimate picture of Rowan, blonde-haired, blue-eyed, and nude in the family bathtub, looking directly at the camera as his mother bathed him. Nearby text read: "We are all . . . subjects of an experiment, with no way to buy your way out, eat your way out or exercise your way out. We are guinea pigs when it comes to the unknown long-term threat these chemicals pose in our bodies and, in particular, our children" (Fischer 2005:2).

This story and the many studies conducted by advocacy organizations suggested that chemical exposures were no longer something that only affected those living in polluted neighborhoods and/or whose jobs brought them into close contact with toxic chemicals. Aided by biomonitoring data, these studies made a strong case that chemical exposures and risks were perhaps more democratically distributed than had once been assumed (see Daemmrich 2008). Douglas Fischer, the author of the *Oakland Tribune* story, made this clear when he wrote, "We are all . . . subjects." Drawing on extant narratives about contamination and the perils associated with the widespread use of industrial chemicals, activists and their allies developed a new vocabulary for talking about this phenomenon. This included phrases such as "toxic trespass," "the pollution in people," and "chemical body burden," all of which were meant to emphasize the disturbing presence of environmental chemicals in human bodies and the urgent need for policy changes.[2] In short, biomonitoring data had become the basis for new discourses and representational practices.

At the same time, in policy arenas and scientific circles the availability of biomonitoring and the production of biomonitoring data were also engendering new debates and provoking new lines of inquiry. During the first decade of this century, several states, including California, adopted new legislation to fund the development of statewide biomonitoring programs. Environmental health scientists also integrated biomonitoring into their ongoing investigations of environmental causes of disease. In California, where I conducted much of my fieldwork, the early 2000s were a time of hope, excitement, and trepidation. For many, a statewide biomonitoring program seemed to provide a path to answering long-standing questions about the unique, and likely quite varied, exposures of Californians. For others, it brought fears of stigmatization.

When I entered the field in 2005, biomonitoring was a hot tool among environmental health scientists and activists, and was a major part of program building. It was also at the center of thorny ethical debates in which actors with different commitments had stakes. Moreover, biomonitoring data were clearly giving rise to the reevaluation of the distribution of chemical exposures and risks, as well as new forms of embodiment and exposure-based identities. All of this made biomonitoring a particularly rich topic for sociological inquiry, but also a challenging one.

Mapping the Biomonitoring Situation

The same year I began my research on biomonitoring, Adele Clarke's book, *Situational Analysis: Grounded Theory after the Postmodern Turn*, was published. As a student in the sociology program at UCSF, I had already learned about grounded theory and developed a particular affinity for Anselm Strauss's social worlds/arenas theory, which was further elaborated by Clarke (1991, 1998, 2003, 2005, 2006; Clarke & Montini 1993; Clarke & Star 2007). Clarke and Montini's (1993) social worlds/arenas analysis of RU486 was especially influential in my approach to studying biomonitoring. This article served as a superb exemplar for how social worlds/arenas analysis could be used to explore the heterogeneous actors and perspectives that coalesce around objects and processes. It also highlighted how such analyses can work to make implicated but silent actors visible. For me, the exciting thing about SA was how it took the systematic approach offered in grounded theory and rerooted this within a social worlds/arenas framework, which assumes the constructedness of objects and processes within multiple social worlds and arenas. I also found the emphasis on nonhuman elements in SA quite valuable in my study of biomonitoring.

During the early stages of data collection, I constructed several "messy" and "ordered" situational maps. The categories Clarke identified for the ordered situational maps often pushed me to think beyond the obvious, a process that helped me see how important particular events, politics, and actors were to the popularity of biomonitoring. Given my tendency to neglect the importance of nonhuman elements, I found the categories "nonhuman elements/actants" and "discursive constructions of nonhuman actants" especially helpful in keeping my analysis open and broad. I was often surprised by how much particular chemicals or instruments mattered and how the confluence of events, concerns, and technical developments shaped the course of biomonitoring. During the early stages of my research, relationships between and among elements were often not clear. However, situational maps are incredibly flexible and gave me a way to hold on to uncertainty and tentative connections during the long process of my data collection and analysis. Looking back at previously constructed maps also gave me a way to reflect on my analysis, and, in times of despair, helped me see that my thinking was, in fact, progressing.

Situational maps, like social worlds/arenas maps, were also fantastic in guiding my data collection. Sometimes this took me down complicated paths with uncertain connections to my project, but mostly the maps pushed me in fruitful directions. On one occasion, after revising a modified social/worlds arenas map, which included symbols for biomonitoring studies, I came to appreciate how incredibly varied the users of biomonitoring were and how biomonitoring actually served to bring these actors together. Not only were government agencies using it, but so, too, were environmental health advocacy organizations (both large and small), industry groups, university-based researchers, media organizations, commercial laboratories, clinicians, and research participants. Identifying these different users and uses helped me refocus and reorient my fieldwork and served as the basis for making difficult and sometimes painful strategic decisions about what to include and leave out of my dissertation.

The two mapping strategies most helpful in my analysis were social worlds/arenas maps and positional maps. My modified social worlds/arenas maps helped me grasp the varied meanings ascribed to biomonitoring in different settings and how this technique enabled the accomplishment of different types of work, ranging from advocacy to population surveillance and from health effects research to individualized risk evaluation. These maps were usually constructed and revised after traditional grounded theory coding. Memoing during and after mapping helped me flesh out what I observed in my maps and sometimes led to remapping.

Though I did not use positional mapping in my dissertation work, I have done so in subsequent research on biomonitoring. Positional maps are probably the most difficult type of map to construct because they require the analyst to focus on positions in discourses, not the individuals or groups who may articulate such positions. They also require plotting these positions in some fashion, usually, but not necessarily, along two axes. I used positional mapping to analyze debates about whether and how to communicate personal biomonitoring data to individuals who participated in biomonitoring research. During the course of my fieldwork, this emerged as one of the most contested issues in the field of biomonitoring. Some felt that all participants had the right to know their personal biomonitoring results, while others argued that without more information on the health consequences of these data, it was better not to provide individual-level results. At one meeting I observed in 2006, this issue turned what had been a cordial dialogue on biomonitoring between scientists, public health officials, and activists into a rather heated exchange.

In the years that followed, several scholarly articles offered explanations for this discord as well as practical solutions for researchers seeking guidance (Brody et al. 2007; Dumez, Van Damme, & Casteleyn 2007; Harrison 2007; Knudsen, Merlo, & Larsen 2008; Morello-Frosch et al. 2009; Sepai et al. 2008; Williams et al. 2008). Most scholars suggested that at the root of differing opinions on the communication of biomonitoring data were competing interpretations of bioethical principles. While this explanation made sense to me, it did not seem to fully capture what I observed in my fieldwork and analyses of texts. What I traced were fundamentally different constructions of biomonitoring data, which I assumed were linked with different positions about whether such data should be shared with research participants.

To explore these possible connections, I went back to my data, recoded transcripts and texts, and then constructed well over a dozen positional maps. This was certainly not an easy process. I especially struggled with the axes of my maps. Several were too vague and did not capture the nuance I identified in my data but had a very hard time putting to words. However, after struggling with these maps for over a month, I finally arrived at what seemed to be the crux of the issue. There were quite divergent positions regarding the *usefulness* of individual-level biomonitoring data. My final map helped me see that three major positions on this issue had been articulated in my data and that several other possibilities were, interestingly, missing from the data. I was also able to see how positions on the usefulness of individual-level biomonitoring data corresponded to positions on the value of communicating these data to research participants. Through this mapping, I identified an important but muted line of contestation that, in my estimation, had considerable bearing on debates about the communication of biomonitoring data to research participants.

Though the mapping strategies in situational analysis are not necessarily intended as finished products, I have found that the maps can travel quite well. In presentations, papers, and books, they invite viewers to ponder and question the analyst's depictions and the analytical decisions on which they are built. They make our thinking more visible and encourage other analysts to question their own assumptions. I have used my project map and positional maps in several presentations to multidisciplinary audiences where they have provoked productive dialogue and questions and in some cases even led me to important revisions.

Conclusion

Situational analysis has provided me with a way of analyzing complexity and heterogeneity that allows for and accepts uncertainty and revision. Perhaps most valuable to me is how the maps have pushed me to see connections between elements that I otherwise would have likely failed to examine. The positional maps, in particular, stretched my analysis. Through the three mapping strategies, I was able to examine the varied meanings of biomonitoring and the worlds and practices through which these meanings were constructed, including muted, but very consequential, lines of contestation.

Notes

1. At the same time, government agencies in several other countries also conducted similar surveys of environmental chemical exposures in their own populations.

2. The term "body burden" had been in use in scientific circles during previous decades, and generally referred to the accumulation of persistent chemicals in bodily tissues. During the first decade of the 2000s, activists and journalists popularized this term and broadened its meaning.

References

Alliance for a Clean and Healthy Maine. 2007. *Body of Evidence: A Study of Pollution in Maine People*. Portland, ME. http://www.cleanandhealthyme.org/bodyofevidencereport/tabid/55/default.aspx (accessed August 5, 2007).

Brody, J. G., R. Morello-Frosch, P. Brown, R. A. Rudel, R. Altman, M. Frye, C. A. Osimo, C. Pérez, and L. M. Seryak. 2007. "Is It Safe?": New Ethics for Reporting Personal Exposures to Environmental Chemicals. *American Journal of Public Health* 97(9):1547–1554.

Centers for Disease Control and Prevention. 2001. *National Report on Human Exposure to Environmental Chemicals*. Atlanta: National Center for Environmental Health. http://www.cdc.gov/exposurereport/ (accessed May 12, 2005).

Centers for Disease Control and Prevention. 2003. *Second National Report on Human Exposure to Environmental Chemicals*. Atlanta: National Center for Environmental Health. http://www.cdc.gov/exposurereport/ (accessed April 11, 2003).

Centers for Disease Control and Prevention. 2005. *National Report on Human Exposure to Environmental Chemicals*. http://www.cdc.gov/exposurereport/ (accessed October 19, 2006).

Centers for Disease Control and Prevention. 2009. *Fourth National Report on Human Exposures to Environmental Chemicals*. http://www.cdc.gov/exposurereport/ (accessed July 3, 2009).

Clarke, A. E. 1991. Social Worlds/Arenas Theory as Organizational Theory. In D. Maines (Ed.), *Social Organization and Social Process: Essays in Honor of Anselm Strauss* (pp. 119–158). New York: Aldine de Gruyter.

Clarke, A. E. 1998. *Disciplining Reproduction: Modernity, American Life Sciences, and the "Problems of Sex."* Berkeley: University of California Press.

Clarke, A. E. 2003. Situational Analyses: Grounded Theory Mapping after the Postmodern Turn. *Symbolic Interaction* 26(4):553–576.

Clarke, A. E. 2005. *Situational Analysis: Grounded Theory after the Postmodern Turn*. Thousand Oaks: Sage.

Clarke, A. E. 2006. Social Worlds. In George Ritzer (Ed.) *The Blackwell Encyclopedia of Sociology* (pp. 4547–4549). Malden, MA: Blackwell.

Clarke, A. E. & T. Montini. 1993. The Many Faces of RU486: Tales of Situated Knowledges and Technological Contestations. *Science, Technology and Human Values* 18(1):42–78.

Clarke, A. E. & S. L. Star. 2008. The Social Worlds/Arenas Framework as a Theory–Methods Package. In E. Hackett, O. Amsterdamska, M. Lynch, & J. Wacjman (Eds.) *Handbook of Science and Technology Studies* (3rd ed., pp. 113–137). Cambridge, MA: MIT Press.

Daemmrich, A. 2008. Risk Frameworks and Biomonitoring: Distributed Regulation of Synthetic Chemicals in Humans. *Environmental History* 13(October):684–694.

Dumez, B., K. Van Damme, & L. Casteleyn. 2007. Research on the Socio–Ethical Impact of Biomarker Use and the Communication Processes in the ECNIS NoE and NewGeneris IP. *International Journal of Hygiene and Environmental Health* 210:263–265.

Fischer, D. 2005. What's in You? *Oakland Tribune*, March 13–15. Series reprinted May 2005, 1–14.

Harrison, M. 2007. Applying Bioethical Principles to Human Biomonitoring. *Environmental Health* 7(Supplement 1 S8).

Houlihan, J. 2006. *Across Generations: Mothers and Daughters*. Washington, DC: Environmental Working Group. http://www.ewg.org/reports/generations (accessed 02/20/07).

Houlihan, J., T. Kropp, R. Wiles, S. Gray, & C. Campbell. 2005. *BodyBurden: The Pollution in Newborns*. Washington, DC: The Environmental Working Group. http://www.ewg.org/reports/bodyburden2/execsumm.php (accessed 11/01/06).

Houlihan, J., R. Wiles, K. Thayer, & S. Gray. 2003. *Body Burden: The Pollution in People*. Washington, DC: Environmental Working Group. http://www.ewg.org/sites/bodybur den1/ (accessed11/01/06).

Knudsen, L. E., D. F. Merlo, & A. D. Larsen. 2008. Workshop on Ethics and Communication in Copenhagen 11–13.3.2007. *Environmental Health* 7(Supplement 1: S1).

Morello-Frosch, R., J. G. Brody, P. Brown, R. Altman, R. A. Rudel, & C. Pérez. 2009. Toxic Ignorance and Right-to-know in Biomonitoring Results Communication: A Survey of Scientists and Study Participants. *Environmental Health* 8:Article 6.

Oregon Environmental Council. 2007. *Pollution in People: A Study of Toxic Chemicals in Oregonians*. Portland. http://www.oeconline.org/our-work/healthier-lives/pollutioninpeople (accessed January 31, 2008).

Schreder, E. 2006. *Pollution in People: A Study of Toxic Chemicals in Washingtonians*. Seattle: Toxic-Free Legacy Coalition. http://pollutioninpeople.org/) (accessed November 11, 2006)

Sepai, O., C. Collier, B. Van Tongelen, & L. Casteleyn. 2008. Human Biomonitoring Data Interpretation and Ethics: Obstacles or Surmountable Challenges? *Environmental Health* 7(Supplement 13).

Williams, B. L., D. B. Barr, J. M. Wright, B. Buckley, & M. S. Magsumbol. 2008. Interpretation of Biomonitoring Data in Clinical Medicine and the Exposure Sciences. *Toxicology and Applied Pharmacology* 233(1):76–80.

CHAPTER EIGHT

GOVERNING THROUGH (IN)SECURITY: A CRITICAL ANALYSIS OF A FEAR-BASED PUBLIC HEALTH CAMPAIGN

Marilou Gagnon, Jean Daniel Jacob, & Dave Holmes

Introduction

Sexually transmitted infections (STIs) have been identified as an important health problem across the globe not only because of their physical manifestations and socioeconomic implications, but also because of our struggle to control outbreaks from a public health perspective. Worldwide, an estimated 340 million curable STIs including Chlamydia, Gonorrhea, Syphilis and Trichomoniasis occur annually (World Health Organization 2007), a reality that disproportionately affects adolescents and young adults aged between 15 and 24 years, thus, highlighting that individuals within this age group are vulnerable to STI infections (Panchaud et al. 2000, Weinstock et al. 2004). Despite remarkable declines of STI rates in the past decades in both Canada and the United States (Weinstock et al. 2004, Center of Disease Control 2007, Public Health Agency of Canada 2007), recent years have shown a gradual increase in incidence for specific infections, including Chlamydia, Syphilis and Gonorrhea. As a Canadian national strategy, STI prevention and control is at the forefront of discussions to address the escalating STI epidemic (MacDonald and Wong 2007).

We have recently engaged in the examination of a public health campaign produced by Quebec's Ministry of Health (Canada) for the prevention of STIs in young adults. Our objective was to critically examine the 2006–2007 prevention campaign entitled 'Condoms: They aren't a luxury'. The purpose of this paper is to engage with the readers on the use of fear in public health campaigns. To set the stage, we introduce the prevention campaign entitled 'Condoms: They aren't a luxury'. Then, drawing on the work of Clarke (2005),

From Gagnon, Marilou, Jean Daniel Jacob, and Dave Holmes. *Critical Public Health*, Volume 20, No. 2, June 2010, 245–256. © Taylor & Francis. Republished in *Situational Analysis in Practice*, by Adele E. Clarke, Carrie Friese, and Rachel Washburn, 270–291. (Taylor & Francis, 2015). All rights reserved.

we explain how the discursive body of the campaign was examined and provide a brief overview of the analytical process. Finally, we expand on the use of fear in public health campaigns by making important connections with the Foucauldian concepts of governmentality and bio-power as well as the non-Foucauldian notion of (in)security. At last, we provide a brief discussion on the application of commercial and advertising principles to public health campaigns.

The Public Health Campaign: "Condoms, They Aren't a Luxury"

In the province of Quebec, the Ministry of Health reaches the population through its various directorates, one of which is the 'Direction Générale de la Santé Publique' (DGSP). Its mandate is to define, promote and update orientations and strategies relative to public health protection and control of infectious diseases, as well as to ensure that these new directions are implemented. As such, the DGSP focuses on improving, protecting and promoting the health and well-being of the population. In this particular directorate, the 'Service de lutte contre les infections transmises sexuellement et par la sang' (SLITSS) is an administrative coordination structure that was established by the DGSP to counter various issues related to the spread of HIV, hepatitis C and other STIs. The SLITSS seeks out various types of expertise, makes use of different experiences and brings together health authorities and professionals to facilitate the implementation of STI prevention activities. It also designs and develops guidelines in the areas of STI prevention, health promotion, screening, testing, health care and services, surveillance, research and development, and expertise.

Every year in the province of Quebec, a new prevention campaign for STIs is launched by the SLITSS as part of the broader mandate and activities of the DGSP and the Ministry of Health (see *Stratégie québécoise de lutte contre l'infection par le VIH et le SIDA, l'infection par le VHC et les ITS—Orientation 2003–2009*). As such, each campaign ensures the maintenance of a communication channel through which the Government can reach the population to achieve disease prevention measures and health promotion goals across the province. In 2006–2007, the SLITSS created 'Condoms: They aren't a luxury' for the prevention of STIs in young adults. This campaign included three types of communication strategies, two of which were selected to perform the analysis: Zoom posters and 'What would you do for pleasure?' web-based messages. The third communication strategy was deactivated from the Ministry of Health website and could not be included in the analysis. Overall, the official objectives of the campaign were to increase the perception of risk linked to sexually transmitted infections and to reaffirm that condom use is the best way to prevent these infections; thus, the statements found on the posters and web-based messages were focused on the consequences of STIs among young adults.

The Zoom posters included four different messages that were written in bold black letters and presented on top of a white canvas. Each of them also displayed the large image of a spotless underwear, the logo of the Ministry of Health and a black text box where the title of the campaign 'Condoms: They aren't a luxury' appeared in bold white letters.[2] Based on the types of underwear presented in the posters, two different sets of messages and images were displayed to reach females (F) and males (M) separately. The following messages were proposed in the Zoom posters:

- **These panties have lived through horror:** Gonorrhea is horrible. It can cause greenish vaginal discharge. Even worse, you might not be able to have sex because it is too painful (F).
- **These boxers have seen suffering:** Gonorrhea can be painful and cause some discomfort to the sexual organs (M).
- **These panties have lived through hell:** Herpes causes painful genital lesions. The pain recurs frequently and is even worse during sexual intercourse (F).
- **This underwear has known fear:** Herpes causes genital lesions and it hurts. The pain recurs frequently and is even worse during sex (M).

To our knowledge, there is limited information on the development and deployment of this prevention campaign. However, we understand that the Zoom posters were developed by a private enterprise that specializes in advertising and marketing. Consequently, we know that these posters were deployed using the established networks of this enterprise with the specific objective of reaching young adults in various settings where they meet sexual partners. These settings included bars, pubs, colleges, universities, restaurants, gyms and so forth.

The second type of communication strategy in the prevention campaign consisted of several web-based messages entitled 'What would you do for pleasure?'[3] Three different versions of the same message were made available through web publicities in which young adults were asked to reassess their desire for pleasure in light of the physical consequences of STIs. The following physical consequences were presented alternatively on a background of human skin and sweat: voiding razor blades, drying off greenish secretions, scratching skin lesions, not having sex anymore, being sterile, experiencing testicular swelling, having brain lesions, living with cardiac insufficiency. A complementary section was also made available at the bottom of the interactive statements to announce the title of the campaign (Condoms: They aren't a luxury) and explain how STIs, such as Chlamydia, Gonorrhea, Herpes, Syphilis, LGV and HPV, can cause permanent physical consequences while being asymptomatic. To our knowledge, there is no information available on the development and diffusion of these web-based messages.

The documents retrieved from this prevention campaign were chosen because they were developed using commercial advertising and marketing strategies; thus, it situated the individual-as-consumer at the nexus of emotional appeal and prescribed conducts. As such, it supported Lupton's (1995) critique of the role played by advertising and mass media in the production of public health campaigns. Furthermore, the compelling words displayed in the Zoom posters and web-based messages (i.e., horror, horrible, suffering, fear, pain, discomfort, permanent physical damages, infertility, etc.) encouraged us to examine the discursive content of the prevention campaign using situational analysis as our method of inquiry. In doing so, we were able to engage in a critical examination of the documents retrieved from the prevention campaign and use mapping strategies to experiment with new ways of conducting discourse analysis.

Method: Situational Analysis

Our perspective is informed by the work of Clarke (2005) regarding situational analysis and its application to discourse materials. Situational analysis is typically integrated to grounded theory research with the objective of 'elucidating the key elements, immaterialities, discourses, structures and conditions that characterized the situation of inquiry' (Clarke 2005, p. xxii). This analytic approach offers three main cartographic exercises that are performed by researchers who wish to examine complex situations of inquiry and 'become stronger at generating the kinds of data in which we can find often invisible issues and silences' (Clarke 2005, p. 76). According to Clarke (2005), these cartographic exercises (situational maps, social worlds/arenas maps, positional maps) can 'deeply situate research projects individually, collectively, organizationally, institutionally, temporally, geographically, materially, discursively, culturally, symbolically, visually, and historically' (p. xxii). There-fore, situational analysis typically 'allows researchers to draw together studies of discourse and agency, action and structure, image, text and context, history and the present moment—to analyze complex situations of inquiry broadly conceived' (Clarke 2005, p. xxii).

For the purpose of this paper, we opted to downscale the situation of inquiry and experiment with the cartographic exercises proposed by Clarke (2005) since they offered a creative and structured analytical process. Our objective was to critically examine the prevention campaign along with the discourse materials located and collected for the project. In order to explore the discursive body of the campaign, we turned to important documents such as the 'Stratégie québécoise de lutte contre l'infection par le VIH et le SIDA, l'infection par le VHC et les ITS—Orientation 2003–2009' and the 'Programme National de Santé Publique 2003-2012'. We also reviewed epidemiological data on sexually transmitted infections and scholarly publications in the field of public health. Finally, we identified that the Zoom posters and the web-based messages would constitute the primary discursive terrain of our analysis.

Using the cartographic exercises proposed by Clarke (2005), we critically examined the prevention campaign (situation of inquiry) using a cluster of key questions:

> What are the discourses in the broader situation? Who (individually and collectively) is involved (supportive, opposed, providing knowledge, materials, money, what else?) in producing these discourses? What and who do these discourses construct? How? What and whom are they in dialogue with/about? What and who do these discourses render invis-ible? How? What material things—nonhuman elements—are involved in the discourses? What are the implicated/silent actors/actants? What were the important discursively constructed elements in the situation? What work do these discourses do in the world? What are some of the contested issues in the discourses? (Clarke 2005, pp. 187–188)

Based on these questions, we created a disorganized situational map to identify all the analytically pertinent elements within the situation of inquiry. We proceeded to write down every one of these elements in a disorganized manner (messy map). Following this brainstorm exercise, we displayed each element onto an organized situational map using the categories provided by Clarke (2005, pp. 97, 193).

The organized map allowed us to situate the prevention campaign within a particular political context. As such, we noted that the campaign is part of a broader governmental strategy to re-sensitize young adults to the risk of contracting a sexually transmitted infection and the physical consequences of becoming infected. The map also demonstrated how the discursive construction of young adults as a de-sensitized and risky population was directly related to the growing incidence of sexually transmitted infections in the province of Quebec. In fact, we noted that the epidemiological data were a key element in the construction of the prevention campaign and the description of its objectives—increase the perception of risk linked to sexually transmitted infections and reaffirm that condom use is the best way to prevent these infections.

The most important feature of the organized map was the identification and reorganization of the major discourses related to the situation of inquiry (Figure 8.1). After considerable examination of the maps and the situation of inquiry (prevention campaign), we chose to focus on fear-based discourse as a way to create a space for critique and resistance. This decision was the starting point of another analytical exercise (relational analysis), which was conducted to investigate the relationship between fear-based discourse and numerous elements contained in the situational maps (including other major discourses). By making connections on paper, we uncovered the inherent assumptions of the campaign whereby the perception of risk is associated with the uptake of a prescribed behavior (condom use) and fear is considered the best way to increase the perception of risk in young adults.

From this perspective, unsafe sex is represented as a form of deviance that takes place when the physical risk is not perceived—the risk of contracting a preventable STI and experiencing horrible, painful, lethal and debilitating physical damages. The perception of risk is, therefore, understood as a prerequisite for the consumption of fear and subsequently, the uptake of a prescribed norm such as condom use. In this sense, fear is used to construct meaning around the experience of contracting an STI by describing the infected body through impact words, debilitating physical symptoms and the social significance of its contagiousness. It is also used to construct meaning around safe sex by describing the condom as the ultimate protecting device and condom use as a rational action for health; one that does not require negotiation, since it should be unquestionably adopted by young adults.

Based on our analysis, fear is inherently political because it is deployed by the state with the clear objective of penetrating the collective and personal

Figure 8.1 Major discourses.

Epidemiology:	Referring to the concepts of incidence, prevalence and probabilities; projections and causalities; statistics on STIs, HIV and HCV.
Public Health:	Referring to the concepts of surveillance, disease control, disease prevention, reportable diseases, contact tracing and screening.
Prevention:	Referring to prevention campaigns; the identification (target) of individuals in the pre-transmission phase; preventing transmission to avoid consequences.
Risk:	Referring to the risk of transmission based on age, gender and sexual activities; statistical risk; risk of experiencing short-term and long-term consequences of STIs; spatial elements of risk; risk of being asymptomatic; risk of not being cured.
Fear:	Referring to terms used to qualify the consequences of contracting an STI such as pain, disgust, horror, horrible, suffering, terror, lived through hell, death and being asymptomatic (you might have it but not know it).
Fatalism:	Referring to the use of extreme vocabulary to re-enforce consequences of STIs including the possibility of not being cured, dying, experiencing intolerable physical repercussions (pain, discharge, lesions, warts, swelling) and experiencing severe repercussions on sexuality, sexual intercourse/performance and sexual organs.
Safe-sex:	Referring to the emphasis attributed to the use of the condom, pleasure, sexual intercourse, sex, sexual organs, making the right choice, responsibility, balancing pleasure and protection.
Moralistic:	Referring to the construction of unprotected sexual activities as dangerously 'immoral' from a health perspective (as opposed to religious or ethical perspectives); condom use as a moral obligation.
Punishment:	Referring to the construction of unsafe sex as deviant (sexual sin); unsafe sex is associated with severe corporal repercussions (short-term and long-term punishment, including death).
Biomedical:	Referring to the introduction of medical terminology to give authority to the campaign, including terms such as: infections, Chlamydia, gonorrhea, LGV, syphilis, HIV/AIDS, herpes, genital warts, symptoms, asymptomatic, cardiac insufficiency, brain lesions, testicular swelling, pain, vaginal discharge, lesions, etc.
Promotional:	Referring to the action of promoting health—discursive strategy which serve to self-promote; provides tangible evidence that the state is doing something about the particular health problem and to promote or to publicize the health problem itself.
Health promotion:	Referring to the concepts of responsibility towards self and others, choice, action, empowerment, 'positive health', self care, personal control, rationality, individualism, mass campaign.
Repression:	Referring to the repressive effects of the campaign, negative repercussions, repression of unsafe sex (discouraging deviant sexual practices).

domains to manage/govern the population and their sexual practices. Unsurprisingly, then, fear is perceived as an effective strategy to create a state of permanent (in)security and manipulate people into becoming calculating, rational and self-interested subjects who avoid the perils of human desires and contagion (Adam 2006, Turner 2008). In the following segment, we will expand on the use of fear in public health campaigns by making important connections with the Foucauldian concepts of governmentality and bio-power as well as the non-Foucauldian notion of (in)security.

Governmentality and the Politics of Fear

The concept of governmentality (Foucault 1979) describes the general mechanisms of society's governance and does not refer specifically to the term government as it is commonly used to designate the organization through which a political unit exercises authority and performs functions (Holmes and Gastaldo 2002). French philosopher Michel Foucault conceptualizes governmentality as a complex system of power relations that binds sovereignty (the state of domination), discipline (disciplinary power) and the government of others and self (government) (Holmes and Gastaldo 2002). In his own terms, Foucault defines governmentality as: 'the ensemble formed by the institutions, procedures, analyses and reflections, the calculations and tactics that allow the exercise of this very specific albeit complex form of power, which has as its target population, as its principal form of knowledge political economy, and as its essential technical means apparatuses of security' (Foucault 1979, p. 20).

The 'governmentalization of the state' (Holmes and Gastaldo 2002, p. 559) relies on a specific *apparatus of security* [*dispositif de sécurité*] composed of many institutions, actors, procedures and techniques that contribute to the maintenance of social order and functioning (Dean 1999). Contained within this apparatus of security, public health campaigns play an important role in social governance because they promote and organize knowledge, norms and social practices, they serve as the basis for the development of an expert discourse, *and* they penetrate the individual's habits of everyday life (Perron et al. 2005). Therefore, public health campaigns such as the one put forward by the government of Quebec (Canada) (and which is part of a new trend in Western countries) must be located within a governmentality framework for it deals directly with matters related to the management of a specific sub-population (young adults) and the regulation of its sexual conducts.

The governmentality framework is of utmost importance to understand that public health campaigns are part of the large-scale operation of bio-power (power over life). In effect, public health campaigns are part of the bio-political axis of bio-power; thus, they are 'concerned with matters of life and death, with birth and propagation, with health and illness, both physical and mental, and with the process that sustain and retard the optimization of the life of a population' (Dean 1999, p. 99). In the interest of health, these campaigns introduce a normalized way of living that reinforces the security of the overall population while capitalizing on the conformity and rationality of each member of that population; thus promoting self-government on behalf of effective social regulation (Oster and Cheek 2008). From this per-spective, bio-politics is concerned with the adoption of healthy choices, healthy desires, healthy lifestyles and healthy conducts by each member of the targeted population (Lupton 1995).

The government of conduct requires an analysis of the technical means (technologies) by which the conducts of individuals are regulated and moni-tored. In the prevention campaign entitled 'Condoms: They aren't a luxury', fear is used as a bio-political technology to govern young adults (as a sub-population) and their sexual conduct. We were able to determine that the prevention campaign is specifically designed to encourage young adults to become calculating, rational and self-regulating subjects who avoid the perils of human desires and contagion (Adam 2006, Turner 2008). As such, the messages call attention to the invasion of the body by sexually transmitted infections with a particular emphasis on contamination, decay, deviance and disgust. Using compelling words to describe the infected body as 'horror of flesh-out-of-control' (p. 120), these messages provoke concerns about bodily integrity, body image, sexual performance and most particularly, the gaze of others (Lupton 1995). Unsurprisingly, then, fear is directly related to the por-trayal of STIs as a form of corporal punishment.

We argue that the prevention campaign primarily reaffirms the moral tale of sexually transmitted infections—'this will happen to *your* body if *you* are not careful' (Lupton 1995, p. 120). It also reinforces the discursive repre-sentation of STIs (and those who contract them) as physically repulsive and socially undesirable. By intensifying the fear of bodily disorder and social repercussions, the prevention campaign suggests that wearing a condom dur-ing sexual intercourse is a practice of self-contained self-control—one that is highly valued in a society where individuals are encouraged to regulate their own lifestyle and modify their risky behaviors (Peterson 1997). In this sense, the use of fear is particularly effective because those who do not adhere to prescribed norms are 'punished through the mechanisms of self-surveillance, evoking feelings of guilt, anxiety and repulsion towards the self, as well as the admonitions of their nearest and dearest for "letting themselves go" or inviting illness' (Lupton 1995, pp. 10–11).

It is likely that the prevention campaign acts as a discursive terrain for deviance amplification by reinforcing the internalized stigma associated with STIs (Nettleton and Bunton 1995). We consider that the prevention campaign emphasizes 'the notion of individual choice [. . .] and draws attention to the fact that [public health] makes people feel responsible and culpable for their health status (Nettleton and Bunton 1995, p. 52). In the event that one is unable to maintain a risk-free existence, STIs (and their physical repercussions) are described as predictable outcomes of bad individual choices, deviant sexual practices and self-negligence. This is an important dimension of the prevention campaign because the governance of a population can only be achieved through the promotion of self-government—the conformity and rationality of each member of that population. As a bio-political technology, fear is productive if each individual consumes fear and is consumed by it; thus, the overall population must be possessed by the impending disaster and its potential consequences on the self. Fear is, therefore, a bio-political technology that creates a state of permanent (in)security and manipulates individuals who buy into this mode of control.

(In)Security and the Consumption of Fear

Fear is [. . .] the most economical expression of the accident-form as subject-form of capital: being as being-virtual, virtuality reduced to the possibility of disaster, disaster commodified, commodification as spectral continuity in the place of threat. When we buy, we are buying off fear and falling, filling the gap with presence-effects. When we consume, we are consuming our own possibility. In possessing, we are possessed, by marketable forces beyond our control. In complicity with capital, a body becomes its own worst enemy.

(Massumi 1993, p. 12)

Under late capitalism, power is both predictive and determining of the disasters identified within the individual, collective and social body (Massumi 1993). In this sense, Massumi (1993) argues that power is a two-fold concept that includes both the prediction of potential threats to the human capital (i.e., surveillance and statistical probability) and the determination of disaster inside particular bodies (i.e., testing) (Massumi 1993). By giving 'disaster a face', power mechanisms that serve to identify disasters produce a socially recognizable content that can be absorbed by the general population and applied to the individual self and body; thus creating a world where the disaster is 'always about to happen and already has (. . .)' (Massumi 1993, p. 22).

In order for public health campaigns to be effective (in a disciplinary sense), they must create 'a space of fear' (Massumi 1993, p. 23). For this reason, the disease must be represented as a probable threat, its consequences on the self must be feared by targeted individuals, and the body must be understood as a potential enemy. As such, fear has wider implication for the ways in which society views 'the body as a site of toxicity, contamination and catastrophe, subject to and needful of a higher surveillance and control' (Lupton 1994, p. 134) and the ways in which society consumes public health warnings about disorders. The prevention campaign put forward by the government of Quebec (Canada) is a great example of this specific mode of control, one that creates a state of permanent (in)security while constructing the body as a hazardous object and condom use as *the* only way to achieve probabilistic security for oneself.

Lupton (1995) has previously suggested that public health campaigns are often created from a social marketing standpoint in which the individual-as-consumer is encouraged to consume a specific product (hereby referring to the public health message and prescribed behaviors) and modify his lifestyle accordingly. From a social marketing standpoint, 'the distinction between the production of health and the consumption of health is collapsed' (Nettleton and Bunton 1995, p. 49)—a process known as the commodification of health. In the interest of health, a plethora of products are implanted in the social domain and valorized in collective perception (Massumi 1993). These products are generally purchased (i.e., anti-aging creams, fat-free products, gym memberships, herbal products, cosmetic interventions, prophylactic medications, condoms) but they can also be distributed en masse to the population (i.e., vaccines).

In the prevention campaign entitled 'Condoms: They aren't a luxury', young adults are encouraged to consume fear—to internalize this marketing product the same way other commodities are incorporated in/to the body. Those who buy into this mode of control are then presented with the promise of ultimate security and persuaded to exercise self-discipline (Lupton 2003). As a result, they are more likely to express anxiety over the invasion of the body by STIs and be consumed with the impeding menace of bodily fluids exchanged during sexual intercourse (Lupton 2003). In this sense, the deployment of fear makes possible the uptake of condom use as the only way to achieve probabilistic security for oneself. Deployed in a permanent state of (in)security, however, condom use is no longer choice but rather a response to the fear of bodily (dis)order and social repercussions. This is particularly concerning because condom use then becomes primarily guided by the fear of corporal punishment and social deviance instead of the motivation to be 'healthy'.

Our position is that young adults are more likely to capture the undertow of the prevention campaign and internalize the invisible messages—hereby referring to the discourses of punishment and moral disgrace surrounding STIs and those who contract them. In this sense, we argue that resistance to/rejection of fear is possible and likely to arise considering that the campaign can be easily identified as a governmental sponsored message and that young adults 'are rarely responsive to overt attempts to coerce them into changing their behavior, unless they have already decided that they wish to do so . . .' (Lupton 1995, p. 124). Based on our analysis, the campaign is constructed to attract those who already want to adopt the prescribed behavior and for that reason, we wonder if the use of fear-based messages in the campaign was no more than 'a cost-effective means of demonstrating that the state considers the issue to be a problem and is working to do something about it' (Lupton 1995, p. 125)—a 'quick fix' solution to its own failures in communicating health messages to young adults.

Final Remarks

In the public health domain, commercial advertising and marketing strategies are commonly used to produce prevention campaigns that command attention and infiltrate the collective imagination by making the image of bad outcomes readily available (Lupton 1995, Sustein 2005). Also known as social marketing, this approach is defined as 'a program-planning process that applies commercial marketing concepts and techniques to promote voluntary behavior change' by facilitating the 'acceptance, rejection, modification, abandonment or maintenance of particular behaviors by groups of individuals, often referred to as the target audience' (Grier and Bryant 2005, p. 321).

We believe that the prevention campaign entitled 'Condoms: They aren't a luxury' is a great example of social marketing because its content was developed and implemented by a private enterprise that specializes in this field and most particularly, in the production of messages that are tailored to discrete target audiences for more effective persuasion (Lupton 1995). Based on our analysis, we consider that the extensive use of fear in the campaign was partly due to the construction of young adults as a risky group, a target audience that needs to be shocked into action in order to abandon its risky sexual behaviors and adopt new safe sex practices.

Along with Stewart and colleagues (2000), we believe that 'as long as any of these identity labels are assumed to produce a particular set of sexual practices, the best-intentioned education and prevention efforts risk being misplaced and, at worst, health-damaging' (p. 420). In this sense, the use of social marketing in the public health domain is a 'quick fix' to much larger issues (such as the STI epidemic) that remain misunderstood and embedded in an array of assumptions that are detrimental to effective health promotion and disease prevention. We argue that the use of social marketing to communicate health raises important questions regarding the 'McDonaldisation' (Turner 1997, p. xviii) of prevention campaigns.

According to Turner (1997), 'McDonaldisation is the application of Fordist production methods and rational managerialism to the fast-food industry which is then extended to all sectors of society' (p. xviii). Based on principles of cheapness, standardization and reliability, fear-based prevention campaigns (such as the one put forward by the government of Quebec) suggest that McDonaldisation is penetrating the health domain (Tuner 1997). From this perspective, the use of fear and the production of prevention campaigns by advertising firms constitute cost-effective solutions to lasting public health issues (such as the STI epidemic in a specific subgroup of the population).

In light of our analysis, we believe that fear is regaining momentum within the public health domain. This particular trend is symptomatic of a broader political context where public health campaigns are inadequately funded and relegated to private enterprises that apply advertising techniques to non-commercial issues such as the socially complex STI epidemic. According to Lupton (1995), this phenomenon is largely based on 'the belief that advertising in the mass media is an effective means of propaganda, able to persuade audiences to take up a desired behavior, whether it be the purchasing of a commodity or the abandonment of a practice believed to undermine the achievement and maintenance of good health' (p. 106).

It is imperative that we maintain an open dialogue on the issues surrounding the STI epidemic and more importantly, on the successes and failures of public health actions in the fight against sexually transmitted infections. We must remain critical of public health campaigns that serve 'to self-promote, to provide tangible evidence that the state is "doing something" about that particular health problem (or is at least spending time and money on producing advertising materials and paying for air-time or column space)' (Lupton 1995, p. 126). This is particularly important given that the effectiveness of public health campaigns remains a contentious issue.

Acknowledgements

Marilou Gagnon would like to acknowledge the financial support of the Canadian Institute of Health Research (CIHR). Jean Daniel Jacob and Dave Holmes would like to acknowledge the financial support of the Social Sciences and Humanities Research Council of Canada (SSHRC).

Notes

1. This section was written based on the information retrieved from www.msss.gouv.qc.ca.

2. http://www.msss.gouv.qc.ca/sujets/prob_sante/itss/index.php?id¼ 83,297,0,0,1,0.

3. http://www.msss.gouv.qc.ca/sujets/prob_sante/itss/index.php?id¼141,273,0,0,1,0.

References

Adam, B. D., 2006. Infectious behaviour: Imputing subjectivity to HIV transmission. *Social Theory & Health*, 4, 168–179.

Center for Disease Control, 2007. Sexually transmitted disease surveillance 2006. Available from: http://www.cdc.gov/std/stats/pdf/introductory-sections.pdf [Accessed 7 Sept 2008].

Clarke, A., 2005. *Situational analysis: Grounded theory after the postmodern turn.* Thousand Oaks, CA: Sage.

Dean, M., 1999. *Governmentality.* Thousand Oaks, CA: Sage.

Foucault, M., 1979. Governmentality. *Ideology and Consciousness*, 6, 5–21.

Grier, S. and Bryant, C.A., 2005. Social Marketing in Public Health. *Annual Review in Public Health*, 26, 319–339.

Holmes, D. and Gastaldo, D., 2002. Nursing as means of governmentality. *Journal of Advanced Nursing Practice*, 38 (6), 557–565.

Lupton, D., 1994. *Moral threats and dangerous desires: AIDS in the news media.* London: Taylor & Francis.

Lupton, D., 1995. *The imperative of health: Public health and the regulated body.* London: Sage.

Lupton, D., 2003. *Medicine as culture.* 2nd ed. London: Sage.

MacDonald, N. and Wong, T., 2007. Canadian guidelines on sexually transmitted infections, 2006. *Canadian Medical Association Journal*, 176 (2), 175–176.

Massumi, B., 1993. *The politics of everyday fear.* Minneapolis, MN: University of Minnesota Press.

Nettleton, S. and Bunton, R., 1995. Sociological critique of health promotion, *In* R. Bunton, S. Nettleton and R. Burrows, eds. *The sociology of health promotion.* London: Routledge, 41–59.

Oster, C. and Cheek, J., 2008. Governing the contagious body: Genital herpes, contagion and technologies of the self. *Health: An Interdisciplinary Journal for the Social Study of Health*, 12 (2), 215–232.

Panchaud, C., Singh, S., and Darroch, J.E., 2000. Sexually transmitted diseases among adolescents in developed countries. *Family Planning Perspectives*, 32 (1), 24–32, 45.

Perron, A., Fluet, C., and Holmes, D., 2005. Agents of care and agents of the state: Bio-power and nursing practice. *Journal of Advanced Nursing Practice*, 50 (5), 536–544.

Peterson, A., 1997. Risk, governance and the new public health. *In* A. Peterson and R. Bunton, eds. *Foucault, health and medicine*. London: Routledge, 187–206.

Public Health Agency of Canada, 2007. Supplement – 2004 Canadian sexually transmitted infections surveillance report. Available from: http://www.phac-aspc.gc.ca/publicat/ccdrr mtc/07pdf/33s1_e.pdf [Accessed 7 Sept 2008].

Stewart, F. J., Mischewski, A., and Smith, A.M.A., 2000. 'I want to do what I want to do': young adults resisting sexual identities. *Critical Public Health*, 10 (4), 409–422.

Sustein, C. R., 2005. *Laws of fear: Beyond the precautionary principle*. Cambridge: Cambridge University Press.

Turner, B. S., 1997. From governmentality to risk: Some reflections on Foucault's contribution to medical sociology, *In* A. Peterson and R. Bunton, eds. *Foucault, health and medicine* (Foreword). London: Routledge, viiii–xxi.

Turner, B. S., 2008. *The body and society*. 3rd ed. London: Sage.

Weinstock, H., Berman, S., and Cates, W., 2004. Sexually transmitted diseases among American youth: Incidence and prevalence estimates, 2000. *Perspectives on Sexual and Reproductive Health*, 36 (1), 6–10.

World Health Organization, 2007. Module 1 – Introduction to STI prevention and control. Available from: http://www.who.int/reproductivehealth/publications/trainingmodules_syndromic_mngt_stis/m1.pdf [Accessed 7 Sept 2008].

Reflection: Allowing Mute Evidence to Be Heard: Using Situational Analysis to Deconstruct a Public Health Campaigns

Marilou Gagnon, Jean Daniel Jacob, & Dave Holmes

Public health campaigns combining both visual and narrative discourses are very common in the field. Every year, agencies develop prevention campaigns on various topics, some targeting large portions of the population (i.e., influenza, obesity, immunization, road safety) and others tailored to specific groups (i.e., adolescents, young adults, women, men) (see, e.g., Pedrana et al. 2014). It is standard practice to use social marketing and advertising strategies to develop these campaigns, crafting their appeal to certain audiences and achieving greater persuasion through the careful combination of visual and narrative elements.

In 2008, we became interested in a prevention campaign created by Quebec's Ministry of Health and Social Services (Canada) for the prevention of sexually transmitted infections (STIs) in young adults. Titled "Condoms: They Aren't a Luxury," it included three types of communication strategies: online messages on syphilis, Zoom posters, and "What would you do for pleasure?" web-based messages. We selected the latter two strategies for our analysis (detailed descriptions appear in our article).

For these reflections, we focus solely on our experience of working with situational analysis (SA). First, we discuss why and how we chose SA. Then, drawing on the work of Clarke (2005) and other authors who have used SA, we describe our mapping process and address the practicalities of doing the actual maps. Last, we share our experience of publishing research findings and reflect on the formatting challenges encountered when it was time to illustrate mapping processes. We conclude with thoughts on SA as a method for analyzing visual and narrative discourses such as those produced by public health agencies.

Experimenting with Situational Analysis

We came to this project with varying degrees of experience with discourse analysis and had previously worked with mute evidence such as nursing notes, legal texts, and institutional policies. Here, we use the term "mute evidence" to differentiate textual and visual data from the type of data that is typically generated in qualitative research when participants speak about their experience in interviews. Mute evidence data tell different stories that can be revealed through the careful analysis of discourses produced by and constituted through texts and images (Clarke 2005). However, to engage in such analysis, one needs to find a suitable approach. This is where SA entered. It was not an approach with which we were already familiar. In fact, none of us had been introduced to this approach in our graduate training. We wanted to try something new and were drawn to the idea of mapping out our ideas as we worked through the process of analyzing discourses. We also felt that the project itself provided an ideal opportunity to learn how to use SA mapping.

SA was attractive for this project because it was not only compatible with our epistemological positions as researchers, but also because it offered practical tools to flesh out our data. It was important for us to find an approach that was consistent with a poststructuralist understanding of discourses and discourse analysis. This was absolutely essential because of the broader provincial context at the time and how it influenced the design of the campaign, the richness of texts and images featured in the campaign, and the importance of paying close attention to elements that were both visible and invisible in the campaign itself. We found the questions listed by Clarke in Chapter 6 to be particularly helpful in keeping the focus of our analysis on discourses. Here are the classic questions that were instrumental to our analysis:

+ What are the discourses in the broader situation?
+ Who (individually and collectively) is involved (supportive, opposed, providing knowledge, materials, money, what else?) in producing these discourses?
+ What and who do these discourses construct? How?
+ What and whom are they in dialogue with/about?
+ What and who do these discourses render invisible? How?
+ What material things—nonhuman elements—are involved in the discourses?
+ What are the implicated/silent actors/actants?
+ What were the important discursively constructed elements in the situation?
+ What work do these discourses do in the world?

◆ What are some of the contested issues in the discourses? (Clarke 2005:187–188)

In retrospect, we can see how experimenting with SA allowed us to work more closely with *all* the discourses rather than immediately focus on a *dominant discourse*. This was consistent with what we were hoping to achieve when we first became interested in the prevention campaign and what it offered from a discursive standpoint.

Our decision to work with SA was also motivated by the fact that it offers practical exercises that researchers can use at their discretion to "map" and "open up" (Clarke 2003:560) their data. According to Clarke (2003:560), such exercises "are not necessarily intended to form final analytic products." We used these exercises to generate maps that became part of our research findings. While this is not always the case for researchers using SA, we wanted to create a space for these maps in the presentation and discussion of our findings. The practical dimensions of SA were particularly helpful in working with mute evidence such as the posters and web messages. As researchers, we were interested in analyzing what was "there" (i.e., words, images, symbols, logos, messages, etc.) *and* what remained "silent" in the campaign (i.e., marketing agencies, young adults, STI testing clinics and services, sexual education, condom negotiation skills, condom usage and accessibility, etc.). We were also interested in working with an approach that allowed us to map out the different elements in the campaign and situate this campaign in broader social, cultural, political, economic, and historical contexts. SA provided the means to achieve these objectives.

Mapping and Deconstructing Discourses

Given that we did not have previous experience of *doing* SA, there was a great deal of trial and error when we first started mapping the campaign. After gathering our data, we began our analysis with multiple versions of disorganized (messy) situational maps drafted on separate pieces of paper. With each version, we added new elements analytically pertinent for the project. It would have been nearly impossible for us to write down all the elements in the first version of the disorganized (messy) map. An electronic copy (in Word format) of the final disorganized (messy) map was made once we felt ready to move to the next step—the organized situational map.

Throughout this process, we took copious notes but did not write memos per se. These notes were useful at the time, but we realized later on that writing memos to document our decision-making process, our struggles, and our ideas would have been more valuable to us. We would therefore highly recommend that researchers interested in doing SA start *memoing* right away and continue this practice throughout the analytical process. We would also recommend that they write memos as part of a paper trail for the analytical process as well as for the research decisions made along the way and the rationales for making such decisions. Finally, we would advise researchers to *digitize* their disorganized (messy) maps and/or find creative ways of mapping directly on a screen using a tablet. In addition to being more interactive and versatile, this format helps keep everything on file and enables working collaboratively with a research team.

Based on our final disorganized (messy) map, we used the categories provided by Clarke (2005:90) to organize the elements identified. The categories were particularly useful to develop an organized map and to add elements that had not been considered up to that point. For example, new political, economic, and temporal elements were added at that stage of the analysis. Because our goal was to focus on discourses, we paid close attention to texts and images. We wrote memos on this particular dimension of the analysis. One of these memos featured a table with a list of all the major discourses identified in the campaign and a brief description of each one. This table was published along with our findings and can be found in the previous chapter. Another memo included reflexive notes and a two-column table. The left column contained prominent words in the campaign posters (i.e., horror, horrible, suffering, hell, fear) and the right column contained a list of physical consequences associated with STIs (i.e., discharge, pain, discomfort). At that stage of the analysis, it became evident to us that the main objective of the campaign was to foster the perception of risk and instill fear in young adults. This was not only fear of contracting an STI but more importantly, fear of experiencing the horrible, painful, and debilitating physical symptoms of STIs. We decided to focus on fear-based discourse for the remainder of our analysis.

At this stage, we developed a relational map to explore relationships between fear-based discourse and all the other elements contained in our disorganized (messy) situational map. This was particularly useful in connecting elements together and thinking about how they interacted together. For example, we were able to make connections on paper between fear-based discourse and marketing and advertising agencies, public health agencies, cost-effectiveness of prevention campaigns, debates on the use of fear in pub-lic health, and the construction of young adults as passive, complacent, and risky. This mapping process helped conceptually link what was becoming the main focus of our analysis (fear-based discourse) and all the other elements in the campaign.

Again, we would recommend *memoing*. Because we were working inten-sively with the data, we did not always see the need to document emerging thoughts and ideas. These were shared within the team and incorporated in the development of the manuscript, but not written as memos. If we were to redo the relational map for this project, we would find a way to *digitize* as well as memo the mapping process so that connections and the nature of these connections can be more clearly delineated.

Over the course of the analysis, we also created a positional map based on all of the major discourses that we identified in the campaign. The process of working on this map was more challenging for us. We struggled with the identification of the two main axes, which made it difficult for us to situ-ate the different positions expressed in the campaign. Our positional map was included in a conference presentation of the findings and it was also incorporated in the original version of the manuscript that was submitted for publication in the fall of 2008. However, we were advised to remove this map from the manuscript for reasons discussed below.

Reflecting back on our experience, we are left wondering if this map was, in fact, relevant and appropriate for the project. As suggested by Clarke (2005), there is no right way of doing SA. Working with a positional map or not is a decision that researchers need to make based on the nature of their project and the reasons for using SA in the first place. Now that we have more experience with SA, we see the value of using positional mapping when analyzing qualitative interview data, for example, or when working with a larger body of "mute evidences." Because our analysis was limited solely to the campaign materials only, it was challenging to map out different posi-tions contained *within* the campaign.

Formatting and Publishing the Findings

As suggested by Clarke (2003), situational maps can be used with various objectives in mind (e.g., opening up the data, doing analytic exercises, reliev-ing analytic paralysis, stimulating thinking, and so forth). Most of the time, the maps are added to an existing research methodology such as grounded theory (see e.g., French & Miller 2012). However, we have seen instances where only SA is used (see e.g., Pérez & Canella 2011). Our experience of attempting to publish findings based on the maps is worth reflecting on here. We briefly discuss two main challenges that arose.

The first challenge has to do with the fact that reviewers may not be familiar with SA and may see the maps as analytic exercises that should not necessarily be shared with readers. This was the case for our positional map. In contrast, we would assert that the maps *should* be shared with the readers because they are integral to how researchers get to their findings. They should also be shared because they contribute to a growing body of knowledge and understanding on the actual process of making situational maps. Furthermore, they can serve as models for those who are interested in using situational maps. Assuming that reviewers (and readers) may not be familiar with SA, it is important for researchers to explain their approach while justifying its relevance and how it works. To illustrate this point, we share the following comment made by our reviewers: "Situational analysis appears innovative, for a public health journal. Nevertheless, this is a complex method which, because recently published, is not well understood and therefore requires considerable explication." Additionally, it is important for researchers to explain *why* maps are important—that these are not just products of brainstorming exercises, but *integral parts of the analysis.*

This leads to our second challenge: the actual publication of the maps within existing constraints on publishing. In the current literature, we have seen authors who were unable or opted not to publish their maps. We have also seen authors select one map (e.g., Carder 2008; Washburn 2013) and others publish all their maps (e.g., Fosket 2014). Among researchers who work with SA, the question of where to publish often arises. Is it better to publish in a journal despite the existing constraints or in a book where there is more room to share working documents and maps? This is an important question to consider, as the popularity of SA is on the rise. We may have to consider publication of additional collections by authors who work with SA to ensure that its application and contribution within qualitative research continue to grow.

Concluding Remarks

In concluding, we would like to reiterate how useful we found SA—especially for the analysis of visual and narratives discourses. Its epistemological and methodological underpinnings clearly guide researchers toward the use of maps as methods of analysis. In turn, the maps allow researchers to produce findings that are consistent with a particular way of constructing knowledge. In closing with this argument, we hope to generate interest in developing more critical qualitative research informed by SA. Undoubtedly, this book will contribute to pushing the conversation forward on this very matter.

References

Carder, P. C. 2008. Managing Medication Management in Assisted Living: A Situational Analysis. *Journal of Ethnographic & Qualitative Research* 3:1–12.

Clarke, A. E. 2003. Situational Analysis: Grounded Theory Mapping after the Postmodern Turn. *Symbolic Interaction* 24(4):553–576.

Clarke, A. E. 2005. *Situational Analysis: Grounded Theory after the Postmodern Turn.* Thousand Oaks, CA: Sage.

Fosket, J. R. 2014. Situating Knowledge. In A. E. Clarke & K. Charmaz (Eds.), *Grounded Theory and Situational Analysis* (pp. 91–110). London: Sage.

French, M. & F. A. Miller. 2012. Leveraging the "Living Laboratory": On the Emergence of the Entrepreneurial Hospital. *Social Science & Medicine* 75:717–724.

Pedrana, A. E., M. E. Hellard, P. Higgs, J. Asselin, C. Batrouney, & M. Stoové. 2014. "No Drama": Key Elements to the Success of an HIV/STI-Prevention Mass Media Campaign. *Qualitative Health Research* 24(5):695–705.

Pérez, M. S. & G. S. Cannella. 2011. Using Situational Analysis for Critical Qualitative Research Purposes. In N. K. Denzin & M. D. Giardina (Eds.), *Qualitative Inquiry and Global Crisis* (pp. 97–117). Walnut Creek, CA: Left Coast Press, Inc.

Washburn, R. 2013. Rethinking the Disclosure Debates: A Situational Analysis of the Multiple Meanings of Human Biomonitoring Data. *Critical Public Health* 23(4):452–465.

CHAPTER NINE

LEVERAGING THE "LIVING LABORATORY": ON THE EMERGENCE OF THE ENTREPRENEURIAL HOSPITAL

Martin French & Fiona Alice Miller

Introduction

The province of Ontario *has identified cancer as an area with unique opportunities for supporting research and innovation.* Exploitation of these opportunities is expected to impact the burden of cancer and also lead to the creation of innovative industries and commercial partnerships (OICR & The Government of Ontario. 2009: 2—emphasis ours).

Unlike most other jurisdictions with individual tertiary care centres, BC manages all cancer patients from first diagnosis to final outcome on a province-wide basis. *With access to a single demographically complex population of uncompromised patients,* our world-class clinicians offer an unprecedented setting in which to evaluate new patient management protocols (LifeSciences BC & The Government of British Columbia. 2006:4—emphasis ours).

The war metaphor once dominated descriptions of cancer (Sontag, 1977/1989: 66); today, however, war is passé. In populations, cancer (and disease in general) is viewed less as battlefield and more as an area of opportunity for research, and perhaps even as a crucible "for the generation of wealth and health" (Rose & Novas, 2005: 456). Thus, for example, in the above quotations, cancer signifies not simply a struggle to be waged, but also an incentive for innovation creation and commercialisation. Drawn from *oncology asset maps*—government-sponsored marketing documents

From French, Martin and Fiona Alice Miller. *Social Science & Medicine*, Volume 75 (2012) 717–724. © Elsevier. Republished in *Situational Analysis in Practice*, by Adele E. Clarke, Carrie Friese, and Rachel Washburn, 292–321. (Taylor & Francis, 2015). All rights reserved.

aimed at accelerating the commercialisation of public-sector life sciences research—these quotations suggest that something more than disease is being transformed into an opportunity; patients, too, are being enrolled to provide an element, as it were, of the material of innovation.

It would be easy enough to dismiss such statements as marketing rhetoric, but we read them here as an invitation to reconsider the "commercial ethos" in contemporary health research and health care. For years, scholars have debated the "commercial ethos" in higher education, and the rise of the entrepreneurial university (as we discuss below). The "entrepreneurial hospital," as we call it, has—by contrast—gone largely unnoticed. Perhaps scholars who have taken note of the commercial ethos in biomedicine have assumed that whatever holds true for universities also holds true for hospitals. However, because its human capital is vested more heavily in health professionals and patients than professors and students, and because it has the capacity to *use* its innovations in clinical settings, the entrepreneurial hospital differs from the entrepreneurial university in important ways.

This article, therefore, emphasises the distinctive features of the entrepreneurial hospital. As it has not yet been subject to sustained empirical attention, we are wary of making premature generalisations—however, to aid our discussion, we propose the following working definition. *An entrepreneurial hospital is one that explicitly seeks to constitute patient populations and care infrastructure as distinctive assets (or resources) in pursuit of entrepreneurial aims.* For example, entrepreneurial hospitals may partner with a pharmaceutical company to conduct a clinical trial of a drug that they could subsequently use in clinical settings. Or, they may seek to connect basic and applied researchers who will develop technology to address particular problems. In many cases, the entrepreneurial hospital will have acquired business acumen and expertise, perhaps concentrated in an in-house technology transfer group. As we have defined it, the concept could be applied equally to public, non-profit hospitals, private, for-profit hospitals, or any hybridization of these organisational configurations.

Our research suggests that the entrepreneurial hospital brings with it new opportunities and challenges for health care, many of which remain under-examined. In this article, we probe its implications using twenty-six semi-structured interviews with key-informants. Our informants, who work in two different, networked organisations within a single *academic health science system* in a Canadian province, describe efforts to assemble and organise resources into unique configurations that will foster biomedical innovation.

The phrase *academic health science system* (Davies, 2008) intends to capture *both* academic health centres—more commonly known in Canada as academic health science centres—*and* the complex constellation of relationships that have grown up around these centres as they have oriented towards the sometimes incommensurate tasks of care, research, education and innovation. We explore these descriptions, focusing on how patients and patient populations might be assets or resources. This exploration reveals that a key task of entrepreneurial hospitals in Canada is to invent and mediate new uses for patient populations and care infrastructure while also reconciling differing "regimes of value" deriving from obligations to *both* improve health *and* generate wealth (Waldby & Mitchell, 2006: 59).

To set up our analysis, we first introduce readers to literature on the entrepreneurial university. We next discuss contextual factors related to the emergence of the entrepreneurial hospital in Canada. Following a brief discussion of method, we then present findings from the analysis of our interview data. We conclude by discussing some implications of the entrepreneurial hospital for care providers, and by calling for more research into its implications for patients, systems of care, and their broader publics.

Academic Context: The Entrepreneurial University and Industry–Academy Relations

In the early 1980s, in conversation with a Mertonian sociology of science preoccupied with assessing normative structures, Henry Etzkowitz (1983) suggested that while opportunities for commercial utilisation of scientific research were frequently available, "the traditional ethos of science did not permit them to erode the boundary between science and private, profit-seeking business" (p. 824). This contrasted deeply, Etzkowitz argued, with the (then) "present situation", where "many academic scientists no longer regard such constraints as necessary or right" (1983: 198). Taking a case-historical approach, Etzkowitz began advancing the idea that scientists—and universities—were becoming more "entrepreneurial" in conjunction with the "growth of a commercial ethos within academia" and "a normative change in science" (1998: 824). Today, Etzkowitz et al. have created a veritable industry around this idea, making the aspirational argument that "the entrepreneurial university" is (and ought to be) evermore "the centre of gravity for economic development, knowledge creation and diffusion in both advanced industrial and developing societies" (Etzkowitz & Viale, 2010: 596).

The idea of the entrepreneurial university occupies a central, and not uncontested, place in contemporary debates about the commercialisation of science (see, among many: Bok, 2003; Colyvas & Powell, 2009; Etzkowitz, Webster, & Healey, 1998; Owen-Smith, 2005a,b; Powell, Owen-Smith, & Colyvas, 2007; Slaughter & Leslie, 1997; Stuart & Ding, 2006). Rothaermel, Agung, and Jiang (2007) identify four major themes in this growing debate, focusing on 1) the nature of the entrepreneurial research university, 2) the productivity of technology transfer offices (TTOs), 3) new firm creation, and 4) networks of innovation. Within and across these themes, much empirical attention has been accorded to entrepreneurial activities in the biomedical sciences.

Some scholars have gone so far as to accord biomedical research a privileged position in the cycle of innovation and academic commercialization, as evinced for example by Rettig's colourful characterisation of this sector as "the spaceship of hope, the mule train of progress" for innovation (1994: 21). While not sharing Rettig's rhetorical aplomb, others have nevertheless signified the importance of biomedicine in the apparent entrepreneurial turn of the university by, for example, taking the presence or absence of a medical school to be a key variable in the measurement of researchers' and universities' proficiency at the commercialization of technology (Chapple, Lockett, Siegel, & Wright, 2005; Estabrooks et al., 2008; Siegel, Waldman, & Link, 2003; Thursby & Thursby, 2002). Some recent scholarship even concentrates analysis solely on universities with medical schools, or solely on biomedical researchers (Bercovitz & Feldman, 2008; Czarnitzki & Toole, 2010), suggesting that biomedical entrepreneurship is becoming a sentinel site for understanding academic entrepreneurship more generally. That universities with medical schools would have captured the attention of scholars examining academic entrepreneurship is not surprising when one considers certain key commercialisation metrics. In the United States, for example, medical schools are thought to account for the majority of university invention disclosures (Bercovitz & Feldman, 2008: Mowery & Ziedonis, 2002). A similar view is evident in scholarship focused on Canada (Herder & Johnston, 2007; Rasmussen, 2008; Read, 2007).

Yet, in spite of this attention to biomedical entrepreneurship, scholars have accorded surprisingly little consideration to the specificity of innovation, commercialisation, and technology transfer activities as these are manifest *in health care organisations*. Indeed, Hicks and Katz's 1996 characterisation of hospital-based research as a "hidden" research system remains trenchant today (Lander & Atkinson-Grosjean, 2011). Although a great deal has been written about the implications and future of the entrepreneurial university, what we call the "entrepreneurial hospital" has been virtually ignored. Accordingly, certain key questions remain under-examined. For example, if the entrepreneurial turn has profound implications for the academic mission of universities, then are there similar implications for the health care mission of hospitals? Likewise, of what significance is it that entrepreneurial hospitals leverage not only students, *but patients*, for innovation, commercialisation, and technology transfer initiatives?

The Emergence of the Entrepreneurial Hospital: Re-imagining Health Care in Canada

The commercial ethos in health care and health research has raised questions not just about the mission of hospitals, but also more generally about the place of health care in a nation's economic portfolio.

Like other core elements of Canadian national identity, health care provision is often conceived of in relation to what it is not. A common trope—invoked by proponents and critics alike—is to distinguish between Canada and the United States (US). And indeed, there are some significant differences. For instance, as of the last US census, some 50 million Americans were without health insurance (De Navas-Walt, Proctor, & Smith, 2011: 23). In Canada, by contrast, the 13 distinct provincial/territorial health systems are entreated by the *Canada Health Act* (CHA) to provide publicly-administered, universal access to medically necessary hospital and physician services (supplemented by an array of other health care services, as insured by individual provinces). As a consequence, Canadian health care has historically been viewed as more inclusive than US health care; its hospital infrastructure has status similar to that of a public good, and the single-payer system provides a measure of insulation from market forces (Marchildon, 2006).

Yet hospitals in Canada are not immune from economic vicissitudes. Like publicly-funded hospitals anywhere, they have had to answer to discourse questioning their performance and accountability, for example as vocalised by supra-national institutions like the World Bank (Preker & Harding, 2003). Additionally, as with many countries, health spending growth in the past decade has exceeded the rate of economic growth, with health spending projected to reach $200 billion in 2011 (CIHI, 2011: v–vii). Meanwhile, hospital utilisation rates have changed, with a decrease in the number of beds, and an increase in the amount of resources consumed by inpatients (CIHI, 2011).

These factors are bound up with a contemporary re-evaluation of the meaning and latent potentialities embedded in health care. In Canada, to the extent that hospitals can facilitate research, they have been positioned as key for addressing the "rather striking contrast" between research strengths in the health sciences and the "weakness of pharmaceutical development" (Canada, COCA, 2006: 9). Such positioning—in Canada and elsewhere—suggests a re-imagining of the role of contemporary hospitals, one that broadens their function beyond care provision, and further beyond ancillary supporters of university-based biomedical research. It is argued that hospitals, if situated within academic health science systems, can help to integrate discovery and care "through reorganization of their key structures and encouragement of cultural change," to emphasise the formation of novel "interfaces" including "effective public-private partnerships" (Dzau et al., 2010: 950).

Meanwhile, leaders in the academic medicine community argue that public expenditures on health care provide not just universally accessible care, but also a platform for "health discovery and innovation [. . .] ensuring that Canadian ideas generate added economic value at home" (Brimacombe, 2005: 61). Similarly, the Conference Board of Canada (CBoC) notes that health care "is at the heart of Canada's national innovation system, both as a contributor of inputs and as an attractor or demander of its outputs" (Canada, CBoC, 2009: 4).

According to The Association of Canadian Academic Healthcare Organizations (ACAHO), its members can leverage their clinical interactions with patients to improve "health and health care for all Canadians *and the country's ability to prosper on a sustained basis*" (ACAHO, 2007: 22—emphasis ours). Similar claims about the need to use "health research as a lever for better health and a stronger economy" are also made by the national agency funding health research (CIHR, 2009: 8; see also CIHR, 2006). Articulated within a larger imaginary that envisions health care as a potential *driver for growth*—advancing both health and wealth (UK,CFST, 2011; see also: Canada, AHSC, 2010; Canada, PPF, 2005; Paige, 2007; UK, BIGT, 2004)—such arguments contextualise the emergence of entrepreneurial hospitals.

Method

To explore health care-oriented and health care-based innovation, the second author is directing a multi-year, multi-site study, which is funded by the

Canadian Institutes of Health Research (CIHR, 81195). The data presented below are embedded within this larger study and were collected by the first author with the aim of undertaking an in-depth examination of such initiatives in different, networked organisations within a single *academic health science system.*

Research conducted in academic health science systems is frequently translational or applied in nature. To facilitate this, patients may be enrolled in studies that aim to develop or validate a technology, such as a novel drug compound or diagnostic assay. Such research often entails the formation of multiple relations with public- and private-sector partners, as well as the movement of patient material, information, ideas, personnel, and so on, within and across organisational boundaries. To help better manage these exchanges, and to nurture health innovation, a health care-based technology transfer office (TTO) was established during the 1990s in one of the organisations we studied. Among other things, this TTO facilitates research contracts, technology screening, intellectual property protection, technology marketing, and start-up assistance for spin-off companies.

We began our exploration by studying organisational histories, strategic plans, and relevant policies. Then, to obtain a descriptive understanding of the everyday work of our study participants, we undertook an interview-based inquiry. In addition, we conducted several hours of participant observation, attending the 2008 and 2009 Alliance for Commercialization of Canadian Technology (ACCF) annual meetings, and conducting site visits to the organisations discussed herein. Field-notes were taken to inform our inquiry, but the analysis presented here concentrates on data from our interview transcripts. Ethics clearance was received from the University of Toronto prior to commencing this inquiry.

The Interviews

Between September 2008 and August 2009, twenty-six semi-structured key-informant interviews were conducted. As noted, our participants work in two different, networked organisations within a single academic health science system in a Canadian province. The majority of participants ($n = 21$) were drawn from the organisation that had established a TTO (Organisation A), while the remainder ($n = 5$), who worked collaboratively with the majority, were employed by a different but connected organisation (Organisation B).

Potential participants were identified through organisational websites and snowball sampling and then mailed a letter of information/consent outlining the details of, and conditions for participation in, our study.

Initially motivated by our interest in the phenomenon of hospital-based TTOs, we began by seeking the views of technology transfer professionals ($n = 5$ of 6). We then cascaded beyond the TTO to capture the views of senior administrators, who had been involved with the development of the on-site TTO, and to whom it reported ($n = 4$ of 8). To understand views of the TTO from the perspective of those who might use its services, we next interviewed selected researchers ($n = 3$) and clinicians ($n = 3$), who had interacted with the TTO and could comment on its mandate and practices.

Then, to better understand issues specific to the commercialisation of genomic or proteomic information, which was seen as an especially promising area of translational research, we focused on informants who used patient information and biomaterial for technology innovation and validation ($n = 3$), as well as administrators, researchers and clinical staff involved in bio-banking initiatives ($n = 8$). Some of these informants (5/11) were employed by Organisation B; however, they were collaborators with our informants from Organisation A.

Interviews, which averaged 1 h in length, were conducted in person ($n = 13$) and by telephone ($n = 13$). Interviews were audio recorded and transcribed verbatim.

The Analysis

Informed by debates over grounded theory and methods (Bryant & Charmaz, 2007), we aimed to iteratively abstract concepts from our interview data in order to generate a lexicon for theorising the developments under review. Our initial interview guide was organised around 4 core questions related to: 1) how technology transfer is fostered within the organisation, 2) what differentiates health care-based technology transfer from technology transfer in universities, 3) whether and how respondents consider the health and health care implications of emerging innovations, and 4) how respondents approach the commercialisation of genome-based innovations (given then-prevalent debates about intellectual property protection for genomics, we asked what it might mean to think of collective, genomic information as *patient* information).

Initial coding and memo-making activities indicated that it would be important to further develop an understanding of our research participants' views concerning how patient information and biomaterial might be mobilised as a resource for technological innovation and commercialisation. Thus, as we moved beyond the TTO to interview additional administrators, researchers and clinical staff ($n = 11$), we gave a stronger emphasis to two core questions concerning: 1) the mission and process of technology transfer and commercialisation within public-sector health care organisations; and 2) how the commercial use of patient information and patient materials, obtained during the course of care, might affect the relationship between patients, health care professionals and systems of care more generally. In these latter interviews, we explicitly asked participants to reflect on excerpts from the oncology asset maps quoted at the outset of this article. By putting these discursive objects into play, we were able to elicit our study participants' reading of the following question, which we took to be implied by the oncology asset maps: what might it mean to think of patients and populations *as* assets? This engagement allowed for a more thickly descriptive, situational analysis (Clarke, 2005) of our participants' views of the entrepreneurial mission and vision adopted by their organisations, and orbiting their everyday practices.

Working collaboratively and iteratively with our data, we first generated the following ways of coding our transcripts: 1) discussion emphasising the collective nature of the resource, 2) stressing proper use while disavowing commodification, 3) leveraging the resource for evidence-based treatment, 4) being compelled to use the resource, 5) mobilising the resource for public benefit, and 6) opening up the question of how best to give back to the public. We applied these codes to our entire dataset and generated the following core concepts, which organise the subsequent presentation of our results, and which suggest some substantive ways of theorising entrepreneurial hospitals: 1) resources that support research aims; and 2) resources that support commercial aims.

Findings

As we shall illustrate, our study participants view patients and patient populations as resources for research. However, they ascribe two rather distinct meanings to this perspective. On the one hand is a meaning that links the value of the resource to the contribution it can make to research that supports improved, more cost-effective care. On the other hand is a meaning that links the value of the resource to its commercial potential. To an extent, these different meanings reflect the different positions held by our study participants within the academic health science system, as well as the differing kinds of relationships these positions make possible with patients. In both cases, there are perceived obligations—seen to stem from public investment in health care—to make proper use of patient populations, and to "give back" to the public-at-large. Yet the ways of "giving back" are several, and not always commensurate. A key (and under-theorised) outcome of this obligation to give back is the resultant *entrepreneurial* search for new ways of mobilising the assets of publicly-funded health care. Our participants broach these conditions and obligations in the context of organisations seeking to leverage extant networks of care and in-house expertise in ways that will add value to publicly-funded health care.

Resources That Support Research Aims

We start with a consideration of the distinctive capacity of the academic health science system to mobilise patient information for research in support of improved clinical care, a capacity stressed especially by those in proximal relation with patients. Our respondents were conscious that the patient population is a resource that health care organisations have "at hand" (BIA-48), and that research was advanced by the capacity to address the needs of patients, which, in turn, make them accessible for research. Yet the research capacity of the academic health science system reflected more than patient need. It also reflected health care arrangements. This was, in the first instance, not simply a collection of patients, but a *population* of patients. Indeed, by serving the "actual demographic" of patients within an entire health region, the academic health science system provided access to what our respondents characterised as, "a population lab" (BIA- 32), or "living laboratory" (BIA-47):

> If you haven't heard that term before—basically [...] I think everybody agrees that you need to have evidence-based treatment—in order to have evidence-based treatment decisions made you have to have evidence. [...] Well, the best evidence you can get is from a population-based, unbiased sampling of the actual demographic you're going to apply the whatever test or treatment to (BIA-47).

Moreover, the "living laboratory" was enabled by the public commitment to universal and accessible care. As one senior administrator noted, research infrastructure was a function of health care arrangements:

> [...] even though the health authority is not directly involved in funding research, such as a granting agency might be doing, [...] they have built a very significant infrastructure of information, for example, the outcomes registry, clinical information etc. [...] So, here we have infrastructure and very knowledgeable people whose mandate is not only for care, but also for research. Of course, care always takes priority for people who are delivering health care, but nevertheless I think for people who are research minded and interested in innovation, they make time to contribute to translational research (BIA-35).

Translational research, in turn, is made possible by the population of patients whose needs make them accessible for research. As an administrator notes, it is precisely because of the public *provision* of comprehensive and accessible care that all, or at least most, of the patient population could be reached for research:

> We have monopoly information on all drugs dispensed with patients [...] even if they're treated externally to the organisation: they're all registered with us for ... [drugs]. So, we have a huge amount of data that allows us to identify patient populations [...]. We can look at incidence and we can track referrals and we can look at drug regimens delivered to see if our treatment policies are actually getting to the patients, that's around access and quality. (BIA-37)

As a result of these service arrangements, respondents were conscious that they were in possession of a "very special" resource—one with a distinctive capacity to improve care. Some respondents argued that failure to take advantage of such an opportunity would be problematic. In the words of an academic physician, the population is "very special and to not take advantage of it would be a huge loss because we can do things here that other people can't do" (BIA-46). A researcher argued in a similar fashion:

> [...] to not use it is actually almost criminal. ... To reach all of the population, to actually penetrate all the different groups—that's hard to

do. You know, it's much easier to run a little study in one centre, but to have a protocol that's applied uniformly [...] that's invaluable (BIA-47).

Thus, once constituted as an opportunity for research, the population seems to demand use. Our participants experience, therefore, a kind of onus to mobilise patient populations in research for discovery, which will hopefully lead to improved treatment outcomes. This is not just about *being able* to use the population in research; it is also about *being*, in some sense, *compelled* to use the population.

In light of this onus to use patient populations as resources, one further point needs to be mentioned. Our study participants were keenly aware of the need to follow policy on ethical conduct in research (CIHR, NSERC, & SSHRC, 2010). Some explicitly vocalised this as both a requirement for, and legitimation of, the use of populations as resources. This position was expressed most directly in discussions of the oncology asset maps, quoted at the outset of this article. As one participant noted, for example, these could have "negative connotations" (BIA-47).

[...] looking at it from the point of view of advertising for drug companies who want to do clinical trials, it's like we're selling the population [...]. That is a bad way to look at it (BIA-47).

For this participant, a better way to look at it would be to see the conditions under which publicly-funded health care research may make patient populations into an asset: "in order for it to be used properly, it has to be overseen with the highest level of ethical review you can imagine because it's the population" (BIA-47).

Here, the process of ethics review is meant to underwrite not just research using human participants, but also research using human populations. "So," our participant continues, "with that caveat, yeah, I think it's, well, there's no question it's an asset" (BIA-47). Others echoed this point, emphasising "informed consent," "privacy legislation" (BIA-37), the dialogic encounter of the "consenting process" (BIA-48), and the importance of maintaining "open communications" (BIA-42) with review boards and other institutional mechanisms of ethics oversight.

To sum up our findings thus far, our study participants recognise in the Canadian academic health science system a research resource that is constituted by patients whose needs make them both accessible to, and valuable for, research. Fundamental to the constitution of this resource is the public, publicly-funded system of care that, through its comprehensive provision of services, has amassed linked datasets on treatments and their outcomes. Utilising this resource to improve care is seen not just as a good idea, but also as a requirement associated with the need to ensure that public monies are being used well. And, overseeing this utilisation is an ethics infrastructure meant to regulate and legitimate research uses.

Resources That Support Commercial Aims

Are there other ways—beyond the kinds of outcomes- and validation-research discussed above—that this resource might be utilised? As we shall now illustrate, study participants working in more distal relation with patients (for example, from within the TTO or in senior administrator positions) take a somewhat more entrepreneurial view of the ways in which patient populations might be resources.

As Miller, Sanders, and Lehoux (2009) argue, a central mandate of TTOs is to build partnerships, research connections and strategic collaborations. For hospital-based technology transfer professionals who are engaged, not in biomedical research per se but rather in efforts to foster the environment in which such research takes place, a considerable surplus value can be realised if the resource can be used to attract partnerships that could benefit patients. Using the example of a collaboration with a pharmaceutical company in clinical trial research, one of our participants observes:

> So, the drug company comes in, for example, to develop a drug with us on a phase I study. If we were to extract information at the molecular level for individual patients both of their DNA as well as the changes to their tumor, we would get a very good understanding as to who's responding to that treatment. We would then be able to advise the drug company as to where we see the best outcomes in terms of patient populations that respond well. This, presumably, would be passed on when it comes to developing phase II and phase III studies and actually improve their likelihood of success. So, all in all, this should benefit everyone (BIA-38).

In this scenario, the resource is leveraged to improve the drug development process. In theory, if the success rate of clinical trials can be improved, then the costs of drug development should come down, as ultimately should the cost of drugs purchased by this health care organisation.

Using the population as a resource for the development of innovative bio-medicine is, in this hospital-based TTO, as much about rationalising medicine as it is about ticking off the traditional commercialisation metrics. For the technology transfer professionals we interviewed, "the goal" driving their efforts to mobilise the resource constituted by their organisation's patient population, "is to have an impact on patient outcome" (BIA-24).

> . . . the hope is a lot of the inventions that we are working on [. . .] can be used to mitigate the cost pressures that our institution is feeling. And, that wouldn't really occur in a university, but here we can say, "wow if this test really works as it says it does, well we could deploy it in the clinic and we'd save a fair amount of cash in terms of these new drugs," because maybe it'll tell you, give the new drugs to this half of the population but not that half of the population (BIA-26).

Long-term savings are as important, in this scenario, as any revenue that might be generated from such transactions. Here, the goal of impacting patient outcomes through controlling health care costs—either upstream in the process of development or downstream in the process of clinical application—helps to mediate the public-private interface in this entrepreneurial hospital.

Research on the entrepreneurial university indicates that TTOs help police the boundary between public organisations and private, for-profit industry (Tuunainen & Knuuttila, 2009). Indeed, our participants are not naive about the power relations and political economy of the interactions they foster and manage:

> . . . no matter how they pose the issue of what their mandate is, the company is there to safeguard shareholder value, right? And, that usually means sales, how much money have you made. [Our organisation] requires access to those companies' drugs in many cases to take care of our shareholders, right? But, if you look at it as shareholders, what our shareholders are interested in is not making money but being treated appropriately (BIA-38).

Mobilising the resource across the public-private divide, therefore, is not just about transacting for long-term savings and the rationalisation of medical care; it is also about managing counter-mandates, those of the hospital, whose mission is to provide care, and those of private-sector interests, whose mission is to make money.

But even here, at this interface between care and commerce, where technology transfer professionals police the boundary between counter-mandates and seek to mobilise patient populations to improve the outcomes of care, we witness not simply an asymmetrical convergence of norms between hospital and industry, but indeed a process of re-interpretation and renormalization (Sanders & Miller, 2010) where the differences between care and research, as well as between resource and commodity, become muted. Why not, for example, ask the question, "to whom is [this resource] actually valuable" (BIA-38)? "Well, it turns out," one of our participant's argues, "there's a huge marketplace south of the border. And, that marketplace suffers from the fact that [. . .] people are insured through different insurers" (BIA-38). Owing to the privatised, fragmented nature of health coverage in the US, our informant argues, care providers are unable to determine the efficacy of treatments on a population-level with the same degree of accuracy available to decision-makers in Canadian academic health science systems. It is precisely this ability to view population health at a higher level of resolution that adds value to the resources that this Canadian entrepreneurial hospital has assembled in the course of care provision. And, it is this ability that has a potentially significant market value, not just in the United States but also globally, wherever populations are segmented according to those who can pay and those who cannot.

Once the resource is "marketised," all manner of opportunities (and challenges) arise. These are apparent if one locates the resource within a broader, speculative calculus, which figures value not merely in terms of financial gain, but also with respect to lost opportunity (Cooper, 2008). Thus, for example, failing to patent an "oncogene" identified during the course of treatment could have a two-fold impact on the organisation's bottom-line. On the one hand it might miss out on a potential revenue stream that could come from licensing this discovery. On the other hand, having left the discovery unprotected and subject to private-sector patents, the organisation might have to pay considerable fees to access whatever subsequent therapies stem from this knowledge. Thinking along these lines, a senior administrator we interviewed offered the following two-fold justification for the entrepreneurial work done by the TTO to mobilise and protect his organisation's distinctive resources:

> with respect to the TTO, there is a strategic piece there that says 'do people who pursue laboratory science and people who treat patients in the clinic, do they actually know how to patent science and turn innovative discovery into something that has legitimate value and can be commercialised'? And, I would say we're pretty sanguine about this. You can't do this because you believe you're going to make money. And, I think the other side of that is you shouldn't also be putting yourself at risk constantly because you don't actually do this properly [...] it's a truism to say scientists in general will give away the shop for a few talks and a few presentations and never realise that they gave away intellectual property. And, whilst we don't mind them talking about it, the issue is that you're giving it to other people who do get commercialise it and might profit from it so why wouldn't we do that? (BIA-30)

Here the value of the resource is configured in terms of commercial potential, a speculative value to be both nurtured and protected. From a more distal perspective, then, entrepreneurial aims extend beyond validation- and outcomes-research towards the economic vicissitudes of the market.

Discussion

Waldby and Mitchell (2006) underscore the key role that health care organisations play in the adjudication and reconciliation of differing regimes of value. Their analysis directs attention to the important custodial work that hospitals undertake as they invent, mediate and manage innovative uses for patient populations and care infrastructure. Drawing from their work, we suggest that entrepreneurial hospitals are positioning themselves as obligatory passage points for biomedical innovation—they strive to broker multiple kinds of access to their unique assets. In so doing, however, they stand to reconfigure embodied social relations in some important ways. This reconfiguration is not well characterised by literature on the entrepreneurial university.

A case in point—there are many, but here we take a particularly well-rounded exemplar—is Krimsky's *Science in the Private Interest*. While articulated with reference to his extensive studies on commercialisation in biomedical science, this text addresses itself to "changes in the culture, norms, and values of academic science", and to the potential contradictions that arise when universities switch from "sources of enlightenment" to "instruments of wealth" (2003: 1-2). Attending to universities and the commercialisation of academic science, Krimsky provides a thorough exploration of important issues related to conflicts of interest, the erosion of ethical standards, the diminishment of public confidence in science, and the commodification of knowledge. However, the university—not the hospital—is the focal point of analysis. As a consequence, issues germane to entrepreneurial hospitals are underemphasised.

For example, the commercial ethos in higher education is said to have transformed the university's mission from the production of knowledge (or, to use Krimsky's term, enlightenment) to the production of wealth. The commercial ethos in health care and health research, however, involves a reconfiguration of the relationship not solely between knowledge and wealth, but also between health and wealth. By connecting wealth to health (or lack thereof), the commercial ethos in health care and health research overcodes the health and disease statuses of populations with potential market value. All manner of implications follow, not least changes in the cultures, norms, and values classically associated with illness and disease. Our interest in this article, however, is with the particular, distinctive capacities cultivated by entrepreneurial hospitals as they endeavour to transform the experience of disease and ill health into a source of potential value. Indeed, building on Waldby and Mitchell (2006), we seek to elucidate the particular embodied social relations that are reconfigured by entrepreneurial hospitals.

If an entrepreneurial hospital may be defined as one that constitutes its patient populations and care infrastructure as distinctive assets (or resources) to be mobilised in pursuit of entrepreneurial aims, then what particular social relations might this activity reconfigure? In Canada, entrepreneurial hospitals derive resources for innovation from a patient population whose needs make them accessible to research, and from an inclusive health care system that—in the course of care provision—has accumulated valuable, population-level information on treatment efficacy. These resources have a value for outcomes- and validation-research. But, they are also seen by our informants to have a potential market value. The twinning of these two different kinds of value is a defining feature of the entrepreneurial hospital in Canada. However, this twinning has knock-on effects. For instance, our informants described an onus to ensure 1) that as many patients as possible are given the opportunity to participate in research, and 2) that patients and their broader publics get some return for their support of the health research and health care enterprise.

A related issue concerns how patients are oriented in this reconfiguration—do they experience an onus to participate in research, a kind of responsibilisation aimed at ensuring that their "unproductive" patient days are paired with "productive" research subject days? And what of the broader health systems that house entrepreneurial hospitals? What benefits do they reap, and what emerging costs are apparent (see, for instance Gilson, 2003, who observes that funding arrangements within health systems influence the level of trust between patient and health care provider)? Finally, what are the implications of this reconfiguration for the broader publics that health care is meant to serve—what "imagined collectives" (Hayden, 2007: 751) are called into being by the entrepreneurial hospital (what kind of collective, for example, must be presupposed to authorise the commodification of assets derived from patient populations)?

To adequately address these questions, more empirical attention to the specificity of entrepreneurial hospitals is required. Just as scholarship on the entrepreneurial university has identified heterogeneous, context-specific organisational forms, processes and practices, so too might we expect to discover salient, context-specific differences across entrepreneurial hospitals. Nonetheless, we venture that entrepreneurial hospitals everywhere are likely to encounter similar opportunities and challenges, especially insofar as they attempt to reconcile incommensurate regimes of value.

Conclusion

In response to myriad problems ranging from micro-level, everyday questions of service provision to macro-level fiscal realities and a re-imagining of health care, entrepreneurial hospitals articulate solutions that push "once sacrosanct" boundaries (Etzkowitz, 1998: 826). This article has showcased how an entrepreneurial hospital is assembling and mobilising its unique resources, sometimes across the public–private divide. In the process, such organisations engage in an entrepreneurial search for new ways of mobilising their resources, *and* for new ways of reconciling differing regimes of value.

What is being transformed by the entrepreneurial hospital? Professional obligations, patient roles, systems of care, and their broader collectivities all stand to be reconfigured. We have begun to explore this transformation by illustrating how an entrepreneurial hospital aspires to leverage its "living laboratory" and the means of care for multiple ends beyond care. However, more research into the entrepreneurial hospital is required to accurately trace its larger implications.

Acknowledgements

We are indebted to the many busy people who agreed to speak with us about their work, and thank the Canadian Institutes of Health Research (CIHR) for funding for this project (81195). Martin French was supported by a Fellowship from the OHR-funded 'Health Care, Technology and Place' Strategic Training Program while conducting this research and now holds a postdoctoral fellowship from the Social Sciences and Humanities Research Council (SSHRC) (756-2010-0741). Fiona A. Miller is supported by a New Investigator Award from the Institute of Health Services and Policy Research of CIHR (80495). Sponsors' support of this work should not imply endorsement of the conclusions, for which the authors retain sole responsibility.

References

Association of Canadian Academic Healthcare Organizations (ACAHO). (2007). *Moving at the speed of discovery: From bench to bedside to discovery.* Ottawa: ACAHO.

Bercovitz, J., & Feldman, M. (2008). Academic entrepreneurship: Organizational change at the individual level. *Organization Science*, 19(1), 69–89.

Bok, D. (2003). *Universities in the marketplace: The commercialization of higher education.* Princeton: Princeton University Press.

Brimacombe, G. (2005). Health, healthcare and nation-building: A three-dimensional approach to innovation in Canada. *Healthcare Quarterly*, 8(3), 65–68.

Bryant, A., & Charmaz, K. (2007). *The Sage handbook of grounded theory.* Thousand Oaks: Sage.

Canada, Academic Health Sciences Centres (AHSC). (2010). *Three missions, one future… optimizing the performance of Canada's academic health sciences centres. A report from the National Task Force on the Future of Canada's Academic Health Sciences Centres.* Ottawa: AHSC.

Canada, Conference Board of Canada (CBoC). (2009). *The heath enterprise: Charting a path for health and innovation.* Toronto: CBoC.

Canada, Council of Canadian Academies (COCA), The Committee on The State of Science & Technology in Canada. (2006). *The state of science & technology in Canada.* Ottawa: COCA.

Canada, Public Policy Forum (PPF). (2005). *From discovery to market: Creating a multi-stakeholder partnership in support of Canada's innovative health industries.* Ottawa: PPF.

Canadian Institute for Health Information (CIHI). (2011). *Health care cost drivers: The facts.* Toronto: CIHI.

Canadian Institutes of Health Research (CIHR). (2006). *CIHR—Catalyst for commercialization.* Ottawa: CIHR.

Canadian Institutes of Health Research (CIHR). (2009). *Health research roadmap: Creating innovative research for better health and healthcare—CIHR's strategic plan 2009–10, 2013–14.* Ottawa: CIHR.

Canadian Institutes of Health Research (CIHR), Natural Sciences and Engineering Research Council of Canada (NSERC), & Social Sciences and Humanities Research Council of Canada (SSHRC). (2010). *TCPS2—Tri-Council Policy Statement: Ethical conduct for research involving humans.* Ottawa: Panel on Research Ethics.

Chapple, W., Lockett, A., Siegel, D., & Wright, M. (2005). Assessing the relative performance of UK university technology transfer offices: Parametric and nonparametric evidence. *Research Policy*, 34(3), 369–384.

Clarke. A. (2005). *Situational analysis: Grounded theory after the postmodern turn.* Thousand Oaks: Sage.

Colyvas, J., & Powell, W. (2009). Measures, memes, and myopia: The challenges and ramifications of sustaining academic entrepreneurship. *Advances in the Study of Entrepreneurship, Innovation & Economic Growth*, 19, 79-112.

Cooper, M. (2008). *Life as surplus: Biotechnology and capitalism in the neoliberal era.* Seattle: University of Washington Press.

Czarnitzki, D., & Toole, A. (2010). Is there a trade-off between academic research and faculty entrepreneurship? Evidence from US NIH supported biomedical researchers. *Economics of Innovation & New Technology*, 19(5), 505–520.

Davies, S. (2008). Academic health centres: What is the agenda for research? *Journal of Health Services Research & Policy*, 13(1), 3–4.

DeNavas-Walt, C., Proctor, B., & Smith, J. (2011). *Income, poverty, and health insurance coverage in the United States: 2010.* Washington, DC: US Government Printing Office. US Census Bureau, Current Population Reports, P60–239.

Dzau, V., Ackerly, D., Sutton-Wallace, P., Merson, M., Williams, R., Krishnan, K., et al. (2010). The role of academic health science systems in the transformation of medicine. *The Lancet*, 375 (9718), 949–953.

Estabrooks, C., Norton, P., Birdsell, J., Newton,. M., Adewale, A., & Thomley, R. (2008). Knowledge translation and research careers: Mode I and mode II activity among health researchers. *Research Policy*, 37(6/7), 1066–1078.

Etzkowitz, H. (1983). Entrepreneurial scientists and entrepreneurial universities in American academic science. *Minerva*, 21(2/3), 198–233.

Etzkowitz, H. (1998). The norms of entrepreneurial science: Cognitive effects of the new university–industry linkages. *Research Policy*, 27(81), 823–833.

Etzkowitz, H., & Viale, R. (2010). Polyvalent knowledge and the entrepreneurial university: A third academic revolution? *Critical Sociology*, 36(4), 595-609.

Etzkowitz, H., Webster, A., & Healey, P. (1998). *Capitalizing knowledge: New intersections of industry and academia.* Albany: State University of New York Press.

Gibson, L. (2003). Trust and the development of health care as a social institution. *Social Science & Medicine*, 56(7), 1453–1468.

Hayden, C. (2007). Taking as giving: Bioscience, exchange, and the politics of benefit-sharing. *Social Studies of Science*, 37(5), 729–758.

Herder, M., & Johnston, J. (2007). *Licensing for knowledge transfer in human genetics research: A study of business models for licensing and technology transfer in human generics patents*. Ottawa: Health Canada.

Hicks, D., & Katz, J. (1996). Hospitals: The hidden research system. *Science & Public Policy*, 23 (5), 297–304.

Krimsky, S. (2003). *Science in the private interest: Has the lure of profits corrupted biomedical research?* Oxford: Rowman & Littlefield.

Lander, B., and Atkinson-Grosjean, J. (2011). Translational science and the hidden research system in universities and academic hospitals: A case study. *Social Science & Medicine*, 72(4), 537–544.

LifeSciences BC & The Government of British Columbia. (2006). *Oncology asset map: Activities, strength, and opportunities*. Vancouver: LifeSciences BC.

Marchildon, G. (2006). *Health systems in transition: Canada*. Toronto: University of Toronto Press.

Miller, F., Sanders, C., & Lehoux, P. (2009). Imagining value, imagining users: Academic technology transfer for health innovation. *Social Science & Medicine*, 68(8). 1481–1488.

Mowery, D., & Ziedonis, A. (2002). Academic patent quality and quantity before and after the Bayh-Dole Act in the United States. *Research Policy*, 31(3), 399–418.

Ontario Institute for Cancer Research (OICR) & The Government of Ontario. (2009). *Unique opportunities—oncology asset map: An analysis of Ontario's R&D excellence and commercialization capacity*. Toronto: Queen's Printer for Ontario.

Owen-Smith, J. (2005a). Commercial imbroglios: Proprietary science and the contemporary university. In K. Moore, & S. Frickel (Eds.), *The new political sociology of science: Institutions, networks, power* (pp. 63–90). Madison: University of Wisconsin Press.

Owen-Smith, J. (2005b). Dockets, deals, and sagas: Commensuration and the rationalization of experience in university licensing. *Social Studies of Science*, 35(1), 69–97.

Paige, C. (2007). The future of health research is hanging in the balance. *Canadian Medical Association Journal*, 177(9), 1057–1058.

Powell, W., Owen-Smith, J., & Colyvas, J. (2007). Innovation and emulation: Lessons from American universities in selling private rights to public knowledge. *Minerva*, 45(2), 121–142.

Preker, A., & Harding, A. (Eds.). (2003). *Innovations in health service delivery: The corporatization of public hospitals*. Washington. DC: The World Bank.

Rasmussen, E. (2008). Government instruments to support the commercialization of university research: Lessons from Canada. *Technovation*, 28(8), 506–517.

Read, C. (2007). Size counts: Outcomes of IP commercialization. *Innovation Analysis Bulletin*, 9(1), 12–13.

Rettig. R. (1994). Medical innovation duels cost containment. *Health Affairs*, 13(3), 7–27.

Rose, N., & Novas, C. (2005). Biological citizenship. In A. Ong & S. Collier (Eds.), *Global assemblages: Technology, politics and ethics as anthropological problems* (pp. 439–463). London: Blackwell.

Rothaermel, F., Agung, S., & Jiang, L. (2007). University entrepreneurship: A taxonomy of the literature. *Industrial & Corporate Change*, 16(4), 691–791.

Sanders, C., & Miller, F. (2010). Reframing norms: Boundary maintenance and partial accommodations in the work of academic technology transfer. *Science & Public Policy*, 37(9), 689–701.

Siegel, D., Waldman. D., & Link, A. (2003). Assessing the impact of organizational practices on the relative productivity of university technology transfer offices: An exploratory study. *Research Policy*. 32(1), 27–48.

Slaughter, S., & Leslie, L. (1997). *Academic capitalism: Policies, policies and the entrepreneurial university*. Baltimore: Johns Hopkins University Press.

Sontag, S. (1977/1989). *Illness as a metaphor and AIDS and its metaphors*. New York: Farrar, Strauss, and Giroux.

Stuart, T., & Ding. W. (2006). When do scientists become entrepreneurs?: The social structural antecedents of commercial activity in the academic life sciences. *American Journal of Sociology*, 112(1), 97–114.

Thursby, J., & Thursby, M. (2002). Who is selling the ivory tower? Sources of growth in university licensing. *Management Science*, 48(1), 90–104.

Tuunainen, J., & Knuuttila, T. (2009). Intermingling academic and business activities: A new direction for science and universities? *Science, Technology & Human Values*, 34 (6), 684–704.

United Kingdom (UK), Bioscience Innovation and Growth Team (BIGT). (2004). *Bioscience 2015: Improving national health, increasing national wealth*. London: Department of Trade and Industry.

United Kingdom (UK), Council for Science and Technology (CFST). (2011). *The NHS as a driver for growth: A report by the Prime Minister's council for science and technology*. London: CFST.

Waldby, C., & Mitchell, R. (2006). *Tissue economies: Blood, organs, and cell-lines in late capitalism*. Durham. NC: Duke.

Reflection: Mapping Maps: Situating Oncology Asset Maps in the Representational Process

Martin French & Fiona Alice Miller

Increasingly, historical, visual, narrative, and other discourse materials and nonhuman material cultural objects of all kinds must be included as elements of our research and subjected to analysis because they are increasingly understood/interpreted as both constitutive of and consequential for the phenomena we study.

(Clarke 2005:145)

In this short reflection, we describe our enrollment of a nonhuman material cultural object—or better, *actant* (Clarke 2005:60–63; see also Latour 1987)—in the representational process of our research. In the course of our fieldwork on innovation, technology transfer, and commercialization initiatives in Canadian health systems, we encountered things called "oncology asset maps," government-sponsored marketing documents aimed at accelerating the commercialization of public-sector life sciences research. Curiously, these discursive actants counted patient populations as assets alongside technological infrastructure and professional expertise. Describing how we enrolled them into our analysis, and specifically the heterogeneous ways our study participants encountered and responded to them, we illustrate the importance of "turning up the volume" on "lesser but still present discourses" in a situation (Clarke 2005:175).

Here, we first briefly recap a main argument of our article, which emphasizes the need for scholarship on the distinctiveness of the entrepreneurial hospital (French & Miller 2012). With reference to our study data, we next reflect on our initial encounter with Clarke's (2005) *Situational Analysis*. For us, situational analysis (SA) helped reconcile divergent methodological assumptions. It also helped us think about how to enroll discursive actants into key-informant interviews.

A Recap of "'Leveraging the Living Laboratory': On the Emergence of the Entrepreneurial Hospital"

For years, scholars have debated the merits and demerits of the entrepreneurial university while the entrepreneurial hospital has gone largely unnoticed. This lack of attention is explained, partly at least, by a tendency in scholarship to treat research-intensive universities and hospitals as similar types of organizations. The rationale underpinning this may be characterized as follows. Research-intensive universities and research-intensive hospitals both perform research; ergo, they are both research organizations. Moreover, many research-intensive hospitals are affiliated with universities; ergo, they are within the university system. Per this rationale, there is no need for a distinctive conceptualization of the entrepreneurial hospital; it is adequately captured in discussions of the entrepreneurial university. In our view, this rationale is mistaken because it overlooks important facets of the health innovation process.

Careful attention to the specific context of the entrepreneurial hospital— the distinctiveness of its particular situation as *both* a site of care *and* as a site of research, technology development and commercialization—reveals several distinguishing characteristics. First, the entrepreneurial hospital is distinguished by the fact that it can use its innovations in clinical settings. A diagnostic test developed from studies of cancer patients, for example, might help the entrepreneurial hospital disburse its cancer treatments in a more targeted and effective way. This is not commonly an innovation-driving dynamic in the entrepreneurial university. Second, and for reasons related to this example, the entrepreneurial hospital is able to count patients among its assets. They form a "living laboratory" of sorts, a population whose medical needs make them available for research, almost on demand, and whose medical information and participation in research can open the door to all kinds of knowledge that would otherwise be inaccessible. For these reasons, the entrepreneurial hospital creates unique potentialities and risks, and merits attention on its own terms.

Accordingly, our article offers an initial conceptualization of the entrepreneurial hospital, which we define as a hospital that explicitly seeks to constitute patient populations and care infrastructure as distinctive assets (or resources) in pursuit of entrepreneurial aims. Our focus is on the different and not always commensurate understandings of the entrepreneurial hospital's assets. As we argue, our study participants view these assets as resources for research, linking their value to the contributions they can make to improved, more cost-effective care. Alongside this understanding has developed the provocative idea that the entrepreneurial hospital's assets themselves might also be a source of commercial potential. As we discovered, a key task of the entrepreneurial hospital is to mediate between these and other novel uses of patient populations and care infrastructure while also reconciling differing understandings of the meaning and potential uses of the hospitals' assets. The distinctiveness and challenging nature of this task is rendered visible by attending to the particular situation of the entrepreneurial hospital.

Study Data

The data we collected and from which we theorized the entrepreneurial hospital were gathered as part of an in-depth examination of innovation, technology transfer, and commercialization initiatives in different, networked organizations within a single academic health science system in a Canadian province.[1] Following a process of ethics review and clearance, our research began with some initial, "scoping interviews" with key informants, a goal of which was to better identify important focal points for subsequent interviews.[2] We also conducted a careful examination of organizational histories, strategic plans, policies, and other grey literature. Such often internal documents can be valuable as they make organizational processes visible (Atkinson & Coffey 2004:56). They are "never inert" but rather "serve as active agents in schemes of human interaction—agents to be recruited, manipulated, scorned or hidden" (Prior 2004:358).

To obtain a descriptive understanding of the everyday work of our study participants, we then undertook sustained observations and interviews. We conducted site visits, touring hospital buildings, offices and laboratories, and attended professional conferences. Between September 2008 and August 2009, we also conducted twenty-six semi-structured, key-informant interviews. Our sample was purposively selected. Potential participants were identified through organizational websites and snowball or chain-referral sampling. The interviews averaged about an hour in length and were conducted in person, by telephone, and were audio recorded and transcribed. The interviews constitute the primary empirical material for the article, while the observational data help provide the ambient, background context of our interpretations.

Encountering Situational Analysis: The Analytic Approach

As is commonplace in grounded theory (GT) approaches, data collection and analysis occurred simultaneously. Our aim was to iteratively abstract concepts from our interview data in order to come up with a lexicon for describing and theorizing the phenomena we were seeing. This is how the concept of the entrepreneurial hospital—which Fiona is to be credited with proposing—emerged.

Our initial interview guide was organized around four core questions. First, how is technology transfer fostered within the organizational settings under analysis? Second, what differentiates health care–based technology transfer from technology transfer in universities? Third, how do study participants consider the health—and health care—implications of emerging innovation, if at all? And fourth, addressing a salient issue at the time, how do study participants view the commercialization of genome-based innovations? As we proceeded with our analysis, it soon became apparent that we needed to develop a further understanding of our participants' views concerning how patient information and biomaterial might be mobilized as resources for technological innovation and commercialization.

In the initial stages of our fieldwork we had encountered oncology asset maps, government-sponsored marketing documents aimed at accelerating the commercialization of public-sector life sciences research. Curiously to us, these asset maps counted patient populations as assets alongside technological infrastructure and professional expertise. We first sought to understand these maps with reference to concepts that would evoke their biopolitical dimensions. Were they bound up with broader efforts to realize a surplus value in vitality, a "biovalue" (Waldby 2000; Waldby & Mitchell 2006)? Were they symptomatic of an emergent form of capitalism in which "biocapital" becomes increasingly central to regimes of accumulation (Sunder Rajan 2006, 2012)? Were they localized formulations of a global discourse promoting the "bioeconomy" (Cooper & Waldby 2014; OECD 2006, 2009)? While these concepts shed light on the broader, macro-level developments that contextualize our case, they did not seem to entirely fit the meso- and micro-level developments we were witnessing. At the least, they were not concepts that resonated with, or were operative within, our study participants' everyday discourse.

In fact, the cognitive distance between the phenomena described by concepts like biovalue, biocapital, and bioeconomy, and the phenomena we were witnessing in our field sites seemed to call for the development of some middle-range concepts. We initially had a challenging time agreeing over how best to characterize our participants' discourse. This impasse of sorts provided a moment to rethink the data we were collecting. It was also an opportunity for us to work through some of the divergent methodological assumptions we each brought to this project. Fiona's experience with GT, and Martin's relative naivety about it, meant that each of us entered the project with different assumptions about how to code, organize, and interpret the data we were gathering. Whereas Fiona had over the course of several past projects developed a highly rigorous system of memoing and coding (e.g., Miller et al. 2009), Martin had approached qualitative data analysis as a bricoleur (e.g., French 2009). At this point in our analytic process we had our initial encounter with SA.

Although we were both familiar with Clarke's work on biomedicalization, and although we had each come across other qualitative research articulated with reference to SA, neither of us had yet had the chance to engage with *Situational Analysis: Grounded Theory after the Postmodern Turn*. As it turned out, this book proved very fruitful for helping us reconcile our differing approaches to GT.

Mapping Maps: Turning Up the Volume on Innovation Discourse

One of the things that Clarke's work helped crystalize for us was the potential to enroll oncology asset maps as actants in our fieldwork as nonhuman actors in the representational process. What we mean by this is that we decided that it would be productive to "turn up the volume" (Clarke 2005:175) of this discourse that was present in the situation we were studying, but that was not necessarily a central feature of the everyday work experiences of our study participants. We decided to reformulate our interview guide so that a particular oncology asset map was an explicit feature of discussion with interview participants.

Although we did not follow exactly the mapping process laid out in *Situational Analysis*—whereby researchers are encouraged to make different types of maps in succession, moving from abstract (messy) maps, to ordered situational maps, to social worlds maps, to positional maps—our iterative approach to data collection and analysis did enable a recursive mapping of the different positions of the discourses and themes that were circulating in the situation we were investigating. For instance, we learned that discourse about the commercialization of heath innovations was central within some organizational nodes (such as the hospital's technology transfer office) but more marginal in other nodes (e.g., a pathology laboratory, or for those working largely in clinical care).

As we progressed through our interviews, we decided to use theoretical sampling to give a stronger emphasis to certain questions. That is, in GT analysis, when you come across something particularly interesting, you can strategically pursue it by seeking out particularly apt informants and/ or changing the interview questions. To do this in our project, we cascaded outward beyond our initial focus on areas of the hospital with a direct connection to technology transfer. We sought participants working in arenas of varying proximity to technology transfer and commercialization initiatives, moving from researchers to clinicians to biobank staff and managers (some of the latter had very little knowledge of the commercial aspirations for banked samples). Next, we put the oncology asset maps into play in our discussions with informants, asking them explicitly to comment on the significance and implications of conceptualizing patients and patient populations as assets.

Our sense is that this effort to turn up the volume on the innovation, technology transfer, and commercialization discourse, even as we increased our distance from its direct participants through our interviews, was greatly aided by enrolling the asset map as an actant in our interviews. Confrontations with the asset map provoked a more head-on and thickly descriptive SA of our participants' views of the entrepreneurial mission and vision of their organizations. These confrontations let us link their descriptions of everyday work practices, the opportunities they pursued and the challenges they wrestled with, to broader social processes and discourses. Furthermore, they let us focus—and this is a crucial, too-often neglected point—on the way people respond to, negotiate with, reposition, and resist ideas that are in play in their situation. This allowed us to emphasize some of the *differences* in our study participants' responses to the question of whether or how patients and populations are assets. It helped us illuminate some of the key, unique work done by the entrepreneurial hospital concerning inventing, negotiating, and mediating new uses of patient populations and care infrastructure. This crucial work of the entrepreneurial hospital is, in our view, key to its distinctiveness within health research and innovation systems—despite its general invisibility in scholarly treatments of the entrepreneurial university.

Conclusion

SA, as we have suggested in this short reflection, helped us describe and theorize the emergence of the entrepreneurial hospital. Importantly, it helped us to think critically about existing social scientific analyses of innovation, and to bridge the gap between macro-level concepts like biovalue, biocapital, and bioeconomy with concepts better tailored to the meso- and micro-level phenomena we were witnessing. Additionally, SA was important for helping us identify and reconcile some of our divergent methodological assumptions. For those new to GT, Clarke's (2005) *Situational Analysis* provides a blueprint for thinking about and undertaking field research. And, for those more experienced with GT approaches, SA offers a range of innovative ways to systematically analyze—and discover concepts—in data.

Acknowledgment

Many thanks are owed to Adele Clarke, not only for providing a sophisticated methodological framework for thinking about our field research, but also for her instrumental role in creating a community of scholars interested in learning about and developing techniques for situational analysis. We also thank Adele for her eagle editorial eye and kind feedback on earlier versions of this essay.

Notes

1. The term "academic health science system" encompasses both academic health centers and the broader constellation of relationships that have grown up around these centers, including relationships, for example, with diagnostic and therapeutic companies and other commercial partners. Research in academic health science systems is frequently translational or applied in nature.

2. Scoping interviews have been described as "loosely-focused and loosely-structured" interviews "designed to evaluate, ground and refine the initial understandings, assumptions and concepts of a research team" (Robertson et al. 2012:517).

References

Atkinson, P. & A. Coffey. 2004. Analyzing Documentary Realities. In D. Silverman (Ed.), *Qualitative Research: Theory, Method, and Practice* (pp. 45–62). London: Sage.

Clarke, A. E. 2005. *Situational Analysis: Grounded Theory after the Postmodern Turn.* Thousand Oaks, CA: Sage.

Cooper, M. & C. Waldby. 2014. *Clinical Labor: Tissue Donors and Research Subjects in the Global Bioeconomy*. Durham, NC: Duke University Press.

French, M. A. 2009. Picturing Public Health Surveillance: Tracing the Material Dimensions of Information in Ontario's Public Health System. Unpublished Ph.D. Dissertation. Kingston, Canada: Queen's University.

French, M. A. & F. A. Miller. 2012. Leveraging the "Living Laboratory": On the Emergence of the Entrepreneurial Hospital. *Social Science & Medicine* 75(4):717–724.

Latour, B. 1987. *Science in Action: How to Follow Scientists and Engineers through Society*. Cambridge, MA: Harvard University Press.

Miller, F. A., C. Sanders, & P. Lehoux. 2009. Imagining Value, Imagining Users: Academic Technology Transfer for Health Innovation. *Social Science and Medicine* 68(8):1481–1488.

Organization for Economic Cooperation and Development (OECD). 2006. *Scoping Document —The Bioeconomy to 2030: Designing a Policy Agenda*. Paris: OECD.

Organization for Economic Cooperation and Development (OECD). 2009. *The Bioeconomy to 2030: Designing a Policy Agenda*. Paris: OECD.

Prior, L. 2004. Documents. In C. Seale, G. Gobo, J. Gubrium, & D. Silverman (Eds.), *Qualitative Research Practice* (pp. 345–361). London: Sage.

Robertson, T., J. Durick, M. Brereton, F. Vetere, S. Howard, & B. Nansen. 2012. Knowing Our Users: Scoping Interviews in Design Research with Ageing Participants. *OZCHI'12*. New York: ACM.

Sunder Rajan, K. 2006. *Biocapital: The Constitution of Postgenomic Life*. Durham, NC: Duke University Press.

Sunder Rajan, K. (Ed). 2012. *Lively Capital: Biotechnologies, Ethics and Governance in Global Markets*. Durham, NC: Duke University Press.

Waldby, C. 2000. *The Visible Human Project: Informatic Bodies and Posthuman Medicine*. London: Routledge.

Waldby, C. & R. Mitchell. 2006. *Tissue Economies: Blood, Organs, and Cell Lines in Late Capitalism*. Durham, NC: Duke University Press.

APPENDIX A

GROUNDED THEORY & SITUATIONAL ANALYSIS WEBSITES

Grounded Theory Sites

http://dne2.ucsf.edu/public/anselmstrauss/index.html
This website is dedicated to the work of Anselm Strauss, one of the founders of grounded theory. The site includes a list of all his publications on grounded theory and "A Personal History of the Development of Grounded Theory" by Strauss. It also offers essays about Anselm Strauss's work, including "On Coming Home and Intellectual Generosity" by Adele E. Clarke and Susan Leigh Star, "Work Sites of an American Interactionist: Anselm L. Strauss, 1917–1996" by Isabelle Baszanger, and "Anselm Strauss's Grounded Theory and the Study of Work" by Roberta Lessor.

www.youtube.com/watch?v=zYIh3387txo
On this YouTube video, Professor Kathy Charmaz, author of *Constructing Grounded Theory* (Sage, 2014), presents a lecture on "The Power and Potential of Grounded Theory."

Situational Analysis Sites

www.situationalanalysis.com
This is the website maintained by Adele E. Clarke, developer of the method of situational analysis. It contains up-to-date lists of publications and dissertations using situational analysis, a list of Clarke's publications on research methods, a searchable and downloadable bibliography from the book *Situational Analysis* (Sage, 2005), and other resources.

www.facebook.com/pages/Situational-Analysis/214734101890718
This Facebook page offers resources about the method, including up-to-date lists of selected exemplars, all known publications and dissertations using situational analysis, and Clarke's publications on methods. It lists past and future seminars and workshops on situational analysis and tells how to contact seminar leaders. The table of contents is posted for the four volumes of *Grounded Theory & Situational Analysis*, edited by Adele E. Clarke and Kathy Charmaz (Sage, 2014), part of the Sage Benchmarks in Social Research Series.

www.qualitative-forschung.de/methodentreffen/archiv/video/closing
lecture_2011/index.html
This is the video of a talk given in English by Adele Clarke at the Berlin
Qualitative Workshops in 2011. There is a long introduction in German by
Prof. Dr. Reiner Keller (University of Augsburg), who arranged for the German
translation of *Situational Analysis*. Clarke's talk and slides are in English.

http://sts.ucdavis.edu/summer-workshop/retreat-2008
This website offers a pdf of Adele Clarke's first paper on situational
analysis: "Situational Analyses: Grounded Theory Mapping after the Postmodern Turn," Special Issue on Theory and Method. *Symbolic Interaction*
26(4):553–576.

http://dne2.ucsf.edu/public/anselmstrauss/social-worlds.html
This page within the website dedicated to Anselm Strauss's life and work
includes a list of his publications on social worlds theory and two articles
about it.

www.researchgate.net/post/What_are_some_examples_of_appling_
the_situational_analysis_approach_to_grounded_theory_in_health_
care_research
This site offers a video of Bryce R. Cassin (University of Western Sydney)
answering the question in the site name. to the Banff Symposium and the
first article by Jan Morse "Tussles, Tensions and Resolutions," and a "Dialog
on Doing Grounded Theory" among all the authors. Source: Jan Morse,
Phyllis N. Stern, Juliet Corbin, Barbara Bowers, Kathy Charmaz, and Adele
E. Clarke. 2009. *Developing Grounded Theory: The Second Generation* (Left
Coast Press, Inc., 2009).

http://nbn-resolving.de/urn:nbn:de:0114-fqs080244
This site offers a review of the book *Situational Analysis*. Source: Tom Mathar
(2008), Making a Mess with Situational Analysis? Review Essay: Adele
Clarke (2005) *Situational Analysis—Grounded Theory after the Postmodern
Turn. Forum Qualitative Sozialforschung/Forum: Qualitative Social Research*
9(2), Art. 4 (accessed January 22, 2015).

APPENDIX B

SELECTED EXEMPLARS OF SITUATIONAL ANALYSIS BY DISCIPLINE

NOTE: The selected exemplars of situational analysis listed here *do not* include those in this volume. Several also fit into multiple categories.

About the Situational Analysis Method in Different Disciplines

den Outer, B., K. Handley, & M. Price. 2012. Situational Analysis and Mapping for Use in Education Research: A Reflexive Methodology? *Studies in Higher Education* 38(10):1504–1521.

Fulton, J. & C. Hayes. 2012. Situational Analysis-Framing Approaches to Interpretive Inquiry in Healthcare Research. *International Journal of Therapy and Rehabilitation* 19(12):662–669.

Newbury, J. 2011. Situational Analysis: Centerless Systems and Human Service Practices. *Child & Youth Services* 32(2):88–107.

Wagner, K. D., P. J. Davidson, R. A. Pollini, S. A. Strathdee, R. Washburn, & L. A. Palinkas. 2012. Reconciling Incongruous Qualitative and Quantitative Findings in Mixed Methods Research: Exemplars from Research with Drug Using Populations. *International Journal of Drug Policy* 23(1):54–61.

Aging Studies

Carder, P. C. 2008. Managing Medication Management in Assisted Living: A Situational Analysis. *Journal of Ethnographic and Qualitative Research* 3:1–12.

Critical Inquiry

Alonso-Yanez, G. & C. Davidsen. 2014. Conservation Science Policies versus Scientific Practice: Evidence from a Mexican Biosphere Reserve. *Human Ecology Review* 20(2):3–29.

Pérez, M. S. & G. S. Cannella. 2013. Situational Analysis as an Avenue for Critical Qualitative Research: Mapping Post-Katrina New Orleans. *Qualitative Inquiry* 19(7):1–13.

Sanders, G. 2009. "Late" Capital: Amusement and Contradiction in the Contemporary Funeral Industry. *Critical Sociology* 35:447–471.

Design Studies

Rodríguez Ramírez, E. R. 2014. Industrial Design Strategies for Eliciting Surprise. *Design Studies* 35:273–e297.

Education Studies

Pérez, M. S. & G. S. Cannella. 2013. Situational Analysis as an Avenue for Critical Qualitative Research: Mapping Post-Katrina New Orleans. *Qualitative Inquiry* 19(7):1–13.

Santoro, N. 2013. "I Really Want to Make a Difference for These Kids but It's Just Too Hard": One Aboriginal Teacher's Experiences of Moving Away, Moving On and Moving Up. *International Journal of Qualitative Studies in Education* 26(8):953–966.

Ethnic Studies

Martinez, A. 2012. Reconsidering Acculturation in Dietary Change Research among Latino Immigrants: Challenging the Preconditions of US Migration. *Ethnicity & Health* 18(2):115–135.

Feminist Research

Eriksson, M. & M. Emmelin. 2013. What Constitutes a Health-enabling Neighborhood? A Grounded Theory Situational Analysis Addressing the Significance of Social Capital and Gender. *Social Science & Medicine* 97:112–123.

Erol, M. 2011. Melting Bones: The Social Construction of Postmenopausal Osteoporosis in Turkey. *Social Science & Medicine* 73:1490–1497.

Khaw, L. 2012. Mapping the Process: An Exemplar of Using Situational Analysis in a Grounded Theory Study. *Journal of Family Theory and Review* 4:138–147.

Lappe, M. 2014. Taking Care: Anticipation, Extraction and the Politics of Temporality in Autism Science. *BioSocieties* 9(3):304–328.

Milwertz, C. & W. Fengxian. 2011. Organizing in the People's Republic of China. *Gender Technology and Development* 15(3):457–483.

Health and Medicine Studies

Eriksson, M. & M. Emmelin. 2013. What Constitutes a Health-enabling Neighborhood? A Grounded Theory Situational Analysis Addressing the Significance of Social Capital and Gender. *Social Science & Medicine* 97:112–123.

Erol, M. 2011. Melting Bones: The Social Construction of Postmenopausal Osteoporosis in Turkey. *Social Science & Medicine* 73:1490–1497.

Lappe, M. 2014. Taking Care: Anticipation, Extraction and the Politics of Temporality in Autism Science. *BioSocieties* 9(3):304–328.

Mathar, T. 2009. Body-identity Trajectories of Preventive Selves. In T. Mathar & Y. J. F. M. Jansen (Eds.) *Health Promotion and Prevention Programmes in Practice: How Patients' Health Practices Are Rationalized, Reconceptualised and Reorganised* (pp. 171–196). Bielefeld, Germany: Verlag.

Library and Information Sciences

Grace, D. & B. Sen. 2013. Community Resilience and the Role of the Public Library. *Library Trends* 61(3):513–541.

Vasconcelos, A., B. Sen, A. Rosa, & D. Ellis. 2012. Elaborations of Grounded Theory in Information Research: Arenas/Social Worlds Theory, Discourse and Situational Analysis. *Library and Information Research* 36(112):120–146.

Nursing

Jacobson, C. H., M. Zlatnik, H. P. Kennedy, & A. Lyndon. 2013. Nurses' Perspectives on the Intersection of Safety and Informed Decision Making in Maternity Care. *JOGNN-Journal of Obstetric Gynecologic and Neonatal Nursing* 42(5):577–587.

Lyndon, A. 2008. Social and Environmental Conditions Creating Fluctuating Agency for Safety in Two Urban Academic Birth Centers. *Journal of Obstetric, Gynecologic and Neonatal Nursing* 37(1):13–23.

Lyndon, A. 2010. Skillful Anticipation: Maternity Nurses' Perspectives on Maintaining Safety. *Quality & Safety in Health Care* 19(5):e8. doi:10.1136/qshc.2007.024547.

Mills, J., K. Francis, & A. Bonner. 2007. The Accidental Mentor: Australian Rural Nurses Developing Supportive Relationships in the Workplace. *Rural and Remote Health* [electronic journal]. http://www.rrh.org.au/articles/subviewaust.asp?ArticleID=842 (accessed January 22, 2015).

Novick, G., L. S. Sadler, K. A. Knafl, N. E. Groce, & H. P. Kennedy. 2012. The Intersection of Everyday Life and Group Prenatal Care for Women in Two Urban Clinics. *Journal of Health Care for the Poor and Underserved* 23(2):589.

Reisenhofer, S. & C. Seibold. 2013. Emergency Healthcare Experiences of Women Living with Intimate Partner Violence *Journal of Clinical Nursing* 22(15–16):2253–2263.

Triamchaisri, S. K., B. E. Mawn, & A. Jintana. 2013. Development of a Home-based Palliative Care Model for People Living with End-stage Renal Disease. *Journal of Hospice & Palliative Nursing* 15(4):E1–E11.

Organization Studies

Alonso-Yanez, G. & C. Davidsen. 2014. Conservation Science Policies versus Scientific Practice: Evidence from a Mexican Biosphere Reserve. *Human Ecology Review* 20(2):3–29.

Fitzgerald, J. 2012. The Messy Politics of "Clean Coal": The Shaping of a Contested Term in Appalachia's Energy Debate. *Organization & Environment* 25(4):437–451.

Sanders, C. B. & S. Henderson. 2013. Police "Empires" and Information Technologies: Uncovering Material and Organisational Barriers to Information Sharing in Canadian Police Services. *Policing and Society* 23(2):243–260.

Postcolonial Studies

Chen, J. 2011. Studying up Harm Reduction Policy: The Office as Assemblage. *International Journal of Drug Policy* 22:471–477.

Milwertz, C. & W. Fengxian. 2011. Organizing in the People's Republic of China. *Gender Technology and Development* 15(3):457–483.

Psychology

Ness, O. & T. Strong. 2013. Learning New Ideas and Practices Together: A Co-operative Inquiry. *Journal of Family Psychotherapy* 24:246–260.

Strong, T., J. Gaete, I. N. Sametband, J. French, & J. Eeson. 2012. Counsellors Respond to the DSM-IV-TR. *Canadian Journal of Counseling and Psychotherapy* 46(2):85–106.

Science and Technology Studies

Alonso-Yanez, G. & C. Davidsen. 2014. Conservation Science Policies versus Scientific Practice: Evidence from a Mexican Biosphere Reserve. *Human Ecology Review* 20(2):3–29.

Fitzgerald, J. 2012. The Messy Politics of "Clean Coal": The Shaping of a Contested Term in Appalachia's Energy Debate. *Organization & Environment* 25(4):437–451.

Friese, C. 2010. Classification Conundrums: Classifying Chimeras and Enacting Species Preservation. *Theory and Society* 39(2):145–172.

Friese, C. 2013. *Cloning Wild Life: Zoos, Captivity and the Future of Endangered Animals.* New York: NYU Press.

Lappe, M. 2014. Taking Care: Anticipation, Extraction and the Politics of Temporality in Autism Science. *BioSocieties* 9(3):304–328.

APPENDIX C

SELECTED EXEMPLARS OF SITUATIONAL ANALYSIS BY MAPPING FOCUS

NOTE: The selected exemplars of situational analysis listed here *do not* include those in this volume. Several also fit into multiple categories.

General Use Of Situational Analysis

Baszanger, I. 2012. One More Chemo or One Too Many? Defining the Limits of Treatment and Innovation in Medical Oncology. *Social Science & Medicine* 75(5):864–872.

Chen, J. S. 2011. Studying up Harm Reduction Policy: The Office as an Assemblage. *International Journal of Drug Policy* 22:471–477.

Davidson, P. J., R. Lozada, P. C. Rosen, A. Macias, M. Gallardo, & R. A. Pollini. 2012. Negotiating Access: Social Barriers to Purchasing Syringes at Pharmacies in Tijuana, Mexico. *International Journal of Drug Policy* 23(4): 286–294.

Eriksson, M. & M. Emmelin. 2013. What Constitutes a Health-enabling Neighborhood? A Grounded Theory Situational Analysis Addressing the Significance of Social Capital and Gender. *Social Science & Medicine* 97:112–123.

Erol, M. 2011. Melting Bones: The Social Construction of Postmenopausal Osteoporosis in Turkey. *Social Science & Medicine* 73:1490–1497.

Multiple Situational Maps In Same Study

Pérez, M. S. & G. S. Cannella. 2013. Situational Analysis as an Avenue for Critical Qualitative Research: Mapping Post-Katrina New Orleans. *Qualitative Inquiry* 19(7):1–13.

Strong, T., J. Gaete, I. N. Sametband, J. French, & J. Eeson. 2012. Counsellors Respond to the DSM-IV-TR. *Canadian Journal of Counseling and Psychotherapy* 46(2):85–106.

Situational Maps Focus

Khaw, L. 2012. Mapping the Process: An Exemplar of Using Situational Analysis in a Grounded Theory Study. *Journal of Family Theory and Review* 4:138–147.

Social Worlds/Arenas Focus

Alonso-Yanez, G. & C. Davidsen. 2014. Conservation Science Policies versus Scientific Practice: Evidence from a Mexican Biosphere Reserve. *Human Ecology Review* 20(2):3–29.

Clarke, A. E. & T. Montini. 1993. The Many Faces of RU486: Tales of Situated Knowledges and Technological Contestations. *Science, Technology & Human Values* 18(1):42–78.

Eriksson, M., L. Dahlgren, & M. Emmelin. 2013. Collective Actors as Driving Forces for Mobilizing Social Capital in a Local Community: What Can Be Learned for Health Promotion? In K. Kiyoshi & H. Westlund (Eds.) *Social Capital and Rural Development in the Knowledge Society* (pp. 273–298). Cheltenham, UK: Edward Elgar.

Grace, D. & B. Sen. 2013. Community Resilience and the Role of the Public Library. *Library Trends* 61 (3):513–541.

Johnson, M., S. Hyysalo, & S. Tamminen. 2010. The Virtuality of Virtual Worlds, or What Can We Learn from Playacting Horse Girls and Marginalized Developers. *Symbolic Interaction* 33(4):603–633.

Licqurish, S. & C. Seibold. 2011. Applying a Contemporary Grounded Theory Methodology. *Nurse Researcher* 18(4):11–16.

Martinez, A. 2012. Reconsidering Acculturation in Dietary Change Research among Latino Immigrants: Challenging the Preconditions of US Migration. *Ethnicity & Health* 18(2):115–135.

Vasconcelos, A., B. Sen, A. Rosa, & D. Ellis. 2012. Elaborations of Grounded Theory in Information Research: Arenas/Social Worlds Theory, Discourse and Situational Analysis. *Library and Information Research* 36(112): 120–146.

Positional Maps Focus

Carder, P. C. 2008. Managing Medication Management in Assisted Living: A Situational Analysis. *Journal of Ethnographic and Qualitative Research* 3:1–12.

Fisher, M. 2014. PTSD in the U.S. Military, and the Politics of Prevalence. *Social Science & Medicine* 115:1–9.

Friese, C. 2010. Classification Conundrums: Classifying Chimeras and Enacting Species Preservation. *Theory and Society* 39(2):145–172.

Discourse Analysis Focus

Sanders, G. 2009. "Late" Capital: Amusement and Contradiction in the Contemporary Funeral Industry. *Critical Sociology* 35:447–471.

INDEX

ABOUT THE EDITORS & CONTRIBUTORS

Editors

Adele E. Clarke (MA, PhD) is professor emerita of sociology and history of health sciences at the University of California, San Francisco, where she also completed her PhD with Anselm Strauss. She has used and taught grounded theory since 1980, and developed situational analysis as an extension. Her book *Situational Analysis: Grounded Theory after the Postmodern Turn* won the Cooley Distinguished Book Award, Society for the Study of Symbolic Interaction. Her research has centered on social, cultural, and historical studies of science, technology, and medicine with emphases on biomedicalization and technologies for women. Her book *Disciplining Reproduction: Modernity, American Life Sciences and the "Problem of Sex"* won the Basker Award, Society for Medical Anthropology, and the Fleck Award, Society for Social Studies of Science. Clarke received the 2013 Bernal Prize for Outstanding Contributions from the Society for Social Studies of Science and the 2015 Reeder Award for Distinguished Contributions to Medical Sociology. Current projects focus on the politics of reproduction and qualitative research methods.

Carrie Friese (PhD) is associate professor of sociology at the London School of Economics and Political Science. Her initial research focused on assisted reproductive technologies for humans and endangered species, including the development of interspecies nuclear transfer (aka cloning) for species preservation in zoos. Her book *Cloning Wild Life: Zoos, Captivity and the Future of Endangered Animals* (NYU Press) appeared in 2013. Friese's new ethnographic research project explores animal husbandry and care in scientific knowledge production, including transnational comparisons of care practices and their regulation. She has used situational analysis across these research projects and has given talks and taught courses on the method across Europe.

Rachel Washburn (PhD) is assistant professor of sociology at Loyola Marymount University in Los Angeles. She used situational analysis in her doctoral research on the politics of human biomonitoring and has continued to do so in subsequent articles on the same topic. Her dissertation, *Measuring the Chemicals Within: The Social Terrain of Human Biomonitoring in the United States*, was awarded the Anselm Strauss Outstanding Qualitative Dissertation Award in 2009. She has given talks and workshops on situational analysis at universities in the United States and Canada. Her current research examines the politics of mid-20th-century science on the human health effects of pesticides.

Contributors

Gaile S. Cannella (MA, PhD) is research professor at Arizona State University and series editor for both "Rethinking Childhoods" and "Critical Qualitative Research" with Peter Lang Publishers. She held the Velma E. Schmidt Endowed Chair in Early Childhood Studies at the University of North Texas and was tenured full professor at Arizona State University and Texas A&M University. Publishing in English, Korean, and Spanish, her books include *Deconstructing Early Childhood Education* and *Critical Qualitative Research Reader* (with Shirley Steinberg). Articles appear in *Qualitative Inquiry, Cultural Studies-Cultural Methodologies*, and other journals.

Martin A. French (PhD) is assistant professor in the Department of Sociology & Anthropology at Concordia University in Montreal, Canada. He completed his PhD in sociology at Queen's University, Kingston, Canada. His research examines the social dimensions of technology with an empirical focus on communications and information technology. It emphasizes the broader social and political contexts of CIT, focusing especially on risk, surveillance, privacy, and social justice.

Marilou Gagnon (RN, ACRN, PhD) is associate professor at the School of Nursing, Faculty of Health Sciences, University of Ottawa, and director of the Unit for Critical Research in Health. Her work is underpinned by critical and sociopolitical approaches. Her program of research focuses on questions related to the body and technology, power and discourses, and social justice. She is currently working on projects on HIV criminalization, HIV-related stigma, HIV testing, and HIV medication side effects.

Dave Holmes (RN, PhD) is professor and University Research Chair in Forensic Nursing in the School of Nursing, Faculty of Health Sciences, University of Ottawa. He completed the PhD in nursing (Montreal, 2002) and a CIHR postdoctoral fellowship in Health Care, Technology and Place in the Faculty of Social Work (Toronto 2003). Most of his work draws on the poststructuralism of Deleuze, Guattari, and Michel Foucault. His research centers on psychiatry, forensic psychiatry, and public health.

Jean Daniel Jacob (RN, PhD) is associate professor and assistant director of undergraduate programs in the School of Nursing, Faculty of Health Sciences, at the University of Ottawa, Canada. His research interests are situated within the field of psychiatry/forensic psychiatry and include topics such as fear, violence, risk, ethics and the sociopolitical aspects of nursing practice.

Fiona A. Miller (PhD) is associate professor in the Institute of Health Policy, Management and Evaluation, director of the Division of Health Policy and Ethics at the Toronto Health Economics and Technology Assessment Collaborative, and a member of the Joint Centre for Bioethics at the University of Toronto. Her program of research centers on health technology policy, including the dynamics of health technology development, assessment, and adoption within systems of health research and health care.

Michelle Salazar Pérez (MS, PhD) is assistant professor of Early Childhood Education at New Mexico State University. From 2007 to 2009, she lived in New Orleans, Louisiana, where she used situational analysis and black feminist thought to examine the impact of disaster capitalism on the public school system post-Katrina. Her work using situational analysis can be found in a number of edited volumes and in the journals *Qualitative Inquiry* and the *International Review of Qualitative Research*.